LATEX INTOLERANCE

Basic Science, Epidemiology,
and Clinical Management

DERMATOLOGY: CLINICAL & BASIC SCIENCE SERIES
Series Editor Howard I. Maibach, M.D.

Published Titles:

Bioengineering of the Skin: Water and the Stratum Corneum, Second Edition
Peter Elsner, Enzo Berardesca, and Howard I. Maibach

Bioengineering of the Skin: Cutaneous Blood Flow and Erythema
Enzo Berardesca, Peter Elsner, and Howard I. Maibach

Bioengineering of the Skin: Methods and Instrumentation
Enzo Berardesca, Peter Elsner, Klaus P. Wilhelm, and Howard I. Maibach

Bioengineering of the Skin: Skin Surface, Imaging, and Analysis
Klaus P. Wilhelm, Peter Elsner, Enzo Berardesca, and Howard I. Maibach

Bioengineering of the Skin: Skin Biomechanics
Peter Elsner, Enzo Berardesca, Klaus-P. Wilhelm, and Howard I. Maibach

Skin Cancer: Mechanisms and Human Relevance
Hasan Mukhtar

Dermatologic Research Techniques
Howard I. Maibach

The Irritant Contact Dermatitis Syndrome
Pieter van der Valk, Pieter Coenrads, and Howard I. Maibach

Human Papillomavirus Infections in Dermatovenereology
Gerd Gross and Geo von Krogh

Contact Urticaria Syndrome
Smita Amin, Arto Lahti, and Howard I. Maibach

Skin Reactions to Drugs
Kirsti Kauppinen, Kristiina Alanko, Matti Hannuksela, and Howard I. Maibach

Dry Skin and Moisturizers: Chemistry and Function
Marie Lodén and Howard I. Maibach

Dermatologic Botany
Javier Avalos and Howard I. Maibach

Hand Eczema, Second Edition
Torkil Menné and Howard I. Maibach

Pesticide Dermatoses
Homero Penagos, Michael O'Malley, and Howard I. Maibach

Nickel and the Skin: Absorption, Immunology, Epidemiology, and Metallurgy
Jurij J. Hostýneck and Howard I. Maibach

The Epidermis in Wound Healing
David T. Rovee and Howard I. Maibach

Protective Gloves for Occupational Use, Second Edition
Anders Boman, Tuula Estlander, Jan E. Wahlberg, and Howard I . Maibach

DERMATOLOGY: CLINICAL & BASIC SCIENCE SERIES

LATEX INTOLERANCE
Basic Science, Epidemiology, and Clinical Management

Edited by
Mahbub M.U. Chowdhury, MBChB, MRCP
Howard I. Maibach, M.D.

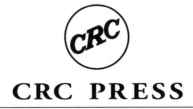

CRC PRESS

Boca Raton   London   New York   Washington, D.C.

Library of Congress Cataloging-in-Publication Data

Latex intolerance : basic science, epidemiology, clinical management / edited by
Mahbub M.U. Chowdhury, Howard I. Maibach.
  p.   cm. — (Dermatology : clinical and basic science)
  Includes bibliographical references and index.
  ISBN 0-8493-1670-7 (alk. paper)
  1. Latex allergy. I. Chowdhury, Mahbub M. U. II. Maibach, Howard I. III.
Dermatology (CRC Press)
  [DNLM: 1. Latex Hypersensitivity. 2. Dermatitis, Allergic Contact. WD L3516 2005]
RL224.L38 2005
616.97′3—dc22   2004051940

Visit the CRC Press Web site at www.crcpress.com

© 2005 by CRC Press LLC

No claim to original U.S. Government works
International Standard Book Number 0-8493-1670-7
Library of Congress Card Number 2004051940
Printed in the United States of America 1 2 3 4 5 6 7 8 9 0
Printed on acid-free paper

Series Preface

Our goal in creating the *Dermatology: Clinical & Basic Science Series* is to present the insights of experts on emerging applied and experimental techniques and theoretical concepts that are, or will be, at the vanguard of dermatology. These books cover new and exciting multidisciplinary areas of cutaneous research, and we want them to be the books every physician will use to become acquainted with new methodologies in skin research. These books can also be given to graduate students and postdoctoral fellows when they are looking for guidance to start a new line of research.

The series consists of books that are edited by experts, with chapters written by the leaders in each particular field. The books are richly illustrated and contain comprehensive bibliographies. Each chapter provides substantial background material relevant to its subject. These books contain detailed tricks of the trade and information regarding where the methods presented can be safely applied. In addition, information on where to buy equipment and helpful web sites for solving both practical and theoretical problems are included.

We are working with these goals in mind. As the books become available, the efforts of the publisher, book editors, and individual authors will contribute to the further development of dermatology research and clinical practice. The extent to which we achieve this goal will be determined by the utility of these books.

Howard I. Maibach, M.D.

Preface

Latex intolerance has become an increasingly important concept and diagnosis. In this textbook, we have aimed to cover all aspects of latex allergy including contact urticaria, irritation, and allergic contact dermatitis. An evidence-based and practical approach has been taken to describe the epidemiology, basic science, clinical presentation, management, and prognosis of the varied manifestations of natural rubber latex intolerance. Other sections including rubber chemical additives and associated problems, hand dermatitis, barrier creams, and medical glove regulations are included to provide relevant background knowledge to readers. Expert contributors from the United Kingdom, Europe, and the United States have provided a balanced international perspective in this first major textbook dedicated to latex intolerance.

We hope dermatologists and other specialists involved in the diagnosis and management of latex intolerance will find this a useful textbook and reference source and welcome any corrections and suggestions for future editions.

Mahbub M.U. Chowdhury
Cardiff, United Kingdom

Howard I. Maibach
San Francisco, United States

The Editors

Mahbub M.U. Chowdhury, MBChB, MRCP(U.K.), is a consultant in occupational dermatology in the Welsh Institute of Dermatology, University Hospital of Wales, Cardiff, United Kingdom. Dr. Chowdhury qualified from Leicester University in 1991 and trained in dermatology in major centers in the United Kingdom including Newcastle, Sunderland, and Cardiff between 1996 and 2001. He has held honorary registrar posts in contact dermatitis and occupational dermatology units in Birmingham and Manchester, U.K. in 2000, and the University of California, San Francisco, U.S. in 2002. He is currently program director for the All Wales Specialist Registrar Training Programme in dermatology and is also the clinical governance and audit lead clinician for dermatology in Cardiff. He is the author of more than 50 papers and book chapters and co-editor of two books. His current research interests include latex allergy and other areas of contact dermatitis and occupational dermatology.

Howard I. Maibach, M.D., is a professor of dermatology at the University of California, San Francisco and has been a long-term contributor to experimental research in dermatopharmacology and to clinical research on contact dermatitis, contact urticaria, and other skin conditions. Dr. Maibach graduated from Tulane University, New Orleans, Louisiana (A.B. and M.D.) and received his research and clinical training at the University of Pennsylvania, Philadelphia. He received an honorary doctorate from the University of Paris Sud in 1988.

Dr. Maibach is a member of the International Contact Dermatitis Research Group, the North American Contact Dermatitis Group, and the European Environmental Contact Dermatitis Group. He is the author, co-author, and/or editor of 1600 publications and 60 volumes.

Contributors

Anil Adisesh
Consultant in Occupational Medicine
Trafford General and Salford Royal
  Hospitals
Manchester, United Kingdom

Harri Alenius
Chief, Laboratory of
  Immunotoxicology
Finnish Institute of Occupational
  Health
Helsinki, Finland

Mahbub M.U. Chowdhury
Consultant in Occupational
  Dermatology
University Hospital of Wales
Cardiff, United Kingdom

Ignatius C. Chua
Department of Clinical Immunology
University Hospital of Wales
Cardiff, United Kingdom

Deborah D. Davis
Technical Director
Medical Products and Services
Cardinal Health
McGraw Park, Illinois

Katja Frisk
FIT Biotech Oyj
Tampere, Finland

Curtis P. Hamann
SmartPractice
Phoenix, Arizona

Graham A. Johnston
Consultant Dermatologist
Leicester Royal Infirmary
Leicester, United Kingdom

Tytti Kärkkäinen
FIT Biotech Oyj
Tampere, Finland

Antti I. Lauerma
Consultant Dermatologist
Finnish Institute of Occupational Health
Helsinki, Finland

Howard I. Maibach
Professor of Dermatology
University of California, San Francisco
Department of Dermatology
San Francisco, California

Nicolas Nicolaou
Specialist Registrar
Department of Dermatology
University Hospital of Wales
Cardiff, United Kingdom

Alison J. Owen
Nurse Practitioner
Department of Clinical Immunology
University Hospital of Wales
Cardiff, United Kingdom

Timo Palosuo
Research Professor
Department of Health and Functional
  Ability
National Public Health Institute
Helsinki, Finland

Hely Reinikka-Railo
Medical Devices Centre
National Agency for Medicines
Helsinki, Finland

Pamela A. Rodgers
SmartPractice
Phoenix, Arizona

Mayanka Singh
Department of Dermatology
University of California, San Francisco
San Francisco, California

Priyanka Singh
Department of Dermatology
University of California, San Francisco
San Francisco, California

Barry N. Statham
Consultant Dermatologist
Singleton Hospital
Swansea, United Kingdom

Natalie M. Stone
Consultant Dermatologist
Royal Gwent Hospital
Newport, United Kingdom

Kim Sullivan
SmartPractice
Phoenix, Arizona

Vesna J. Tomazic-Jezic
Immunologist
FDA, Center for Devices and
 Radiological Health
Rockville, Maryland

Sarah H. Wakelin
Consultant Dermatologist
St. Mary's Hospital
London, United Kingdom

Paul E. Williams
Consultant Clinical Immunologist
University Hospital of Wales
Cardiff, United Kingdom

Tanya D. Wright
Senior Dietician
Amersham General Hospital
Amersham, United Kingdom

Hongbo Zhai
Department of Dermatology
University of California, San Francisco
San Francisco, California

Contents

Chapter 1 Epidemiology of Latex Allergy 1

Barry N. Statham

Chapter 2 Allergenic Proteins.. 15

Harri Alenius and Timo Palosuo

Chapter 3 Chemical Additives 27

Curtis P. Hamann, Pamela A. Rodgers, and Kim Sullivan

Chapter 4 Natural Rubber Latex Allergy: Clinical Manifestations................... 57

Ignatius C. Chua, Alison J. Owen, and Paul E. Williams

Chapter 5 Natural Rubber Latex Allergy and Allergens: *In Vitro* Testing 67

Vesna J. Tomazic-Jezic

Chapter 6 New Developments in Measuring Allergens in Natural Rubber
Latex Products.. 87

Katja Frisk, Tytti Kärkkäinen, Hely Reinikka-Railo, and Timo Palosuo

Chapter 7 Contact Urticaria: Clinical Manifestations 97

Sarah H. Wakelin

Chapter 8 Contact Urticaria Syndrome: Predictive Testing 107

Antti I. Lauerma and Howard I. Maibach

Chapter 9 Contact Urticaria Syndrome: Prognosis 113

Sarah H. Wakelin

Chapter 10 Allergic Contact Dermatitis: Clinical Manifestations 119

Natalie M. Stone

Chapter 11 Allergic Contact Dermatitis: Tests...127

Natalie M. Stone

Chapter 12 Allergic Contact Dermatitis: Prognosis...133

Natalie M. Stone

Chapter 13 Latex-Fruit Syndrome 135

Tanya D. Wright

Chapter 14 Irritant Dermatitis Due to Occlusive Gloves: Clinical
Manifestations 141

*Priyanka Singh, Mayanka Singh, Mahbub M.U. Chowdhury, and
Howard I. Maibach*

Chapter 15 Irritation Dermatitis Due to Occlusive Gloves: Predictive
Testing 147

*Mayanka Singh, Priyanka Singh, Mahbub M.U. Chowdhury, and
Howard I. Maibach*

Chapter 16 Management of Hand Dermatitis 151

Graham A. Johnston, Nicolas Nicolaou, and Mahbub M.U. Chowdhury

Chapter 17 Barrier Creams/Moisturizers...165

Hongbo Zhai, Mahbub M.U. Chowdhury, and Howard I. Maibach

Chapter 18 Occlusive Effects: Man vs. Animal 177

Hongbo Zhai, Mahbub M.U. Chowdhury, and Howard I. Maibach

Chapter 19 Medical Glove Regulation: History and Future of Safety..............189

Deborah D. Davis

Chapter 20 Occupational Health Management of Latex Allergy.......................205

Anil Adisesh

Chapter 21 Management of Rubber-Based Allergies in Dentistry 211

Curtis P. Hamann, Pamela A. Rodgers, and Kim Sullivan

Chapter 22 Management of Latex Allergy: Allergist's Perspective 249

Ignatius C. Chua, Alison J. Owen, and Paul E. Williams

Index 261

1 Epidemiology of Latex Allergy

Barry N. Statham

CONTENTS

I. Introduction 1
II. Epidemiological Study Determinants 2
    A. Latex Allergy versus Hypersensitivity 2
    B. Recruitment of the Study Population 2
    C. Allergy Prevalence in "Normal Population" 2
    D. Identification of Latex-Related Symptoms 3
    E. Strengths and Weaknesses of Diagnostic Tests 3
III. Risk Factors and Latex Allergy 4
    A. Atopic Diathesis 5
    B. Hand Dermatitis 5
    C. Multiple Operations and/or Indwelling Latex 6
    D. Latex Glove Exposure 7
    E. Latex and Food Allergy 7
IV. Prevalence in Occupational Subgroups 8
V. Incidence of Latex Sensitization or Allergy 8
VI. Changing Trends of Latex Sensitivity after Latex Exposure Alteration 8
VII. Conclusions 10
References 11

I. INTRODUCTION

Many studies have attempted to address the question of the prevalence of latex allergy with the reported rates varying widely. Before examining the studies in detail it is important to consider the sources of error that, to a certain extent, all studies share.

These inconsistencies can be broadly divided into a number of categories as follows:

- Definition of allergy versus hypersensitivity
- Recruitment of study population
- Knowledge of allergy prevalence in "normal population"

0-8493-1670-7/05/$0.00+$1.50
© 2005 by CRC Press LLC

- Identification of latex related symptoms
- Strengths and weaknesses of diagnostic tests

II. EPIDEMIOLOGICAL STUDY DETERMINANTS

A. LATEX ALLERGY VERSUS HYPERSENSITIVITY

Fundamental to the investigation and management of all allergy is the separation of those individuals who possess the ability to mount an allergic response to an allergen in terms of measurable IgE specific to that allergen or produce a positive skin prick test (SPT). Many individuals who test positive with either of these methods have no clinical history compatible with allergy nor can a positive response be demonstrated on allergen exposure. These individuals are best defined as sensitized rather than allergic. The implications of sensitization in terms of future potential to show a clinical reaction are unknown.

B. RECRUITMENT OF THE STUDY POPULATION

The perfect epidemiological study would first clearly define the population to be studied and a suitable reference population for comparison. All of the study population would participate and records would contain detailed clinical information and a comprehensive history of exposure to the allergen. Finally, all participants would be investigated using identical diagnostic tests with 100% sensitivity and specificity.

The reality, of course, is often significantly removed from this ideal. Patient recruitment is often the most difficult to standardize. Awareness of latex allergy and its possible implication for future employment was substantially heightened following the publication by the Food and Drug Administration (FDA) of a bulletin warning of the risk associated with the use of natural rubber latex (NRL) medical devices.[1] Many glove users are symptomatic on exposure to latex leading to an entirely understandable concern that they may have developed latex allergy.

These factors have had a significant effect on recruitment to epidemiological studies. Patients fearing possible loss of employment have been very reluctant to come forward to participate in a study that may lead to loss of employment. At the same time many individuals who had nonspecific symptoms on glove exposure may have believed that they had acquired latex allergy and been more willing to take part in an investigation that would answer their suspicions. These factors are almost certain to have distorted population sampling in any epidemiological study.

C. ALLERGY PREVALENCE IN "NORMAL POPULATION"

Accurate knowledge of the background prevalence in the normal population is fundamental to epidemiological investigation but often it is difficult to define and thoroughly investigate a representative sample. One group often used for this purpose is the blood donor, although this group may be far from representative of normality. Saxon tested 1997 blood donations for latex specific IgE, finding positive results in 5.4 to 7.6%.[2]

Among patients hospitalized for routine surgery investigated by Turjanmaa, only 1 out of 804 patients (0.12%) were positive.[3] Another reference group used by Gautrin were apprentices around the start of their training, with prevalence of latex sensitization at 0.6%.[4] Chaiear in a study of latex allergy in the Malaysian rubber industry found no cases of latex sensitivity in 144 students tested as a control population.[5] Each of these studies used a latex SPT as the diagnostic procedure.

D. IDENTIFICATION OF LATEX-RELATED SYMPTOMS

The symptoms of latex allergy are well known as part of the symptom complex defined as contact urticaria syndrome.[6] These symptoms range from localized contact urticaria through to generalised urticaria with or without rhinoconjunctivitis, to asthma and anaphylaxis. The history of the typical highly latex allergic individual leaves little room for doubt. However, the history can also be very misleading with false positive and false negative diagnoses equally common. Hamilton and coworkers found that 15% of patients originally classified as "latex sensitized" on the basis of the clinical history were reclassified as not sensitized on the basis of negative SPT to multiple latex allergens and a negative two stage latex challenge procedure.[7,8]

Difficulty in correlating symptoms and allergic status is compounded by the fact that many subjects are symptomatic on latex exposure. Glove-related symptoms have been reported in up to 72% of glove wearers with hand dermatitis and 33% of those without.[9] Symptoms are not confined to glove wearers. Among children on long-term mechanical ventilation, 38% were symptomatic on latex exposure but almost half (45%) of these were negative to latex on IgE testing.[10]

While contact urticaria, rhinoconjunctivitis, asthma, and anaphylaxis on latex exposure are all highly suggestive of latex allergy, Turjanmaa found 10% of patients had nonspecific irritation at the site of latex exposure and 2% had no symptoms at the site of latex exposure.[3] From 1990, Turjanmaa has screened all patients being tested for inhalant allergens to a latex SPT. Those who tested positive without a clinical history supporting latex allergy were submitted to a latex glove challenge to confirm latex allergy.[11] Among those diagnosed with latex allergy, 18% of health-care workers and 37% of nonhealthcare workers could not recall symptoms associated with latex exposure, with an additional 46 cases of latex allergy diagnosed in this way (28% of total number of cases).

E. STRENGTHS AND WEAKNESSES OF DIAGNOSTIC TESTS

It is clear that the symptoms of latex exposure are not, in many cases, sufficiently reliable to allow a confident diagnosis of latex allergy. The tests used to support the clinical diagnosis also vary in their sensitivity and specificity. Many investigators regard the SPT as the most reliable investigation but varying preparations are in use for the latex allergen and differing criteria used to delineate a positive result.

Glove eluates have been used by many investigators.[12,13,14,9] Different sources of gloves have been used often without specifying the latex protein content that can vary by as much as 1000-fold between different brands.[15] Commercially prepared latex allergen preparations for skin testing are available in many countries (not in

TABLE 1.1

Comparison of Positive Tests by IgE and SPT and Challenge Test Result

Study Population (Number)	IgE + ve	SPT + ve	Challenge Tested	Challenge Tests	Reference
Spina bifida (159)	80 (50.3%)	77/159 (48.4%) raw latex 31/159 (19.5%) Stellergenes	159	55 + ve (34.6% = latex allergy)	Niggemann[17]
Anaesthesiologists (168)	14 (8%)	17/154 (11%) Greer	21 (total number with either test + ve)	4 + ve (2.4% = latex allergy) 17 – ve (10.1% = latex sensitized)	Brown[18]

Note: + ve = positive; – ve = negative.

the U.S.). These offer greater standardization and quoted values for sensitivity and specificity are approaching 100% and 96% respectively.[9]

While the majority of authors regard a SPT test as positive when the wheal diameter is 3 mm compared with the negative control, others set the standard at 50% of the positive control. In this area small differences can have a significant impact on the number of positive tests.[13] Tarlo found 4.7% of a population sensitized with a 3 mm detection limit compared with 11% when the limit was set at 2 mm.[16] Niggemann applied both 3 mm compared to negative control and 60% of the positive control as minimum diagnostic criteria,[17] while Brown set the limit of 2 mm compared with the negative control.[18]

Table 1.1 illustrates the differing results for prevalence rates of latex allergy when groups are tested by a variety of investigations including challenge tests.

The IgE specific to latex is reported in most studies as being less sensitive and less specific than the SPT. The sensitivity values for the two commonly used investigations range from 74.8% (CAP-Pharmacia) and 86.9% for the alaSTAT assay with specificity at 93.8% and 85.2% respectively.[19] Earlier studies were often performed with less accurate antibody assays so it is not possible to directly compare values between current and earlier studies.

Yeang, using a mathematical model, illustrates the potential for substantial overdiagnosis of latex sensitivity using tests with a low specificity in populations where the true prevalence of latex allergy is low.[20] Table 1.2 strikingly illustrates the risk of reliance on serological testing as a sole diagnostic tool.

III. RISK FACTORS AND LATEX ALLERGY

In addition to the differences in methodology used to identify latex allergy/sensitization and recruitment of a suitable study population there are a variety of factors that determine the susceptibility of an individual to latex allergy. Epidemiological

TABLE 1.2
Outcome of *In Vitro* Tests Based on a Sensitivity of 86.9% and Specificity of 85.2%[20]

True Prevalence (%)	True Positives (per hundred)	False Positives (per hundred)	Total Positives (per hundred)	Underestimate or Overestimate
100	86.9	0.00	86.9	0.87
50	43.45	7.40	50.85	1.02
10	8.69	13.32	22.01	2.20
5	4.35	14.06	18.41	3.68
1	0.87	14.65	15.52	15.52
0.5	0.43	14.73	15.16	30.32

Note: In this model the specificity of an investigation has a disproportionate impact on the reliability of the outcome compared with the sensitivity.

studies of those with latex allergy can help to delineate these associations. The following factors are often linked to latex allergy:

- Atopic diathesis
- Presence of hand dermatitis in glove wearers
- Multiple episodes of surgery and/or prolonged exposure to indwelling latex
- Use of latex gloves, especially for occupationally acquired allergy
- Coexistence of food allergy

A. ATOPIC DIATHESIS

The susceptibility of atopics to mount IgE mediated reactions is mirrored in the high prevalence of atopy reported in many studies. Turjanmaa reported atopy in 72% of healthcare workers and 83% of nonhealthcare workers diagnosed with latex allergy.[13] Konrad found a history of atopic disorders in 14/16 (87%) latex sensitized individuals compared with 26/85 (31%) nonsensitized staff.[21] Ylitalo identified atopy in 97% of children with latex allergy who had not undergone multiple episodes of surgery.[22]

A wide range of figures is available illustrating the risk of latex allergy in atopic individuals. Monteret-Vautrin tested patients attending an allergy clinic to latex and common inhalant allergens clearly demonstrating the synergistic effect of exposure and atopy as risk factors in latex allergy, as illustrated in Table 1.3.[23] In the same study, only 2/14 children with spina bifida without atopy were sensitized compared with 6/11 with both atopy and spina bifida.

B. HAND DERMATITIS

Occupations involving frequent use of latex gloves are also those where hand dermatitis is often encountered. The dermatitis is often multifactorial in its causation. Irritant dermatitis compounded by type IV contact allergies may both contribute to

TABLE 1.3
Effects of Atopy and Latex Exposure
on the Prevalence of Latex Allergy

Atopy	Latex Exposure	Number Tested	Latex Positive
No	No	272	0.37%
No	Yes	73	6.8%
Yes	No	180	9.4%
Yes	Yes	44	36.4%

the damaged skin barrier that in turn enhances penetration of the allergen, increasing the risk of sensitization.

Hand dermatitis was found at the time of presentation of the latex allergy in 41% of healthcare workers and 34% of nonhealthcare workers among 160 patients with latex allergy in Finland.[11] Konrad identified hand dermatitis in 5/16 (31%) latex-sensitized healthcare workers compared with 23/85 (27%) nonsensitized latex staff.[21]

C. MULTIPLE OPERATIONS AND/OR INDWELLING LATEX

Repeated episodes of surgery with or without long-term exposure to latex are a common feature in several reports with a high prevalence of latex exposure. Table 1.4 illustrates the prevalence of latex allergy in this high risk group. A study, by Capriles-Hulett from Venezuela, of affected patients not sharing this pattern showed less latex exposure as measured by fewer operations and no use of latex catheters.[24] There is also a striking variation in the reported incidence of anaphylaxis with 1.2% in Niggemann's group compared with 31% reported by Konz, suggesting that patient selection may have skewed the distribution of latex allergic cases in some studies.[17, 25]

TABLE 1.4
Studies of Latex Allergy in Populations with Long-Term Latex Exposure

Study Group	Number	Sp IgE	SPT	Symptoms or Provocation	Reference
Ventilated children	57	28.8%	ND	71% of + ve test	Nakamura[10]
Spinal cord injury (adult)	15	47%	ND	Not given	Monasterio[26]
Spina bifida	159	**55%**	**55%**	62% of + ve test	Niggemann[17]
Spina bifida	36	64%	ND	Not given	Konz[25]
Spinal cord injury	50	2	ND	Not given	Konz[25]
Spina bifida	93	ND	4.3%	75% of + ve test	Capriles-Hulett[24]

Note: + ve = positive; **either test positive**; ND = not done.

D. LATEX GLOVE EXPOSURE

The rapid increase in glove usage in the healthcare setting following the appearance of hepatitis and HIV has been suggested as a major factor responsible for the emergence of latex allergy in healthcare professionals. Evidence for the role of latex gloves as a source of sensitization to latex comes from a number of studies. It is largely indirect and, at least in part, contradictory.

First, studies have compared the prevalence of latex allergy in glove users and controls. Turjanmaa identified 15 of 512 (2.9%) of hospital workers to be latex allergic compared with 1/130 (0.8%) control subjects. Also a higher prevalence of allergy was found in surgical specialities (6.2%), where more intense exposure would be expected, compared with those in nonsurgical areas (1.6%).[13]

Garabrant in a study based on data gathered as part of the Third National Health and Nutrition Examination Survey (NHANES III) examined the rates of latex sensitization across a wide range of occupations including healthcare.[27] The conclusions included the unexpected finding that healthcare workers not currently using gloves were at increased risk of latex allergy compared with current glove users, especially in the presence of a history of childhood atopy. Wartenberg questions the use of data gathered in this survey in terms of its reliability and sensitivity in separating real differences from confounding variables in such large population studies; this study should be interpreted with caution in view of these potential difficulties.[28]

Page examined hospital clinical and administrative staff finding an overall prevalence of sensitization of 6.2% by latex specific IgE testing, with no difference between those occupationally exposed to latex gloves compared with nonusers.[29]

Bollinger found 5.9% of 476 employees in nonpatient care jobs to have positive latex specific IgE compared with 8.6% of 1304 employees with direct patient care roles.[30]

The common weakness of each of these studies is the lack of information regarding other sources of latex exposure that may have initiated the allergy and the latex protein content of the gloves in use at the time of the studies. The available evidence supports a weak role for latex gloves as an initiator of latex allergy; these studies are not sufficiently robust in their design to allow separation of the relative effects of exposure and an atopic background.

E. LATEX AND FOOD ALLERGY

Allergy to foods and latex frequently coincide due to cross-reacting epitopes shared by many plant materials. Many foods have on occasion been associated. Posch found positive SPT reactions to foods in 68% of latex allergic adults.[31] The foods found to be positive were avocado, banana, sweet pepper, potato, kiwi, and tomato in descending frequency. However, the majority of those with positive tests were not symptomatic. Kim found 21% symptomatic food allergy, confirmed by SPT in patients with latex allergy. Symptoms ranged from local oral irritation to anaphylaxis in some patients.[32] For further details refer to Chapter 13.

IV. PREVALENCE IN OCCUPATIONAL SUBGROUPS

Table 1.5 shows a representative sample of the available publications reporting the prevalence of latex allergy in those occupationally exposed to latex. At first inspection there is a large variation in reported figures with the range from 0.5 to 24%. Closer examination reveals that some studies have reported the prevalence figures as they relate to the group of participants[33,36] rather than to the entire population at risk.[35,18] Other studies have only investigated symptomatic individuals[37,38,39] or subgroups with very intense exposure to latex gloves.[18,37] Some studies have separated latex sensitized from latex allergic cases by their history alone,[38] while others have performed challenge or use testing to help to separate these subgroups.[13,18] In some studies, no attempt at separation has occurred. [36]

In addition, it is very probable that certain groups have been exposed to gloves high in latex protein levels over an extended time period while others have fortuitously been provided with gloves with far lower latex protein content. Thus not all of the variation between published studies need be due to methodological differences.

V. INCIDENCE OF LATEX SENSITIZATION OR ALLERGY

In comparison with the number of studies of the prevalence of latex allergy in various populations, there are few studies of the incidence rates. Gautrin prospectively studied three groups of apprentices entering training in animal health technology, pastry making, and dental hygiene technology. [4] The study examined the presence of latex positivity on SPT at or around enrollment into training and at follow-up 8 to 44 months into training. There were significantly more cases of latex allergy arising in the dental hygiene technicians compared to the other two groups, with only the dental hygiene technicians having significant exposure to latex gloves during training. At the time of entry into training, none of the 110 dental hygiene students were positive to latex; by the time of follow-up 7 were sensitized, at 2.5% per person year.

A Finnish study of the incidence of contact urticaria to latex during a 6-year period (1991–1996) provides a unique insight into the incidence rate of contact urticaria in various occupational groups.[41] The lowest rates identified were for managerial workers at 0.01 per 10,000 employed worker years to 0.5 for cleaners, 1.3 for healthcare workers in general, and 11.8 for dental assistants. The incidence of latex induced contact urticaria annually, by occupation, remained stable during the period. Clearly, heightened awareness of latex allergy in healthcare employees influenced the reporting of contact urticaria in this group.

VI. CHANGING TRENDS OF LATEX SENSITIVITY AFTER LATEX EXPOSURE ALTERATION

In an attempt to reduce the risk to staff of acquiring latex allergy through glove exposure, many organizations have implemented policies that replace the use of

TABLE 1.5
Prevalence of Latex Allergy in Various Occupational Settings

Study Population	Year of Study	Total Size of Cohort	Number Tested	Positive (% of Total Cohort)	Test Performed	Reference
Hospital and dental staff	1994	250	202	3.5% (2.7%)	SPT + IgE	Wransjo[9]
Lab staff (Netherlands)	1998	98	66	8.3% (5.1%)	SPT + IgE	De Groot[14]
Construction workers (Spain)	1996–2000	230	54	7%	SPT+ IgE	Conde-Salazar[13]
Operating theatre staff (Australia)	2001	169	102	1% (0.6%)	IgE	Hack[34]
Surgical and lab staff (Finland)	1987	Not given	512	2.9%	SPT + use test	Turjanmaa[13]
Rubber tapping (Malaysia)	2001	475	314	1.3% (0.8%)	SPT-Stellergene	Chaiear[5]
Glove manufacture (Malaysia)	2001	783	480	1.7% (1%)	SPT-Stellergene	Chaiear
Students (Control) (Malaysia)	2001	144	144	0%	SPT-Stellergene	Chaiear
Anaesthetic staff (Switzerland)	1997	117	101	15.8% (13.7%)	SPT-glove +IgE	Konrad[21]
Hospital employees (U.S.)	1995	1967	156	24% (1.9%) 19% (1.5%)-symptomatic	SPT-multiple +IgE	Kim[35]
Hospital glove users (U.S.)	2000	255	239	6.1% (6.1%)	IgE	Page[29]
Hospital nonglove users (U.S.)	2000	254	239	6.3% (6.3%)	IgE	Page
Hospital employees (U.S.)	1999	1795	1795	8%	IgE SPT (72 only)	Bollinger[30]
Hospital E.R. (U.S.)	1996	915	381	6% (2.5%)	IgE	Kaczmarek[36]
Anaesthetic staff (U.S.)	1998	171	168	10.1% sensitized, 2.4% allergic	IgE, SPT (Greer) Challenge test	Brown[18]
Health workers (Wales, U.K.)	1998–2000	5548	257	0.6%	SPT-ALK If symptomatic	Chowdhury[37]
Health workers (U.K.)	1999–2000	5600	115	0.5% (0.3%)	IgE, SPT If symptomatic	Poole[38]
Health workers (U.K.)	1995	867	57	0.9% (0.9%)	SPT-glove If symptomatic	Handfield-Jones[39]
O.R. nurses (France)	1991	258	197	10.7% (7.8%)	SPT-Stellergene	Lagier[40]
Primary care hospital (Belgium)	1995	289	273	5% (4.5%)	SPT-Stellergene	Vandenplas[12]

powdered, high protein latex gloves with gloves that are powder free and low in protein content. A number of publications appear to support these measures.

Sussman examined the rate of SPT conversion in two groups of healthcare workers; one exposed to powdered latex gloves and the other exclusively to powder-free protein-poor latex gloves.[42] Initial analysis identified an identical 1% annual incidence of latex conversion in both groups. At a later date, the two individuals in the powder-free, protein-poor group who had converted were reexamined and found to be SPT negative suggesting that they had been wrongly classified at first examination.[43]

Tarlo studied the number of workers presenting to occupational health or allergy clinics in an Ontario hospital.[44] The number of cases rose annually from 1988 (1 case) to 1998 (6 cases). Following the introduction of a worker education program in 1994, 45 sensitized workers were identified. In 1997, powder-free low protein latex gloves were introduced with no cases identified in 1999.

Allmers examined latex specific IgE levels in latex sensitized healthcare workers after switching to powder free, low protein gloves. In 5 of 7, the IgE levels halved within 1 year of changing exposure and in all 7 a highly significant fall occurred, mirrored by a fall in latex aeroallergens to undetectable levels within 24 hours of removing powdered gloves from the environment.[45] In another study, Allmers identified the number of new cases of latex allergy reported to a German insurance company. The cases of occupational asthma due to latex declined steadily after the replacement of powdered latex gloves in the German healthcare setting.[46]

Levy examined the prevalence of latex allergy in French and English dental students who had been exposed to exclusively powdered gloves with moderately high (335–635µg/g) extractable protein levels or powder-free protein poor gloves (< 25µg/g).[47] None of the 93 students exclusively using powder-free protein poor gloves were sensitized compared with 11/96 (11.5%) in those exposed to the powdered higher protein gloves.

Saary found the prevalence of latex sensitivity among staff and dental students fell between 1995 and 2000 (a period when the use of latex gloves changed from high protein powdered gloves to low protein powder-free gloves) from 10 to 3%. All cases identified in 2000 were among staff not tested in the 1995 study, i.e., it is possible that some cases of sensitization may have arisen prior to the change in glove use. No cases were found in the group of dental students trained exclusively after the change in glove exposure. The same study identified a significant change in the incidence of rhinoconjunctivitis (from 12 to 0% in 1995 and 2000 respectively).[48]

VII. CONCLUSIONS

The evidence presented gives some insight into the underlying factors that may trigger latex allergy. Changes in the level of exposure to latex allergens during the 1980s and early 1990s, together with heightened awareness, both played a significant part in bringing latex allergy to prominence. Much less is known concerning the background prevalence in the population outside of certain high risk subgroups. Excluding the healthcare professions, few other occupational groups have been studied in detail. Encouraging evidence now suggests that strategies that limit the use of latex gloves to powder-free low protein brands may be reducing the incidence of occupational sensitization to latex.

Further study is needed in many areas to increase our understanding of latex allergy and extend the benefits of allergy prevention strategies to the wider population. The prevalence of latex allergy outside of the high-risk groups is likely to be very low, but nonetheless significant numbers of people are affected. Given that the diagnosis of latex allergy may not be clear cut from the clinical history, these individuals are easily missed, placing them at risk especially in the healthcare setting.

Further refinement of investigative techniques will help separate those that are sensitized from those that have clinical allergy. Ongoing surveillance of sensitized individuals is needed to determine the factors that may precipitate the onset of allergy and to improve the guidance given to this group.

REFERENCES

1. Anon., Allergic reactions to latex-containing devices, *FDA Med. Bull.*, 21, 1, 1991.
2. Saxon, A. et al., Prevalence of IgE to natural rubber latex in unselected blood donors and performance characteristics of AlaSTAT testing, *Ann. Allergy Asthma Immunol.*, 84, 199, 2000.
3. Turjanmaa, K. et al., Natural rubber latex allergy — The European experience, *Immunol. Allergy Clinics N. Am.*, 15, 71, 1995.
4. Gautrin, D. et al., Incidence and determinants of IgE-mediated sensitization in apprentices: A prospective study, *Am. J. Respir. Crit. Care Med.*, 162, 1222, 2000.
5. Chaiear, S. et al., Sensitisation to natural rubber latex: An epidemiological study of workers exposed during tapping and glove manufacture in Thailand, *Occup. Environ. Med.*, 58, 386, 2001.
6. Amin, S. and Maibach, H.I., Contact urticaria syndrome, *Am. J. Contact Dermatitis*, 8, 15, 1997.
7. Hamilton, R.G. et al., Diagnosis of natural rubber latex allergy: Multi-centre latex skin testing efficacy study, *J. Allergy Clin. Immunol.*, 102, 482, 1998.
8. Hamilton, R.G. and Adkinson F., Natural rubber latex skin testing reagents: Safety and diagnostic accuracy of nonammoniated latex, ammoniated latex and latex rubber glove extracts, *J. Allergy Clin. Immunol.*, 98, 872, 1996.
9. Wransjo, K., Osterman, K., and van Hage-Hamsten, M., Glove related skin symptoms among operating theatre and dental care unit personnel (II): Clinical examination and laboratory findings indicating latex allergy, *Contact Dermatitis*, 30, 139, 1994.
10. Nakamura, C.T. et al., Latex allergy in children on home mechanical ventilation, *Chest*, 117, 1000, 2000.
11. Turjanmaa, K. et al., Long-term outcome of 160 adult patients with natural rubber latex allergy, *J. Allergy Clin. Immunol.*, 110, S70, 2002.
12. Vandenplas, O. et al., Prevalence of occupational asthma due to latex among hospital personnel, *Am. J. Respir. Crit. Care Med.*, 151, 54, 1995.
13. Turjanmaa, K., Incidence of immediate allergy to latex gloves in hospital personnel, *Contact Dermatitis*, 17, 270, 1987.
14. De Groot, H. et al., Prevalence of natural rubber latex allergy (Type I and Type IV) in laboratory workers in the Netherlands, *Contact Dermatitis*, 38,159, 1998.

15. Palosuo, T., Turjanmaa, K., and Reinikka-Railo, H., Allergen content of latex gloves: A market surveillance study of medical gloves used in Finland in 1997, *National Agency for Medicines,* 1997.

16. Tarlo, S.M. et al., Occupational asthma caused by latex in a surgical glove manufacturing plant, *J. Allergy Clin. Immunol.,* 85, 625, 1990.

17. Niggemann, B. et al., Latex provocation tests in patients with spina bifida: Who is at risk of becoming symptomatic? *J. Allergy Clin. Immunol.,* 102, 665, 1998.

18. Brown, R.H., Schauble, J.F., and Hamilton, R.G., Prevalence of latex allergy among anesthesiologists: Identification of sensitized but asymptomatic individuals, *Anesthesiology,* 89, 292, 1998.

19. Yman, L. et al., Clinical efficacy of UniCAP specific IgE, *J. Allergy Clin. Immunol.,* 97, 234, 1996 (abstract).

20. Yeang, H.Y., Prevalence of latex allergy may be vastly overestimated when determined by *in vitro* assays, *Ann. Allergy Asthma Immunol.,* 84, 628, 2000.

21. Konrad, C. et al., The prevalence of latex sensitivity among anaesthesiology staff, *Anaesth. Analg.,* 84, 629, 1997.

22. Ylitalo, L. et al., Natural rubber latex allergy in children who had not undergone surgery and children who had undergone multiple operations, *J. Allergy Clin. Immunol.,* 100, 606, 1997.

23. Monteret-Vautrin, D.A. et al., Prospective study of risk factors in natural rubber latex hypersensitivity, *J. Allergy Clin. Immunol.,* 92, 668,1993.

24. Capriles-Hulett, A. et al., Very low frequency of latex and fruit allergy in patients with spina bifida from Venezuela: Influence of socioeconomic factors, *Ann. Allergy Asthma Immunol.,* 75, 62, 1995.

25. Konz, K.R. et al., Comparison of latex hypersensitivity among patients with neurologic defects, *J. Allergy Clin. Immunol.,* 95, 950, 1995.

26. Monasterio, E.A. et al., Latex allergy in adults with spinal cord injury: A pilot investigation, *J. of Spinal Cord Medicine,* 23, 6, 2000.

27. Garabrant, D.H. et al., Latex sensitisation in health care workers and in the U.S. general population, *Am. J. Epidemiology,* 153, 512, 2001.

28. Wartenberg, D. and Buckler, G., Invited commentary: Assessing latex sensitisation using data from NHANES III, *Am. J. Epidemiology,* 153, 523, 2001.

29. Page, E.H. et al., Natural rubber latex: Glove use, sensitisation and airborne and latent dust concentrations at a Denver hospital, *J. O. E. M.,* 42, 613, 2000.

30. Bollinger, M.E. et al., A hospital-based screening program for natural rubber latex allergy, *Ann. Allergy Asthma Immunol.,* 8, 560, 2002.

31. Posch, A. et al., Latex allergens, *Clin. Exp. Allergy,* 28, 134, 1998.

32. Kim, K.T. and Hussain, H., Prevalence of food allergy in 137 latex-allergic patients, *Allergy Asthma Proc.,* 20, 95, 1999.

33. Conde-Salazar, L. et al., Latex allergy among construction workers, *Contact Dermatitis,* 47, 154, 2002.

34. Hack, M.E., The prevalence of latex allergy in operating theatre staff, *Anaesth. Intensive Care,* 29, 43, 2001.

35. Kim, K.T., Wellmeyer, E.K., and Miller, K.V., Minimum prevalence of latex hypersensitivity in health care workers, *Allergy and Asthma Proc.,* 20, 387, 1999.

36. Kaczmarek, R.G. et al., Prevalence of latex-specific IgE antibodies in hospital personnel, *Ann. Allergy Asthma Immunol.,* 76, 51, 1996.

37. Chowdhury, M.M.U. and Statham, B.N., Natural rubber latex allergy in a Welsh healthcare population, *Br. J. Dermatol.,* 148, 737, 2003.

38. Poole, C.J.M. and Nagendran, V., Low prevalence of clinical latex allergy in U.K. health care workers: A cross-sectional study, *Occup. Med.,* 51, 510, 2001.
39. Handfield-Jones, S.E., Latex allergy in health-care workers in an English district general hospital, *Br. J. Dermatol.,* 138, 273, 1998.
40. Lagier, F. et al., Prevalence of latex allergy in operating room nurses, *J. Allergy Clin. Immunol.,* 90, 319, 1992.
41. Jolanki, R. et al., Incidence rates of occupational contact urticaria caused by natural rubber latex, *Contact Dermatitis,* 40, 329, 1999.
42. Sussman, G.L. et al., Incidence of latex sensitization among latex glove users, *J. Allergy Clin. Immunol.,* 101, 171, 1998.
43. Sussman, G.L., Liss, G.M., and Wasserman S., Update on the Hamilton, Ontario latex sensitization study, *J. Allergy Clin. Immunol.,* 102, 333, 1998.
44. Tarlo, S.M. et al., Outcomes of a natural rubber latex control program in an Ontario teaching hospital, *J. Allergy Clin. Immunol.,* 108, 628, 2001.
45. Allmers, H. et al., Reduction of latex aeroallergens and latex specific IgE antibodies in sensitized workers after removal of powdered natural rubber latex gloves in a hospital, *J. Allergy Clin. Immunol.,* 102, 841, 1998.
46. Allmers, H., Schmengler, J., and Skudlik, C., Primary prevention of natural rubber latex allergy in the German health care system through education and intervention, *J. Allergy Clin. Immunol.,* 110, 318, 2002.
47. Levy, D.A. et al., Powder-free protein-poor natural rubber latex gloves and latex sensitisation, *J. Am. Med. Assoc.,* 281, 988, 1999.
48. Sarry, J.M. et al., Changes in rates of natural rubber latex sensitivity among dental school students and staff members after changes in latex gloves, *J. Allergy Clin. Immunol.,* 109, 131, 2002.

2 Allergenic Proteins

Harri Alenius and Timo Palosuo

CONTENTS

I. Introduction 15
II. Allergenic NRL Proteins 16
    A. Hev b 1 (Rubber Elongation Factor) 16
    B. Hev b 2 (1,3-β-glucanase) 16
    C. Hev b 3 (22-27 kD rubber particle protein) 18
    D. Hev b 4 (50-57 kD microhelix protein complex) 18
    E. Hev b 5 (acidic NRL protein; 16 kD pI 3.5) 18
    F. Hev b 6.01 (prohevein), Hev b 6.02 (hevein), and Hev b 6.03
       (prohevein C-domain) 19
    G. Hev b 7 (46 kD patatin-like protein) 19
    H. Hev b 8 (profilin) 19
    I. Hev b 9 (enolase) 20
    J. Hev b 10 (manganese superoxide dismutase; MnSOD) 20
    K. Hev b 11 (Class 1 chitinase) 20
    L. Hev b 12 20
    M. Hev b 13 20
    N. Other NRL Allergens 21
III. IgE-Binding Epitopes of NRL Allergens 21
IV. T-Cell Epitopes of NRL Allergens 22
V. Allergens in NRL Products 23
VI. Future Aspects 24
References 24

I. INTRODUCTION

Natural rubber latex (NRL) is the intracellular exudate obtained from the rubber tree, *Hevea brasiliensis*. Its main constituent, other than water, is natural rubber, the polymeric hydrocarbon *cis*-polyisoprene. NRL contains several proteins that are involved in various plant functions. Protein content of fresh liquid latex is estimated to be approximately 1 to 2%.[1]

Hevein is the predominant protein in NRL and is involved in the coagulation of natural rubber by bridging rubber particles via *N*-acetyl-ᴅ-glucosamine residues and the 22-kD receptor protein present on the surface of the rubber particles.[2] Hevein may also play a role in the protection of rubber tree wounds by inhibiting the growth of chitin-containing fungi and defending the attacks of insects. Other proteins involved in the rubber biosynthesis are rubber elongation factor[3] and small rubber particle protein,[4] which are both tightly bound to the surface of rubber particles. NRL also contains several other proteins that play roles in defense systems of the plant (e.g., class 1 and class 2 chitinases, beta-1,3-glucanases, and hevamines) and in other plant functions (e.g., profilins, enolases, esterases, and lipid transfer proteins).

Consensus exists that proteins or peptides eluting from manufactured NRL products are responsible for the sensitization processes in NRL allergy. Of more than 250 different polypeptides detected from NRL, only about one-fourth are suggested to be IgE binding allergens.[5] Knowledge of the causative allergens is required to develop reliable diagnosis of NRL allergy and to develop methods for determination of allergenicity of NRL products.

II. ALLERGENIC NRL PROTEINS

Substantial progress has been made in recent years in the purification and molecular characterization of NRL allergens, which has facilitated the assessment of their significance. The WHO/IUIS (International Union of Immunological Societes) Allergen Nomenclature Committee (www.allergen.org) lists 13 NRL allergens characterized at the molecular level (Table 2.1). Several important NRL allergens have been characterized, cloned and produced by recombinant DNA techniques. Recently, also B-cell and T-cell epitopes of a few NRL allergens have been determined. Three-dimensional structure is known only for one of the WHO/IUIS designated NRL allergens, i.e., hevein (Hev b 6.02), rendering possible studies of conformational B-cell epitopes.[6]

A. Hev b 1 (Rubber Elongation Factor)

Rubber elongation factor (Hev b 1) was the first NRL allergen characterized at molecular level.[3] Hev b 1 is a 137-amino acid (aa) long hydrophobic protein that also has a tetrameric form with a molecular mass of 58 kD. It can be purified from the rubber particle fraction of the liquid latex of the rubber tree, and the molecule has also been produced as recombinant protein in bacteria and plant cells.[7] IgE antibodies to Hev b 1 have been common (50 to 80%) in children with spina bifida (SB) or other congenital anomalies. However, authors have reported highly varying prevalence figures for adult NRL allergic patients (frequencies ranging from 0 to 100%). Consensus exists that Hev b 1 is a major allergen in patients with SB but depending on antibody assays used and populations studied, different views have persisted as to its significance in adults and in NRL-allergic patients with no history of multiple surgery.

B. Hev b 2 (1,3-β-glucanase)

Alenius et al. isolated and purified a 36-kD NRL protein that showed high homology to several plant endo-1,3-β-glucanases in sequence analysis.[8] Purified 1,3-β-gluca-

TABLE 2.1
NRL Allergens

Allergen	Trivial Name	Mol.wt. (kDa)	Length (Amino Acids)	Function	Significance as NRL Allergen	Accession No.
Hev b 1	Rubber elongation factor	14.6	138	Biosynthesis of polyisoprene	Minor/major**	X56535
Hev b 2	1,3-β-glucanase	35.1	374	Defence protein (PRP)	Major?***	U22147
Hev b 3	Small rubber particle protein	22.3	204	Coagulation of latex?	Minor/major**	AJ223388, AF051317
Hev b 4	Microhelix complex	50–57	N/A*	Structural protein	Minor?***	N/A
Hev b 5	Acidic NRL protein	16	151	Structural protein?	Major	U42640, U51361
Hev b 6.01	Prohevein	20	187	PRP, coagulation of latex	Major	M36986
Hev b 6.02	Mature hevein	4.7	43			
Hev b 6.03	Prohevein C-domain	14	138			
Hev b 7	Patatin homologue	42.9	388	Defence protein	Minor	U80598, AJ223038
Hev b 8	Profilin	14	131	Cytoskeletal actin-binding protein	Minor	AJ132397, Y15402
Hev b 9	Enolase	47.6	445	Enzyme	Minor	AJ132580
Hev b 10	Mn superoxide dismutase	22.9	206	Enzyme	Minor	AJ249148, L11707
Hev b 11w	Class 1 chitinase	30	295	Defence protein	Minor	AJ238579
Hev b 12	Lipid transfer protein	9.3	92	Enzyme	Minor	AY057860
Hev b 13	Early nodule-specific protein	43	N/A*	Esterase	Major?***	P83269

* N/A: not available
** Minor for HCW, major for SB
*** Significance not fully established

nase bound IgE from 21% of NRL-allergic patient (n=29) sera. Subsequently, Sunderasan et al. isolated a basic-1,3-β-glucanase from *Hevea* latex that was designated as Hev b 2 in the IUIS allergen nomenclature. [9] Depending on the methods used, IgE-binding in ELISA assays to purified Hev b 2 varied between 20 to 61% in NRL allergic patients, but only 2/29 patients reacted to recombinant Hev b 2 in skin prick testing (SPT).[9–11] However, in another recent study, using SPT a 63% reactivity to native purified Hev b 2 was reported, suggesting that Hev b 2 is an important NRL allergen.[12] Caution should however be exercised in interpreting these results, which should be confirmed using scrupulously purified natural proteins. The current data available suggests that Hev b 2 is a significant NRL allergen, but additional studies are needed to assess its factual importance.

C. HEV b 3 (22-27 kD RUBBER PARTICLE PROTEIN)

A 27-kD NRL allergen associated with patients with SB was first described in 1993 by Alenius et al.[13] This 27-kD allergen bound IgE from 83% of U.S. and 67% of Finnish SB patients and it showed partial sequence homology to Hev b 1. Subsequently, Lu et al. isolated from NRL, a 23-kD protein that revealed 45% similarity with Hev b 1 and shared identical sequence motifs with the 27-kD protein.[14] Later, Yeang et al. isolated a 24-kD protein from small rubber particles that was similarly recognized by IgE from NRL allergic patients with SB and was named as Hev b 3.[15] Recently, a cDNA clone encoding a 204 amino acid NRL protein (22.3-kD; pI 4.6) and showing 47% identity to Hev b 1 was described by Wagner et al.[16] All published amino acid sequences of fragments of the 27-kD, the 23-kD NRL and the 24-kD allergens fit into the deduced amino acid sequence of the rHev b 3. In immunoblotting, 83% of the NRL allergic patients with SB revealed IgE binding to rHev b 3. These findings suggest that Hev b 3 is a highly important allergen for patients with SB.

D. HEV b 4 (50-57 kD MICROHELIX PROTEIN COMPLEX)

An acidic 50- through 57-kD NRL protein that was bound by IgE in serum from one NRL allergic patient was identified and named as Hev b 4 by Sunderasan et al. in 1995.[9] N-terminal sequencing revealed no homology to any known sequences available in the data banks. This allergen has not yet been cloned and expressed. Kurup et al. reported in 2000, IgE responses to purified Hev b 4 by two different RAST assays and by an ELISA method.[10] Depending on the IgE assay used, Hev b 4 was shown to bind IgE from 23 to 65% of healthcare workers (HCW) (n=31) and from 30 to 77% of the patients with SB (n=13) suggesting that Hev b 4 is a major NRL allergen. However, in their study, also 6 to 20% of the control subjects without evidence of NRL allergy showed IgE binding to Hev b 4. Further studies are needed to evaluate the precise role of Hev b 4 as an NRL allergen.

E. HEV b 5 (ACIDIC NRL PROTEIN; 16 kD pI 3.5)

Hev b 5 was cloned simultaneously by Slater et al. and Akasawa et al. in 1996.[17,18] Hev b 5 (163 aa) is one of the most acidic proteins in the laticifer cells of the rubber tree, and is exceptionally rich in glutamic acid. Hev b 5 shows high sequence homology

(46%) to kiwi fruit protein pKIWI501. In the study of Slater et al. 56% of SB patients (n=57) and 92% of HCW (n=13) with NRL allergy had IgE to Hev b 5. Similarly, IgE from more than 50% of adult NRL allergic patients reacted with Hev b 5 in the study by Akasawa et al. More recently, Yip et al. [11] showed that 18/29 (62%) of NRL allergic patients reacted to recombinant Hev b 5 in SPT and a reactivity of similar magnitude (65%) was obtained also by Bernstein et al.[12] These results indicate that Hev b 5 is a highly significant allergen for both HCW and patients with SB.

F. HEV b 6.01 (PROHEVEIN), HEV b 6.02 (HEVEIN), AND HEV b 6.03 (PROHEVEIN C-DOMAIN)

Hevein is synthesized as a precursor protein (187 aa; also known as prohevein) that is processed into aminoterminal hevein (43 aa) and the carboxyterminal domain (138-aa C-domain).[19] Hevein domain shows high homology to several chitin-binding proteins, whereas the C-domain is highly homologous to wound-inducible proteins. Hevein has been produced as recombinant protein in insect cells[20] and prohevein in bacterial cells.[21]

Alenius et al. reported that 69% of NRL-allergic patients (n=56) had IgE antibodies to purified prohevein, whereas 21% of these patients had IgE against the purified prohevein C-domain.[22] Moreover, 56% of 45 NRL-allergic patient sera showed IgE antibodies to purified N-terminal hevein domain. Essentially similar results were reported by the study of Banerjee et al. in 1997, where 84% of HCW sera (n=25) exhibited IgE binding to recombinant prohevein.[23] Recombinant hevein showed IgE binding with 88% sera whereas 40% of these patients had IgE to recombinant prohevein C-domain. In the study of Chen et al., purified hevein gave positive SPT reactions in 81% patients (n=21) with NRL allergy.[24] All the available data indicate that prohevein and its N-terminal hevein domain are major NRL allergens.

G. HEV b 7 (46 kD PATATIN-LIKE PROTEIN)

Beezhold et al. reported that IgE in sera from 22% NRL allergic patients (n=29) bound to a 46-kD NRL protein.[25] Hev b 7 has been cloned and shown to have 39 to 42% homology with patatin from potato. More recently, Kurup et al. measured IgE responses to purified Hev b 7 by different assays (two RAST assays and ELISA) and found that, depending on the method used, 15 to 77% of the NRL allergic patients, including HCWs and SB patients, had IgE antibodies to purified Hev b 7.[10] Recombinant Hev b 7 expressed in *Pichia pastoris* was shown to bind IgE from 4 sera of 36 (11%) latex allergic patients,[26] while Yip et al.[11] noted positive SPT reactions in 12/29 (41%) latex allergic patients to a recombinant Hev b 7 produced in bacterial cells. A similar rate of positivity (45%) was reported by Bernstein et al.[12] in SPT using purified natural Hev b 7. Currently, Hev b 7 is considered to be a minor NRL allergen in most publications.

H. HEV b 8 (PROFILIN)

Profilins, ubiquitously present in various plants, are frequently identified as IgE binding proteins. Vallier et al. demonstrated that NRL profilin (Hev b 8) bound IgE in sera from 2/19 (11%) NRL allergic patients.[27] A more recent study by Rihs et al. using recombinant Hev b 8 as an antigen found that IgE antibodies from 5/25 (20%) NRL allergic patient sera recognized this recombinant protein.[28] Hev b 8 appears to represent a minor NRL allergen, and is presumed to be very thermolabile, and therefore unlikely to be present in manufactured rubber products.

I. HEV b 9 (ENOLASE)

Wagner et al. described recently the cloning from *Hevea* latex of a 1651 basepair (bp) cDNA encoding a protein of 445 amino acids (47.6 kD; pI 5.6).[29] The Hev b 9 displays 62% identity with Cla h 6, the enolase of the mold *C. herbarum*, and 60% identity with Alt a 5, the enolase of the *A. alternata*. Sixteen out of 110 NRL allergic patients (14.5%) showed IgE binding to rHev b 9 suggesting that Hev b 9 is a minor NRL allergen.

J. HEV b 10 (MANGANESE SUPEROXIDE DISMUTASE; MnSOD)

A *Hevea* latex MnSOD consisting of 206 amino acid residues was cloned and expressed in *E. coli* by Wagner et al.[30] The allergen was designated as Hev b 10. In immunoblotting, latex- as well as *A. fumigatus*-allergic patients revealed IgE binding to rHev b 10. Cross-reactivity to Asp f 6, the MnSOD from *A. fumigatus*, and human MnSOD was determined by inhibition of IgE binding to these MnSODs by rHev b 10. Hev b 10 is a new cross-reactive allergen of *H. brasiliensis,* which belongs to the 'latex-mold' group of latex allergens.

K. HEV b 11 (CLASS 1 CHITINASE)

Cloning and expression of a Class 1 chitinase (295 aa) from *Hevea* latex was reported to the list of the Allergen Nomenclature Committee by O'Riordain et al.[31] Of 57 NRL allergic patients, 10 (19%) recognized the recombinant Hev b 11. More recently, Rihs et al. cloned and expressed recombinant Class 1 chitinase from *Hevea brasiliensis* leaves.[32] This recombinant protein (rHev b 11.0102) was shown to contain an N-terminal hevein-like domain with 56% homology to hevein. IgE binding to rHev b 11.0102 was seen in 17/58 (29%) sera of NRL allergic patients, suggesting that despite its high homology to hevein, Hev b 11 is a minor NRL allergen.

L. HEV b 12

When searching for additional putatively cross-reacting allergens in NRL, Beezhold et al. cloned and expressed in bacterial cells a lipid transfer protein that was named as Hev b 12.[33] Nine of 37 (24%) NRL allergic patients had IgE recognizing the rHev b 12.

M. HEV b 13

Yeang et al. recently isolated an allergen from NRL that showed homology to early nodule-specific protein of soy bean, *Glycine max*.[34] This protein was designated as

Hev b 13 and was reported by Bernstein et al. to give positive SPT reaction in 63% of NRL allergic patients tested.[12] Further studies are needed to assess the significance of Hev b 13 as a new NRL allergen.

N. Other NRL Allergens

Certain other allergens, like hevamine and prenyl transferase, have been reported to bind IgE antibodies and can thus be classified as allergens. Their possible significance in NRL allergy remains to be elucidated.

In conclusion, consensus exists that Hev b 1 and Hev b 3 are major allergens for pediatric patients with SB or other congenital anomalies requiring multiple surgical operations at an early age. Hev b 5 and Hev b 6.01 (prohevein) and Hev b 6.02 (N-terminal hevein-domain of prohevein) are major allergens for both adult and pediatric patients, irrespective of their surgical histories.[35] Overall significance of Hev b 2, Hev b 4, Hev b 7 and Hev b 13 as NRL allergens is still somewhat controversial and needs further clarification.

III. IGE-BINDING EPITOPES OF NRL ALLERGENS

The knowledge of IgE-binding epitopes of allergens (i.e. IgE-binding structures on the surface of an allergen) is important in the design of specific therapies for immediate type allergy. Linear IgE binding epitopes of several NRL allergens have been described and just recently, also conformational IgE epitopes have been reported.

IgE binding sites on Hev b 1 have been analyzed using synthetic overlapping peptides covering the entire Hev b 1 sequence.[36] IgE binding epitopes were located in the C-terminal segment (121–137) and in segments with amino acid residues of 30–49 and 46–64. Banerjee et al. synthesized overlapping decapeptides of prohevein (Hev b 6.01) and identified two major linear IgE-binding epitopes (residues 19–24 and 25–37) in the N-terminal hevein domain (Hev b 6.02) and 3 epitopes in the C-domain (Hev b 6.03) (aa 60–66, 98–103, 164–172).[23] Essentially similar results were reported by Beezhold et al.[37] who identified two linear IgE epitopes in the hevein domain (residues 13–24 and 29–36) and 4 in the C-domain. In another study, Beezhold et al. synthesized octapeptides spanning the entire Hev b 5 protein and detected 6 IgE-binding regions (aa 15-22, 28-32, 50-56, 76-81, 90-95 and 132-139).[38] Investigation of linear IgE binding regions of the two homologous NRL allergens, Hev b 1 and Hev b 3, have been previously described.[39] The authors found 8 IgE binding epitopes for Hev b 1 and 11 for Hev b 3, identified by sera from NRL allergic patients with SB.

A combination of linear peptide mapping strategy and mutational IgE analysis was recently used in the study by Beezhold et al.[40] Eleven linear IgE epitopes were identified in Hev b 5 by SPOT analysis. Subsequently, alanine substitutions to selected synthetic peptides was used to identify the important amino acids for IgE binding. Site-directed mutagenesis was used to replace the crucial amino acids with alanine in a recombinant Hev b 5 mutant. Mutants with amino acid substitutions in single epitopes failed to reduce IgE binding, but simultaneous changes in 8 epitopes (simultaneous mutation of 14 selected amino acids) resulted in a 4500-fold reduction in IgE binding. Mutants with reduced IgE-binding activity may prove to be valuable reagents for immunotherapy.

A novel approach to the localization and reconstruction of conformational IgE-binding epitope regions of hevein (Hev b 6.02), has been recently described by Karisola et al.[6] An antimicrobial protein (AMP) from the amaranth, *Amaranthus caudatus*, was used as an immunologically silent adaptor molecule to which terminal or central parts of hevein were fused. Hevein and AMP share a structurally identical core region, but have different N-terminal and C-terminal regions. Only 1/16 hevein-allergic patients showed weak IgE binding to purified AMP. Chimeric AMP with the hevein N-terminus (aa 1-11) was recognized by IgE from 14 (88%) patients and the AMP-chimera with the hevein C-terminus (aa 32–43) by 6 (38%) of the patients. When both the N-terminal and C-terminal regions of hevein were fused with the AMP core, IgE from all 16 patients bound to the chimera. In contrast, only two patients showed IgE to the AMP chimera containing hevein core region (aa 12–31). These results suggest that the IgE-binding ability of hevein is almost exclusively determined by its N-terminal and C-terminal regions, which seem to contain conformational epitopes not detectable by linear IgE epitope analysis. The chimera-based epitope mapping strategy may provide a valuable tool for defining structural epitopes and selecting critical amino acids for site-directed mutagenesis.

Amino acid residues of hevein molecule (Hev b 6.02) that interact critically with IgE have been recently identified using site-specific mutations.[41] Twenty-nine hevein mutants were designed and produced by a baculovirus expression system in insect cells and tested by IgE inhibition-ELISA using sera from 26 latex allergic patients. Six potential IgE-interacting residues of hevein (Arg5, Lys10, Glu29, Tyr30, His35, and Gln38) were identified and characterized further. Based on these six residues, two triple mutants (HD3A, HD3B) and a hevein mutant where all six residues were mutated (HD6), were designed, modelled, and produced. The IgE-binding affinity of the mutants decreased by 100- through 10,000-fold as compared to that of recombinant hevein. Skin prick test reactivity of the triple mutant HD3A was drastically reduced and that of the six-residue mutant HD6 was completely abolished in all patients. Hevein with highly reduced ability to bind IgE should provide a valuable candidate molecule for immunotherapy of NRL allergy and is anticipated to have a low risk of systemic side effects.

IV. T-CELL EPITOPES OF NRL ALLERGENS

Specific IgE response to protein allergens requires the activation of B cells by T-helper 2 cells (Th2) that respond to the same allergen. Knowledge of the T-cell epitopes of allergens (i.e. linear regions of allergens that interact in the context of MHC class II molecules with their specific receptor on the surface of T-cells) is important in the design of effective strategies for allergen specific immunotherapy.

T-cell reactive regions of Hev b 1 have been characterized by Raulf-Heimsoth et al.[42] Nine overlapping peptides with 17 or 19 amino acid lengths covering the complete sequence of Hev b 1 were used for T-cell epitope mapping. Peripheral blood mononuclear cells (PBMCs) of NRL allergic patients and healthy subjects were stimulated with the synthetic peptides. Positive proliferation responses induced by one or more peptides were detected in the PBMCs of 10/14 NRL allergic patients and in 2/8 NRL-exposed nonallergic subjects. More than 65% of patients' PBMCs responded to the peptides aa 31–49 and aa 91–109.

T-cell epitope mapping of Hev b 5 was described by de Silva et al.[43] NRL specific T-cell lines derived from 6 NRL-allergic healthcare workers were generated and screened for proliferative response to overlapping 20 amino acid length peptides of Hev b 5. T-cell reactivity to one or more Hev b 5 peptides was identified in 5 patients. Peptide aa 46–65 induced T-cell proliferation in all of these 5 patients. Peptide aa 109–128 stimulated T cells from 3 of these patients. Proliferative responses were accompanied by substantial IL-5 secretion and minimal IFN-gamma secretion, indicating a Th2-dominant cytokine profile.

Characterization of T-cell responses of Hev b 3 was recently reported by Bohle et al.[44] T cell reactivity was investigated in NRL-allergic SB patients using Hev b 3 specific T-cell lines and clones. All T-cell clones were CD3/CD4-positive and expressed the alphabeta TCR. Twelve of 21 T-cell clones were classified as Th2-like, 2 of 21 were Th1-like, and 7 of 21 belonged to a Th0-like subset according to their cytokine production pattern. Nine T-cell stimulating peptides were determined out of 52 overlapping 12 amino acid length peptides covering the complete amino acid sequence of Hev b 3. Half of the patients exhibited T-cell reactivity to the peptide aa 103–114 suggesting its status as the dominant T-cell epitope.

T-cell epitopes of Hev b 6 have been recently investigated.[45] Ten NRL-allergic glove users and 6 non-NRL-allergic atopic control subjects were examined. NRL specific short-term oligoclonal T-cell lines were generated from PBMC of NRL-allergic subjects. These lines were tested for proliferative responses to overlapping 20 amino acid-length peptides of the Hev b 6.01 molecule. T-cell proliferation assays showed that NRL specific T-cell lines from all subjects responded to one or more peptide, with greatest frequency of reactivity to peptides Hev b 6 p(10-29) and Hev b 6 p(19-38) in the hevein domain.

V. ALLERGENS IN NRL PRODUCTS

Knowledge about the presence of the specific NRL allergens in the NRL gloves and other manufactured rubber products is rapidly increasing but still scanty. A large number of allergens have been identified in the source material for rubber products, whereas at present, only a limited number of NRL allergens or their fragments have been unequivocally demonstrated in NRL products. Hev b 1 was the first allergen extracted from NRL gloves[3] and large amounts of immunologically active Hev b 6.02 have previously been purified from a highly allergenic glove brand.[22] Current evidence strongly suggests that Hev b 6.02 and Hev b 5 are responsible for a major part of latex allergen levels in currently marketed medical gloves.[46,47] Preliminary data by Yeang et al. suggest that Hev b 2 can also be present in NRL gloves.[48] It should be noted that exact information of the molecular forms in which the allergenic proteins reside in manufactured products is only available for Hev b 6.02[22] and for Hev b 1.[3]

It is clear that these rubber product–associated proteins are those that sensitize people and produce symptoms in latex allergic patients. Other NRL proteins, not resisting the harsh conditions of rubber manufacture, may play roles as cross-reacting allergens, e.g., in the latex-fruit syndrome. The selection of relevant allergens for diagnostic test materials for SPT and serum IgE assays is of crucial importance for optimal specificity and sensitivity of the tests. Currently, the situation is far from ideal as the available test reagents contain uncharacterized and nonstandardized mixtures of proteins, the vast majority of which appear to be irrelevant for allergy to rubber products. This has led to difficulties in assessing "sensitivity" to NRL (occurrence of IgE antibodies to NRL allergens), in particular, in the general population where clinical allergy to NRL is less than 1%.[49,50] It is therefore likely that results from a large number of epidemiological studies have vastly overestimated the frequency of "true" sensitization to proteins derived from the manufactured NRL products.

VI. FUTURE ASPECTS

Knowledge of the whole spectrum of clinically relevant NRL allergens will help researchers to develop more specific in vivo and in vitro tests for diagnostic purposes and the production of pure allergens could provide tools for immunotherapy. Future studies will undoubtedly be focused on the analysis of immunodominant IgE epitopes in the allergen molecules and on possibilities to modify or destroy them to decrease their allergenic potential. These reagents are anticipated to have a low risk of systemic side effects when used in immunotherapy.

Recent research has brought specific methods for quantifying allergenic proteins of NRL in medical and other gloves, and this progress has already led governmental authorities in certain countries to inform the consumers on allergen levels of glove brands in the market. The international rubber manufacturers could also benefit from these new methods which are expected to help the development of less allergenic gloves and other NRL products.

REFERENCES

1. Jacob, J.L., d'Auzac, J., and Prevot, J.C., The composition of natural latex from *Hevea brasiliensis, Clin. Rev. Allergy,* 11, 325, 1993.
2. Gidrol, X. et al., Hevein, a lectin-like protein from *Hevea brasiliensis* (rubber tree) is involved in the coagulation of latex, *J. Biol. Chem.,* 269, 9278, 1994.
3. Czuppon, A.B. et al., The rubber elongation factor of rubber trees (*Hevea brasiliensis*) is the major allergen in latex, *J. Allergy Clin. Immunol.,* 92, 690, 1993.
4. Oh, S.K. et al., Isolation, characterization, and functional analysis of a novel cDNA clone encoding a small rubber particle protein from *Hevea brasiliensis, J. Biol. Chem.,* 274, 17132, 1999.
5. Alenius, H. et al., Latex allergy: Frequent occurrence of IgE antibodies to a cluster of 11 latex proteins in patients with spina bifida and histories of anaphylaxis, *J. Lab. Clin. Med.,* 123, 712, 1994.
6. Karisola, P. et al., The major conformational IgE-binding epitopes of hevein (Hev b 6.02) are identified by a novel chimera-based allergen epitope mapping strategy, *J. Biol. Chem.,* 277, 22656, 2002.

7. Breiteneder, H. et al., Rapid production of recombinant allergens in *Nicotiana benthamiana* and their impact on diagnosis and therapy, *Int. Arch. Allergy Immunol.,* 124, 48, 2001.

8. Alenius, H. et al., Prohevein from the rubber tree (*Hevea brasiliensis*) is a major latex allergen, *Clin. Exp. Allergy,* 25, 659, 1995.

9. Sunderasan, E. et al., Latex B-serum β-1,3-glucanase (Hev b II) and a component of the microhelix (Hev b IV) are major latex allergens, *J. Nat. Rubber Res.,* 10, 82, 1995.

10. Kurup, V.P. et al., Detection of immunoglobulin antibodies in the sera of patients using purified latex allergens, *Clin. Exp. Allergy,* 30, 359, 2000.

11. Yip, L. et al., Skin prick test reactivity to recombinant latex allergens, *Int. Arch. Allergy Immunol.,* 121, 292, 2000.

12. Bernstein, D.I. et al., In vivo sensitization to purified *Hevea brasiliensis* proteins in health care workers sensitized to natural rubber latex, *J. Allergy Clin. Immunol.,* 111, 610, 2003.

13. Alenius, H. et al., IgE reactivity to 14-kD and 27-kD natural rubber proteins in latex-allergic children with spina bifida and other congenital anomalies, *Int. Arch. Allergy Immunol.,* 102, 61, 1993.

14. Lu, L.J. et al., Characterization of a major latex allergen associated with hypersensitivity in spina bifida patients, *J. Immunol.,* 155, 2721, 1995.

15. Yeang, H.Y. et al., Amino acid sequence similarity of Hev b 3 to two previously reported 27- and 23-kDa latex proteins allergenic to spina bifida patients, *Allergy,* 53, 513, 1998.

16. Wagner, B. et al., Cloning, expression, and characterization of recombinant Hev b 3, a *Hevea brasiliensis* protein associated with latex allergy in patients with spina bifida, *J. Allergy Clin. Immunol.,* 104, 1084, 1999.

17. Slater, J.E. et al., Identification, cloning, and sequence of a major allergen (Hev b 5) from natural rubber latex (*Hevea brasiliensis*), *J. Biol. Chem.,* 271, 25394, 1996.

18. Akasawa, A. et al., A novel acidic allergen, Hev b 5, in latex. Purification, cloning and characterization, *J. Biol. Chem.,* 271, 25389, 1996.

19. Broekaert, I. et al., Wound-induced accumulation of mRNA containing a hevein sequence in laticifers of rubber tree (*Hevea brasiliensis*), *Proc. Natl. Acad. Sci. U.S.A.,* 87, 7633, 1990.

20. Airenne, K.J. et al., Avidin is a promising tag for fusion proteins produced in baculovirus-infected insect cells, *Protein Expr. Purif.,* 17, 139, 1999.

21. Rozynek, P., Posch, A., and Baur, X., Cloning, expression and characterization of the major latex allergen prohevein, *Clin. Exp. Allergy,* 28, 1418, 1998.

22. Alenius, H. et al., The main IgE-binding epitope of a major latex allergen, prohevein, is present in its N-terminal 43-amino acid fragment, hevein, *J. Immunol.,* 156, 1618, 1996.

23. Banerjee, B. et al., IgE from latex-allergic patients binds to cloned and expressed B cell epitopes of prohevein, *J. Immunol.,* 159, 5724, 1997.

24. Chen, Z. et al., Isolation and identification of hevein as a major IgE-binding polypeptide in *Hevea* latex, *J. Allergy Clin. Immunol.,* 99, 402, 1997.

25. Beezhold, D.H. et al., Identification of a 46-kD latex protein allergen in health care workers, *Clin. Exp. Immunol.,* 98, 408, 1994.

26. Sowka, S. et al., cDNA cloning of the 43-kDa latex allergen Hev b 7 with sequence similarity to patatins and its expression in the yeast *Pichia pastoris, Eur. J. Biochem.,* 255, 213, 1998.

27. Vallier, P. et al., Identification of profilin as an IgE-binding component in latex from *Hevea brasiliensis*: Clinical implications, *Clin. Exp. Allergy,* 25, 332, 1995.

28. Rihs, H.P. et al., PCR-based cloning, isolation, and IgE-binding properties of recombinant latex profilin (rHev b 8), *Allergy,* 55, 712, 2000.
29. Wagner, S. et al., Hev b 9, an enolase and a new cross-reactive allergen from hevea latex and molds. Purification, characterization, cloning and expression, *Eur. J. Biochem.,* 267, 7006, 2000.
30. Wagner, S. et al., Identification of a *Hevea brasiliensis* latex manganese superoxide dismutase (Hev b 10) as a cross-reactive allergen, *Int. Arch. Allergy Immunol.,* 125, 120, 2001.
31. O'Riordain, G. et al., Cloning and molecular characterization of the *Hevea brasiliensis* allergen Hev b 11, a class I chitinase, *Clin. Exp. Allergy,* 32, 455, 2002.
32. Rihs, H.P. et al., Molecular cloning, purification, and IgE-binding of a recombinant class I chitinase from *Hevea brasiliensis* leaves (rHev b 11.0102), *Allergy,* 58, 246, 2003.
33. Beezhold, D.H. et al., Lipid transfer protein from *Hevea brasiliensis* (Hev b 12), a cross-reactive latex protein, *Ann. Allergy Asthma Immunol.,* 90, 439, 2003.
34. Yeang, H.Y. et al., Allergenic proteins of natural rubber latex, *Methods,* 27, 32, 2002.
35. Alenius, H., Turjanmaa, K., and Palosuo, T., Natural rubber latex allergy, *Occup. Environ. Med.,* 59, 419, 2002.
36. Chen, H.D., Chen, C.L., and Huang, S.W., Characterization of latex allergens and correlation of serum IgE/IgG antibody ratio with clinical symptoms, *Allergy Asthma Proc.,* 17, 143, 1996.
37. Beezhold, D.H., Kostyal, D.A., and Sussman, G.L., IgE epitope analysis of the hevein preprotein; a major latex allergen, *Clin. Exp. Immunol.,* 108, 114, 1997.
38. Beezhold, D.H. et al., Human IgE-binding epitopes of the latex allergen Hev b 5, *J. Allergy Clin. Immunol.,* 103, 1166, 1999.
39. Banerjee, B. et al., Unique and shared IgE epitopes of Hev b 1 and Hev b 3 in latex allergy, *Mol. Immunol.,* 37, 789, 2000.
40. Beezhold, D.H., Hickey, V.L., and Sussman, G.L., Mutational analysis of the IgE epitopes in the latex allergen Hev b 5, *J. Allergy Clin. Immunol.,* 107, 1069, 2001.
41. Karisola, P. et al., Construction of hevein (Hev b 6.02) with reduced allergenicity for immunotherapy of latex allergy by co-mutation of six amino acid residues on the conformational IgE epitope, *J. Immunol.,* 172, 2621, 2004.
42. Raulf-Heimsoth, M. et al., Analysis of T-cell reactive regions and HLA-DR4 binding motifs on the latex allergen Hev b 1 (rubber elongation factor), *Clin. Exp. Allergy,* 28, 339, 1998.
43. de Silva, H.D. et al., Human T-cell epitopes of the latex allergen Hev b 5 in health care workers, *J. Allergy Clin. Immunol.,* 105, 1017, 2000.
44. Bohle, B. et al., Characterization of T cell responses to Hev b 3, an allergen associated with latex allergy in spina bifida patients, *J. Immunol.,* 164, 4393, 2000.
45. de Silva, H.D. et al., The hevein domain of the major latex glove allergen Hev b 6 contains dominant T-cell reactive sites, *J. Clin. Exp. Allergy,* 2004, in press.
46. Palosuo, T., Alenius, H., and Turjanmaa, K., Quantitation of latex allergens, *Methods,* 27, 52, 2002.
47. Sutherland, M.F. et al., Specific monoclonal antibodies and human immunoglobulin E show that Hev b 5 is an abundant allergen in high protein powdered latex gloves, *Clin. Exp. Allergy,* 32, 583, 2002.
48. Yeang, H. et al., Hev b 2 and Hev b 3 content in natural rubber latex and latex gloves., *J. Allergy Clin. Immunol.,* 107, S118, 2001.
49. Turjanmaa, K. et al., Natural rubber latex allergy, *Allergy,* 51, 593, 1996.
50. Liss, G.M. and Sussman, G.L., Latex sensitization: occupational versus general population prevalence rates, *Am. J. Ind. Med.,* 35, 196, 1999.

3 Chemical Additives

Curtis P. Hamann, Pamela A. Rodgers,
and Kim Sullivan

CONTENTS

I. Introduction...28
II. Manufacture of Rubber..28
    A. History of Rubber Manufacturing...28
    B. Manufacturing Processes..29
        1. Harvesting and Processing of Natural Rubber 30
        2. Centrifugation...30
        3. Compounding 31
        4. Dipping Technology 31
        5. Vulcanization and Prevulcanization 32
        6. Leaching 33
        7. Drying...33
        8. Chlorination..33
        9. Surface Coatings 34
    C. Rubber and Rubberlike Elastomers 34
        1. Natural Rubber Polyisoprene 36
        2. Nitrile...37
        3. Neoprene...37
        4. Polyvinyl Chloride 38
        5. Polyurethanes 38
        6. Styrene-Based Elastomers..39
        7. Synthetic Polyisoprene...39
        8. Other Rubberlike Elastomers 40
III. Rubber Compounding..40
    A. Chemical Additives 41
        1. Vulcanizing Agents and Accelerators 41
        2. Antidegradants..44
        3. Pigments, Fragrances, and Flavorants 46
        4. Processing Aids 47
        5. Releasing Agents and Lubricants...47
    B. Allergenicity of Rubber Additives 47
        1. Vulcanization Agents and Accelerators 48
        2. Antidegradants..49
        3. Other Additives...49
        4. Release Agents and Lubricants...50

0-8493-1670-7/05/$0.00+$1.50
© 2005 by CRC Press LLC

IV.   Conclusions and Future Developments...50
References..51

I. INTRODUCTION

In the 1890s, the surgeons W. S. Halsted and J. C. Bloodgood popularized the use of natural rubber surgical gloves.[1,2] Initially used to protect the hands of a surgical assistant from harsh disinfectants, rubber gloves were soon worn by the entire surgical team to reduce postoperative infections. Eventually, however, rubber gloves themselves became known as a source of dermatitis in healthcare and other occupations. In 1927 and 1933, Downing described electrical linemen and factory workers with symptoms consistent with type IV allergies to natural rubber.[1,3] In 1934, Prosser-White reported allergic responses to the vulcanizing accelerator hexamethylenetetramine, and additional cases of contact allergies to guanidines and benzothiazoles were subsequently reported by Bonnevie and Marcussen.[4,5]

In healthcare, construction, and food processing occupations, natural and synthetic rubber products are ubiquitous. Used in many industries, these products range from rubber vial stoppers to rubber components in tools and equipment including rubber gloves. Unfortunately, both natural and synthetic rubbers have the ability to cause both allergic and irritant reactions.

Healthcare workers appear to have the greater risk for the development of contact allergies to chemical allergens, including those found in rubber gloves.[6] This probably reflects their repeated use of rubber gloves, exposure to potentially allergenic chemicals, as well as poor skin health due to frequent handwashing.[7] The resulting skin disease can remain undiagnosed and unresolved for an average of 3 years or more.[8,9] A recent case report by Beltrami et al. sadly illustrated this point. A healthcare worker with chronically broken and abraded skin on her hands contracted HIV and HCV from an infected patient.[10] While insufficient barrier precautions also contributed to the problem, the critical role of occupational skin disease was underestimated.

Research in occupational dermatology has shown that contact allergies to rubber processing chemicals are common in healthcare, as well as food processing, construction, and industrial workers.[11,12] These rubber-based hand dermatoses can be effectively diagnosed and managed once workers and physicians obtain an adequate understanding of the chemicals in gloves and other rubber products. This latter issue of education has been identified as a critical factor in the prognosis of occupational skin disease.[13] Therefore, to aid in the understanding of rubber allergies, this chapter reviews the chemical composition and manufacturing permutations of natural and synthetic rubbers.

II. MANUFACTURE OF RUBBER

A. HISTORY OF RUBBER MANUFACTURING

Rubber has been utilized since at least 1600 B.C., according to studies of ancient Mesoamerican rubber balls, figurines, bands, paint, and medicines.[14] During these prehistoric days of rubber manufacture, latex rubber was harvested from the *Castilla* plant and modified by the natural solubilizers and plasticizers contained in a coharvested climbing vine. This crude, naturally 'compounded' rubber was then molded into the bouncing balls that graced Mesoamerican ball courts and subsequent treasure troves of Spanish conquistadors. As Spain and France increased their presence in the New World, more rubber-based products made their way back to Europe. However, it would take over 100 years before Europeans would take full advantage of these observations.

Rubberized goods became more popular in the early 1800s due to the use of new solvents and the development of the Hancock mastication process.[15,16] However, the use of crude natural rubber was still limited by temperature-dependent changes: it turned sticky when warm and rigid when cold. Charles Goodyear discovered that reacting sulfur and natural rubber together under heat created a product with great elasticity and strength, and without stickiness. He patented the vulcanization process in 1839, founding the modern rubber industry.

With the rapid development of the tire and automobile industry at the end of the 19th century, rubber manufacturing increased and accelerated the demand for natural rubber. Wild *Hevea* trees scattered throughout the Amazonian forest were still the prime source of natural rubber, driving a South American rubber boom.[17] However, this industry was plagued with corrupt business practices, inefficient harvesting, and labor problems. In anticipation of the growing demand for rubber, British industrialists expanded cultivation of natural rubber to Asia. By the end of the 19th century, *Hevea brasiliensis* seedlings were distributed throughout Asia and rubber plantations had developed.[17,18] New horticultural methods were soon applied to the Asian *Hevea* plantations, including a harvesting technique known as excision tapping. When combined with modern trait selection, rubber production advanced significantly. As a result, by the late-1930s natural rubber production had risen above 1 million tonnes, with Asian plantations as the predominant source.

In the early 1900s, the value of organic vulcanization accelerators was also discovered.[19] Organic compounds such as aniline, nitrobenzene, and various peroxides greatly reduced vulcanization time, temperature requirements, and enhanced the properties of rubber. When activated by zinc oxide, vulcanization processes again improved. Subsequent introduction of mercaptobenzothiazole, carbamates, thiurams, and sulfenamides fueled the growing rubber industry and many are still in use today.

Global events impacted the rubber industry again during World War II when Asian rubber plantations were isolated or destroyed. This natural rubber shortage spurred the U.S. government to establish programs to research and develop synthetic rubbers as well as explore alternative natural rubber sources.[20,21] As a result, synthetic rubber production has increased and today dominates the market.

B. Manufacturing Processes

Generally, rubbers and rubberlike elastomers begin their manufacturing process in a liquid form, either aqueous or solvent based. Although many rubber polymers can be processed in either dry or liquid forms, many products are manufactured from dry rubber sources. In fact, most natural rubber is exported to product manufacturers as dried slabs known as crepe rubber.[18] This crepe rubber is extensively processed with heat, water, and/or solvents before being used in the manufacture of dry-rubber goods such as tires, hoses, and shoes.

By comparison, dipped, foamed, and some molded products are manufactured from liquid rubber. Technically known as 'latex', it is best defined as "a stable dispersion of a polymeric substance in an essentially aqueous medium."[15] Therefore, latex can be derived from either natural or synthetic rubber polymers. Products derived from liquid rubber sources include thin-film products such as gloves, which are frequently associated with allergic reactions.

In general, a similar chemical compounding, vulcanization, and overall manufacturing process is utilized for gloves made of natural and synthetic rubber materials. Over 200 different chemical compounds, including ammonia, accelerators, stabilizers, and antidegradants are added to natural and synthetic rubber during processing. These chemicals are added to preserve, stabilize, and cure the rubber; improve the manufacturing process and product characteristics; and prevent the degradation of finished goods. To better understand the sources and uses of chemical allergens in rubber products, it is important to review key aspects of rubber manufacturing particularly as it relates to thin-film rubbers.

1. Harvesting and Processing of Natural Rubber

Natural rubber latex (NRL) is commercially harvested from the *Hevea brasiliensis* tree using excision tapping to release the milky cytoplasm of the laticifer cells.[22] This crude latex contains approximately 60% water and 35% rubber.[23,24] The remainder is composed of lipids (fats, waxes, sterols, and phospholipids), inositols and carbohydrates, resins, tannins, alkaloids, metals (potassium, magnesium, copper, iron, sodium, calcium, and phosphate), and well over 200 polypeptides and proteins. The majority (~ 60%) of these proteins are bound to the rubber particles.

Crude NRL is perishable; it coagulates and spoils unless preservatives are added in the field. According to current practices, ammonia is usually added at a low concentration (0.2%) with secondary preservatives to stabilize rubber particles prior to manufacturing.[22] These secondary preservatives can include zinc oxide, sodium pentachlorophenate, tetramethylthiuram disulfide, sodium dimethyldithiocarbamate, and boric acid.[25–27] These chemicals prevent coagulation and sequester impurities. They also hydrolyze proteins and lipids, which further stabilize the crude NRL.[22,23]

2. Centrifugation

Before further processing, liquid NRL is centrifuged to reduce water content, concentrate the rubber, and remove contaminants such as bark, dirt, and insects.[23,28] Surfactants may be used to displace hydrophobic proteins from the rubber particles. During routine factory centrifugation (~ 6000 rpm), crude NRL separates into upper and lower phases. The upper concentrated phase (~ 60% rubber content) is collected for further processing, excluding lower serum phase which contains the more water-soluble extractable proteins.[23] Multiple centrifugations of crude NRL can result in significant reductions in extractable protein content.[29,30]

Ultracentrifugation (~ 30,000 rpm), separates crude NRL into three layers. The uppermost layer contains the hydrocarbon rubber particles and associated insoluble proteins, which represent approximately 27% of the total available proteins.[22,23] The majority of extractable proteins are found in the aqueous middle fraction, or C-serum, and in the bottom fraction, or B-serum. These water-soluble proteins represent 48 and 25%, respectively, of the total protein available. Some of these C and B water-soluble serum proteins are likely retained and decanted with the rubber phase following a typical lower speed centrifugation.

3. Compounding

Natural and synthetic rubbers are amended with chemicals to produce the required durability, flexibility, and strength. Through the process known as compounding, chemicals are added to improve manufacturing efficiency as well as finished product performance. During this process, approximately 5 lbs of chemicals are added for every 100 lbs of rubber.[15,25,31] Much greater amounts can be added to products such as tires, which may contain more chemical additives than rubber.[31]

Of the different chemical additives, 90% are vulcanization accelerators and antidegradants, the latter of which includes antioxidants and antioxonants.[15,31] Other compounding agents include processing aids such as plasticizers, blowing agents, coagulants, and lubricants. Pigments, fragrances, flavorants, and agents designed to enhance product hydrophilicity may be added to improve aesthetic appeal or comfort. After the addition of compounding chemicals, the liquid latex is allowed to "mature," often for several days.[23] During this time, the chemicals intersperse throughout the latex, stabilizing, solubilizing, protecting, and reacting with the rubber particles.

4. Dipping Technology

The majority of thin-film devices (e.g., condoms, gloves, diaphragms, balloons, nipples, bathing caps, football bladders, toys, pacifiers) are manufactured by dipping formers or molds into compounded liquid latex derived from either synthetic or natural rubber. The formers and molds can be made of porcelain, glass, metal, plastic, or plaster. They move by batch or continuous production through various dipping and leaching tanks, ovens, and processing areas (Figure 3.1).

The formers are coated with a thin film of the liquid latex by one of several dipping methods.[22,27] Coagulant dipping is the most common process used for manufacturing rubber gloves. The hand-shaped glove former is initially immersed in a coagulant solution, and then dried prior to immersion in liquid latex. The coagulant typically consists of calcium salt solutions (e.g., calcium nitrate and calcium carbonate), although magnesium, or zinc salt solutions may also be used. It is thought that the coating of positively charged ions in these salts may attract the negatively charged rubber molecules. After dipping, the latex film on the former surface is dried and allowed to harden through a process known as gelation.

Other dipping variants include straight dipping and heat-sensitive dipping.[25,27] Straight dipping involves immersing an untreated former in liquid latex, and withdrawing it slowly. The latex that adheres is subsequently dried and vulcanized.

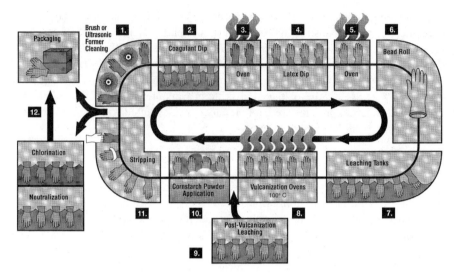

FIGURE 3.1 Manufacturing process for coagulant-dipped gloves. Glove formers are cleaned (1), then dipped in a coagulant such as calcium nitrate (2), and dried (3). The coagulant-coated formers are then dipped (4) into the compounded latex and rotated into low temperature ovens (5) for gel formation. After the cuff bead is formed, (6) the wet-gel latex-coated formers rotate through tanks (7) for prevulcanization leaching to remove soluble chemicals and proteins. Surface coatings may also be applied at this stage. Finally, the latex gloves are vulcanized (8) before passing on to a possible on-line postcure leaching (9) or application of surface coatings such as cornstarch (10). The glove is stripped from the formers (11) prior to packaging, off-line chlorination and neutralization, or additional off-line treatments (12). (From Hamann, C. P. and Sullivan, K., 1996. With permission.) [32]

Heat-sensitive dipping involves immersing heated formers into liquid latex compounded with a temperature-sensitive gelling agent such as a polypropylene glycol.[23]

5.   Vulcanization and Prevulcanization

Vulcanization is defined as a change in the chemical structure of rubber that causes its elastic properties to be conferred, reestablished, improved, or extended.[15,33] In general this change occurs by establishing chemical cross-links between the polymer chains. Vulcanization can be accomplished using sulfur-based or sulfur-independent chemical systems as discussed below in greater detail. Many different techniques range from the use of compression molding to liquid cure methods, and most involve elevated temperatures.[34] The production of thin-film articles such as gloves utilize an open cure method with hot air ovens that are used to both dry and vulcanize the rubber product.

Prevulcanization is based on the same chemical principles as vulcanization, but is conducted at a lower temperature and can result in an incomplete cure.[27] Prevulcanized latex, synthetic or natural rubber, is heated with the appropriate vulcanizing agents and accelerators prior to dipping. Prevulcanization can be used alone to simplify the manufacturing process or used to supplement oven-based vulcanization.

6. Leaching

Dipped products are usually leached to remove water-soluble materials such as salts, residual chemicals, and water-soluble proteins.[23,30,35] Leaching involves washing the product in a tank of heated water that is replenished regularly. Under controlled conditions, leaching can be very effective in removing extractable proteins from natural rubber, as well as residual chemicals from both natural and synthetic rubber products. Factors such as soft or hard water, movement or flow rate, duration, temperature, and rate of water exchange all contribute to the efficacy of the leaching process.[23,35,36]

On-line *wet-gel* leaching is carried out with the product still on the formers, usually before vulcanizing. Wet gel leaching involves soaking the coagulated (and possibly prevulcanized) latex gel while still on the former.[22] On-line leaching may also be conducted after vulcanization, referred to as *post cure* or *dry film* leaching. Usually dry film leaching is conducted off-line and takes longer, depending upon product thickness. On-line wet-gel leaching is more commonly utilized, and can improve a product's physical properties.[22,37] For removal of large water-soluble surface proteins, the best results are obtained using both processes.

7. Drying

After dipping, the formers are withdrawn and rotated into ovens for drying. The drying process can significantly affect the surface concentration of solubilized proteins or chemicals. Due to heat, water evaporates from the outside surface of the latex film on the formers.[36] An osmotic gradient drives water-soluble proteins and chemicals to this outside surface. When products such as gloves are then inverted upon removal from the formers, this outside surface becomes the *skin side* surface and now contains a potentially higher surface concentration of chemical and protein allergens.[23,36]

8. Chlorination

Chlorination can be performed on either natural or synthetic rubbers and is principally used to remove cornstarch when a powder-free or reduced-powder product is required.[22,38] Unfortunately, if not carefully controlled, chlorination can undermine the physical properties of rubber. At low concentrations of chlorine (0.1%), the tensile strength and surface integrity of the rubber film are maintained.[39] But as the concentration of chlorine increases, more of the polyisoprene is chlorinated, destabilizing the polymer's structure and increasing its susceptibility to oxidation. As a result, tensile strength and resistance to aging diminishes, the surface cracks and yellows, and the products' shelf life and integrity are compromised.

In addition to removing cornstarch powder, chlorination increases the slipperiness of natural and synthetic rubber surfaces, creating a unique texture. As the glove surface is chlorinated, carbonium ions can form leading to internal cross-linking, cyclization, and oxidation of the polyisoprene.[39] This halogenation causes the rubber surface to be more slippery and less sticky.[40] The increased washing required also diminishes the extractable protein content of natural rubber films, and probably the residual chemical content of all rubbers.[36] Chlorine also reportedly decreases the aqueous solubility of surface NRL proteins by reacting with the amine groups.[39] The acidic pH of the process may further reduce the aqueous solubility of surface NRL proteins.[36]

The chlorination process can be costly in materials and water resources, and presents operational challenges. During chlorination, rubber products such as gloves are exposed to a solution containing free chlorine such as acidified hypochlorite, organic chlorinating agents, or water treated with chlorine gas.[22,38] After neutralization with ammonia, sodium thiosulphate, or sodium bicarbonate, the products are rinsed repeatedly and dried. Although chlorination can be performed on- or off-line, open tanks of chlorine corrode equipment and are hazardous. Therefore, off-line processes are more common and usually involve industrial-scale washing machines. Regardless of the method, the wastewater that is generated must also be appropriately treated to avoid contaminating local water resources and ecosystems, an increasing concern in countries with rapid industrial growth.[39]

9. Surface Coatings

Powdered lubricants such as cornstarch can be applied to gloves on or off the production line. The simplest process involves the on-line dipping of latex-coated formers through a powder slurry tank, after which they are dried and the powdered product stripped from the former.[22] Latex-coated formers may also undergo on-line post cure leaching, and subsequently be dipped into the powder slurry and dried. Alternatively, the rubber products can be stripped from their formers, and subsequently washed, dried and powdered off-line.

For powder-free gloves, coatings on the inner surface of the glove improve donnability and comfort. Some coatings can be applied on-line before the final oven drying. Alternatively, they may be applied prior to vulcanization, but after gelation of the thin-film latex. They are applied on-line by dipping the primed or unprimed latex-coated former into the coating. This technique applies the coating selectively to the surface that will ultimately become the inside of the glove. Alternatively, stripped finished rubber gloves may be treated with a coating material during batch washing, but this process is less uniform and can apply coating material to the inside and outside surfaces.[22]

C. RUBBER AND RUBBERLIKE ELASTOMERS

Rubbers and rubberlike compounds belong to a larger class of molecules known as elastomers. Rubber polymers are generally made up of large molecules arranged in repeating sequences in long, stringlike chains (Table 3.1). Their fundamental unifying characteristic is the ability to stretch and return to their original shape. This permanent elasticity is based on chemical cross-links between the chains.[41] Each polymer may also have unique properties, such as low electrical conductivity and resistance to chemicals, environmental factors, and corrosion.[15]

Any artificially produced substance that resembles natural rubber in essential chemical and physical properties can be called a synthetic rubber. The most common

TABLE 3.1
Common Rubber Polymers and Rubberlike Elastomeric Polymers

Name	Chemical Structure

Polyisoprene
(*cis* 1,4 isomer)

$$\left[\begin{array}{c} CH_2 \\ \diagdown \\ CH_3 \end{array} C = C \begin{array}{c} CH_2 \\ \diagup \\ H \end{array}\right]_n$$

Nitrile
(acrylonitrile and *trans* 1,4 butadiene)

$$\left[\begin{array}{c} \quad\quad H_2 \quad\quad C\equiv N \\ \quad\quad C \quad\quad | \\ H \quad\quad\quad CH \\ C = C \quad C \\ CH_2 \quad H \quad H_2 \end{array}\right]_n$$

Neoprene
(*trans* 1,4 polychloroprene)

$$\left[\begin{array}{c} CH_2 \quad\quad H \\ \diagdown \quad\quad \diagup \\ Cl \quad C = C \quad CH_2 \end{array}\right]_n$$

Polyvinyl chloride

$$\left[\begin{array}{c} CH_2 - CH \\ | \\ Cl \end{array}\right]_n$$

Polyurethane
(P = polyether or polyester groups;
R = aliphatic or aromatic groups)

$$HO\left[\begin{array}{c} O \quad\quad\quad\quad O \\ \| \quad\quad\quad\quad \| \\ C - N - R - N - C \\ P - O \quad H \quad\quad H \quad O \end{array} POH\right]_x$$

Styrene-butadiene

$$\left[\begin{array}{c} H \quad H \\ C = C \\ (CH_2 \quad CH_2-)_n - (CH - CH_2 -) \end{array}\right]_x$$

Styrene-isoprene

$$\left[\begin{array}{c} CH_3 \quad H \\ C = C \\ (CH_2 \quad CH_2-)_n - (CH - CH_2 -) \end{array}\right]_x$$

Silicone (or polysiloxane)

$$\left[\begin{array}{c} CH_3 \\ | \\ Si - O \\ | \\ CH_3 \end{array}\right]_n$$

synthetic rubber polymers used today are derived from isoprene, butadiene, ethylene, styrene, chloroprene, and acrylonitrile. Although their chemistry is diverse, many synthetic rubbers are vulcanized and require compounding agents similar to those required for natural rubber. Unless the synthetic rubber is blended with natural rubber, it does not contain the protein allergens that are responsible for a type I NRL hypersensitivity.

Unlike vulcanized natural or synthetic rubbers, thermoplastic elastomers behave as if they are chemically cross-linked, but only at normal temperatures.[41] They obtain their final physical properties after heating and cooling, or after solvent evaporation. As a result, thermoplastic elastomers have a mix of thermoplastic and rubberlike properties.[42] Probably the most commonly used thermoplastic elastomers in thin-film applications include polyvinyl chloride (PVC), polyurethane block copolymers and polystyrene block copolymers. Other thermoplastic elastomers include polyester block copolymers, polyamide block copolymers, and polypropylene/ethylene propylene blends. As with other nonvulcanized thermoplastics, they generally do not contain the same compounding chemicals as natural and synthetic rubbers.

1. Natural Rubber Polyisoprene

Natural rubber latex (NRL) can be isolated from more than 2000 species of trees, shrubs, or vines.[43] In these plants, wounds exude a milky protective fluid that defends against further invasion by bacteria, fungi, insects, and animals. This NRL contains polyisoprene, which can exist as two stereoisomers: *cis* and *trans* (Table 3.1). The *cis*-stereoisomer is of greater commercial importance due to its superior elasticity and resilience.[41] The *Hevea brasilensis* trees of the Euphorbiacea family produce a high molecular weight linear *cis*-1,4-polyisoprene and currently supply about 90% of all natural rubber.[15,43]

Natural rubber polyisoprene has a structural formula of $[C_5H_8]_n$, where the n equals several thousand.[15] It is insoluble in water, alkalis, and weak acids but soluble in carbon disulfide and several petroleum based solvents such as naphtha, benzene, gasoline, and chlorinated hydrocarbons. Like other unsaturated rubber polymers, natural rubber polyisoprene is susceptible to oxidative damage by chemical and environmental agents. It is usually compounded with vulcanizing agents and accelerators, as well as antidegradants to protect the unsaturated carbon bonds in its polymer chains.

Other natural rubbers, such as gutta-percha, balata, and chicle, have largely been replaced commercially by synthetic rubbers.[43,44] Gutta-percha is harvested by solvent extraction of leaves and branches from the *Palaquium gutta* tree of the Sapotaceae family.[44] It contains a lower molecular weight *trans*-polyisoprene, which has a rigid crystalline structure after heating and cooling and is not vulcanized.[45] Historically, gutta-percha was used in postmortem exam gloves, undersea telegraph cables, and golf balls.[2,45] Today, it is primarily used to produce endodontic points for obturating root canals.[44] Despite their botanical origins, gutta-percha endodontic points apparently contain no detectable allergenic proteins that cross-react with NRL.[44,46]

Other natural rubbers include balata, chicle, and guayule rubbers.[43] The infrequently used balata rubber is obtained by tapping the *Mimusops balata* trees. Chicle rubber — a mixture of *cis* and *trans* configurations — is obtained by tapping several species, including the South American *Sapodilla* tree and the Asian *Jelutong* tree. Guayule rubber is an alternative source of predominantly *cis*-polyisoprene that has been harvested commercially, albeit principally during the 1940s shortage of natural *Hevea* rubber.[43] Recent research suggests that guayule rubber contains no allergenic proteins that cross-react with NRL.[47]

2. Nitrile

Developed in the 1930s, nitrile is a polymer of butadiene and acrylonitrile.[48] There are many different types of nitrile, with varying acrylonitrile and butadiene content and polymer branching (Table 3.1). Depending on the type, nitrile may contain a third difunctional monomer or bound antioxidant. Nitrile may be used alone or blended with other rubbers and other elastomers.[48,49] It is generally considered resistant to oils and solvents. As a result, nitrile is often used in the production of automotive parts, fuel hoses, diaphragms, seals, gaskets, O-rings, cements, adhesives, shoes, conveyor belts, flooring, cables, weather stripping, waterproofing, and thicker chemically resistant industrial gloves. Nitrile and nitrile-blends are also used to make thin-film medical grade gloves.

Vulcanized nitrile has good tensile strength but may be less elastic than natural rubber. Many nitrile curing systems are based on thiurams and peroxides with thiazoles or sulfenamides as a secondary accelerator.[48,49] Zinc oxide and stearic acid may also be added as vulcanization activators. Nitrile rubber requires protection from ozone and oxidation and thus wax protective coatings or resistant polymers are sometimes added. Plasticizers, fillers, and pigments can also be used in the compounding mix.

3. Neoprene

Developed in 1931, neoprene became one of the first successful synthetic rubbers.[15,50] It has good mechanical strength, low flammability, and is resistant to chemical, oxidative, and environmental damage. As a result, neoprene may be blended with natural or synthetic rubbers to improve their resistance to oil, environmental ozone, and weathering.[18,51,52] There are many different types of neoprene and neoprene blends with varying properties. This diversity is useful in the production of dipped, molded, extruded, and foamed objects, including protective gloves, belts, hoses, bearings, seals, stoppers, wet suits, shoes, roof coatings, adhesives, and protective coatings on cable, cord, wire, and clothing.

Neoprene is composed of 2-chlorobutadiene (or chloroprene) monomers that are polymerized in a predominantly *trans*-polychloroprene configuration (Table 3.1).[52,53] Polymerization, compounding, and vulcanization conditions can all influence the finished properties of neoprene. Zinc and magnesium oxides are frequently used as vulcanizing agents, with organic sulfur-based accelerators such as dialkydithiocarbamates, and thiuram disulfides, as well as mixtures of thioureas and diphenylguanidine. Cross-links are formed mainly at the tertiary allylic chlorines. Antioxidants such as the hindered bis-phenols are required to protect the chlorinated and unsaturated neoprene polymer from oxidative damage. Other potential additives include phthalate and sebacate plasticizers, oils, pigments, and fillers such as calcium carbonate.[52]

4. Polyvinyl Chloride

While not technically considered a rubber, polyvinyl chloride (PVC) can be manufactured as a thermoplastic elastomer with rubberlike properties.[54] First synthesized in 1835, the PVC polymer is produced from vinyl chloride monomers (Table 3.1). PVC can be extruded, rolled, molded, blown, thermoformed, or dipped, depending upon its compounding and resin content.[55] Emulsions of PVC polymers can be blended with polyurethanes, styrenes, and other monomers such as vinyl acetate, acrylates, and olefins. Generally, PVC has good resistance to inorganic acids, alkalis, water, and oxidation. Due to its versatility and low cost, PVC is utilized in many products, including blood bags, bottles, house siding, packaging, tubing, upholstery, pipes, coatings, toys, shoes, gloves, bumpers, and floor coverings.

Like other thermoplastics, PVC is not vulcanized. For dipped manufacturing applications, PVC is usually polymerized as an emulsion and then compounded with plasticizers to form a suspension known as a plastisol.[54,56] The physical properties of the finished product are affected by the plasticizers and stabilizers chosen, as well as the polymerization temperature. Plasticizers in PVC typically include phthalate esters such as diethyl hexyl diisodecyl and isononyl, butyl, and butyl benzyl.[54] Nonphthalate PVC plasticizers include esters of sebacates, adipates, citrates, phosphates, and glycols. Epoxidized soybean or linseed oil is often added as a secondary plasticizer, acting also as a lubricant and emulsion stabilizer.

PVC may also contain stabilizers, fillers, pigments, and flow/impact modifiers.[54] Added thermostabilizers can include metal salts or soaps such as calcium or lead stearates, octyltin-thioglycolate, magnesium, and barium, some of which may also function as processing aids. Calcium carbonate, clay, silica, glass fibers, graphite, and other mineral microfibers can be used as fillers. Added inorganic pigments include titanium dioxide, sulfates, sulfides, iron, lead, chromium, and cadmium. Organic pigments based on phthalocyanines and azo compounds may also be used to add color to a product.

In recent years the potential toxicity of PVC products has been questioned.[55] Concerns have been raised about the potential leaching of phthalate plasticizers from PVC products such as medical tubing blood bags, and subsequent patient exposure.[57,58] The commonly used plasticizer, di-(2-ethylhexyl) phthalate can be hazardous to certain populations, and may be carcinogenic under certain circumstances.[57] While the significance and interpretation of these findings is still debated, alternative plasticizers and thermoplastic elastomers (e.g., styrene block copolymers and polyurethanes) are now more frequently utilized.

5. Polyurethanes

Polyurethanes can be molded, foamed, cast, injected, milled, extruded, coated, and blended with other elastomers.[59,60] They are found in a variety of products, including foams, caulks, adhesives, gaskets, binders, footwear, gloves, prostheses, material coatings, and biomedical devices. In general, they are considered to have good tensile strength, oil resistance, and abrasion resistance. As with other synthetic elastomers, the finished properties of polyurethane vary with its composition and chemical additives.

Discovered in the late 1930s, polyurethanes consist of aromatic or aliphatic polyisocyanates that are reacted with macroglycols and chain extenders (Table 3.1). Polyurethane chains are stabilized by hydrogen bonds.[59] Unlike covalent sulfur-based cross-links, these highly elastic "virtual cross-links" deteriorate at elevated temperatures. In this characteristic, polyurethanes are similar to the thermoplastic styrene-based block copolymers.[60] However, polyurethane chains can be chemically cross-linked with organic peroxides or sulfur-based vulcanizing agents to increase their stability.[59] Softening agents or plasticizers (e.g., phthalates) may be added to improve material processing, and product performance.

6. Styrene-Based Elastomers

Styrene-based elastomers include both synthetic rubber and thermoplastic formulations. The most common is styrene-butadiene rubber (Table 3.1), which comprises over half the world's synthetic rubber production.[61] It was one of the synthetic rubbers developed in response to limited natural *Hevea* rubber resources. This polymer's composition varies by the styrene–butadiene ratio, the content of chemical additives, and the method of polymerization. Like other vulcanized rubbers, styrene-butadiene rubbers are compounded with accelerators, antidegradants, fillers, extenders, and other processing agents. Approximately three-quarters of the styrene-butadiene rubber made is used to produce tires, with the remainder going to the manufacture of footwear, mechanical parts, hoses, belts, adhesives, sponges and foams, waterproofing, carpet-back coatings, and construction equipment.

Styrene-based thermoplastic block copolymers (Table 3.1) include styrene-butadiene styrene (SBS), styrene-isoprene styrene (SIS), and styrene-ethylene-butylene styrene (SEBS).[42,60] These block copolymers may be used to manufacture medical grade gloves, condoms, catheters, blood bags, and components for medical equipment. While styrene-based thermoplastic block copolymers generally have good tensile strength and elongation, their resistance to heat and solvents can be limited.

Like other thermoplastics, styrene-based thermoplastic block copolymers are not vulcanized. These block copolymers are prepared by emulsion polymerization and solvent evaporation. Polymer strength is based on cross-chain attraction of the styrene regions, which anchor the elastic copolymer segments.[42] Styrene-isoprene derivatives with unsaturated carbon bonds often contain antidegradants such as dithiocarbamates or hindered phenols to minimize oxidation damage. Styrene-based thermoplastic elastomers may also contain plasticizers (e.g., phthalates) as processing aids and softening agents. By comparison to vulcanized natural and synthetic rubbers, these elastomers utilize few of the same allergenic chemicals.

7. Synthetic Polyisoprene

Polyisoprene was successfully synthesized in 1950.[62] Today, the majority of synthetic polyisoprene polymers produced are in the *cis*-1,4 configuration, but *trans*-

polyisoprene is also available. Vulcanized synthetic polyisoprene is generally similar to natural rubber with high tensile strength and resilience. It also contains the same compounding agents as natural rubber, including vulcanizing agents, accelerators, and antidegradants. Synthetic polyisoprene may be found in surgical gloves, shoes, tires, rubber bands, baby bottle nipples, cut threads, erasers, sponges, pharmaceutical supplies, sports equipment, and hoses.

8. Other Rubberlike Elastomers

Silicone rubber can be molded, extruded, and bonded to other materials. It is used for coatings, adhesives, sealants, gaskets, molded parts, automotive and industrial products, medical and dental products, and tubing.[63] Silicone rubber (or polysiloxane) is based on a polymeric string of silicon and oxygen atoms (Table 3.1).[15] The unsaturated polymer backbone is a flexible structure that tolerates temperature extremes, oxidation, and corrosive conditions. The physical properties of silicone vary with side-chain composition, which can include methyl, phenyl, vinyl, and even fluoride substituents. Silicone rubber is often chemically cross-linked (but not vulcanized) using organic peroxides at elevated temperatures. It does not contain the typical sulfur-based vulcanization accelerators.

Polybutadiene is the second most common synthetic rubber. It is frequently blended with other rubber polymers such as polystyrene or acrylonitrile. Polybutadiene is vulcanized, using sulfenamide-based accelerators, thiurams, or guanidines.[62] Because of its superior resistance to abrasion, impact and ozone, it is used to produce tire treads, conveyor belts, golf ball cores, and ABS pipe.

Butyl rubber is also found primarily in the tire industry and is highly resistant to heat, oxidation, chemicals, gas permeation, and moisture. Other applications include adhesives, coatings (including industrial gloves), air cushions, conveyor belts, high-temperature hoses, inner tubes, O-rings, gaskets, and bellows. Prepared from polymerization of isobutylene with butadiene or isoprene, butyl rubber requires vulcanization and contains multiple compounding agents.[18]

Ethylene propylene, one of the fastest-growing general-purpose elastomers, is widely used for consumer, automotive, electrical, and construction products.[64,65] It is valued for its excellent resistance to water, oxidation, and heat. These properties are based largely on its saturated polymer backbone, which is derived from the polymerization of ethylene and propylene. Alone, ethylene propylene (abbreviated as EPM) is considered a thermoplastic elastomer and is not vulcanized. However, it is commonly polymerized with a third polymer that is vulcanizable. These rubberlike polymers (abbreviated EPDM) frequently contain thiazoles combined with thiurams or dithocarbamates, as well as plasticizing oils and fatty-acid lubricants.

III. RUBBER COMPOUNDING

Before natural or synthetic rubber polymers are manufactured into products, they are amended with chemicals that influence their physical properties. This process, known as compounding, involves many different organic and inorganic chemicals. Historically, the first compounding agents were inorganic oxides of lead and other metals used in conjunction with inorganic sulfur.[19,33,66] These were soon augmented by organic accelerators, initiating an era of improvements in rubber vulcanization. Today, vulcanization accelerators and antidegradants account for the majority of the chemicals added to rubber.[15] The choice of chemical additives varies with the type of rubber polymer and manufacturing process.

Rubber compounding chemicals are also potential sources of allergic and irritant reactions for workers in healthcare, construction, and food industries. Skin moisture and oils may extract residual chemicals from the glove or other rubber product, exposing the worker's skin. Over time, this repeated chemical exposure can result in the development of an allergy to a specific chemical or even a family of structurally related chemicals. Therefore, it is important to understand the frequency with which these chemicals are utilized in the rubber industry, and their relative potency as allergens. This information should also be evaluated with an appreciation of the manufacturing process, which affects the potential availability of these chemicals in the finished products.

A. CHEMICAL ADDITIVES

1. Vulcanizing Agents and Accelerators

Vulcanizing agents are required for the permanent chemical cross-links between and across polymer chains. Accelerators generally facilitate cross-linking at lower temperatures and higher rates, and may modify the length and number of the cross-links.[15,33,66] The choice of vulcanizing agent and accelerator varies with the type of rubber polymer, manufacturing process, and desired finished properties. There is sometimes little distinction between vulcanizing agents and accelerators.[67] Some chemicals can function in multiple capacities. For example, zinc oxide can be an accelerator, vulcanizing agent, filler, and pigment. Although the specific chemistry varies, accelerators often participate directly in cross-link formation. Some compounds can completely supplant the need for inorganic sulfur.[15,67]

Some of the commonly used vulcanizing agents and accelerators include inorganic sulfur (rhombic and amorphous forms), sulfur-containing organic chemicals, peroxides and metal oxides (Table 3.2).[31,67,68] Secondary accelerators or activators are often combined with primary accelerators to potentiate their effects.[15] At elevated temperatures, these compounds generate sulfhydryl radicals that react with rubber polymers and create sulfur (S_x) cross-links.[34] Roughly half of sulfur-based organic accelerators used today are sulfenamides, while thiazoles, dithiocarbamates, and thiuram sulfides constitute most of the remainder.[31] Other specialty sulfur-based compounds include xanthates, thiophosphates, and dithiodimorpholine.

These sulfur-based organic accelerators are highly reactive and are categorized by their different abilities to increase the rate of vulcanization.[31,68] Thiuram sulfides, dithiocarbamates, and xanthates are considered *fast* or *ultra-fast accelerators*. Examples of *moderate accelerators* include sulfenamides, benzothiazoles, and thiophosphates. By comparison, thiourea derivatives are considered *slow accelerators*.

Not all vulcanization agents and accelerators depend on sulfur-based mechanisms. Sulfur independent vulcanization agents can include peroxides, difunctional

TABLE 3.2
Vulcanizing Accelerators Found in Natural and Synthetic Rubbers

Thiurams	Chemical Structure
Tetramethylthiuram disulfide (TMTD) CAS# 137-26-8	CH_3—N(—CH_3)—C(=S)—S—S—C(=S)—N(—CH_3)—CH_3
Tetramethylthiuram monosulfide (TMTM) CAS# 97-74-5	CH_3—N(—CH_3)—C(=S)—S—C(=S)—N(—CH_3)—CH_3
Tetraethylthiuram disulfide (TETD) CAS# 97-77-8	C_2H_5—N(—C_2H_5)—C(=S)—S—S—C(=S)—N(—C_2H_5)—C_2H_5
Dipentamethylenethiuram tetrasulfide (PTT) CAS# 120-54-7	(piperidine)N—C(=S)—S—S—S—S—C(=S)—N(piperidine)

Carbamates	Chemical Structure
Zinc dibutyldithiocarbamate (ZDBC) CAS #136-23-2	$[C_4H_9$—N(—C_4H_9)—C(=S)—S$]_2$Zn
Zinc diethyldithiocarbamate (ZDEC) CAS# 14324-55-1	$[C_2H_5$—N(—C_2H_5)—C(=S)—S$]_2$Zn
Zinc dimethyldithiocarbamate (ZDMC) CAS# 137-30-4	$[CH_3$—N(—CH_3)—C(=S)—S$]_2$Zn
Zinc pentamethylene-dithiocarbamate (ZPD) CAS# 13878-54-1	$[$(piperidine)N—C(=S)—S$]_2$Zn

TABLE 3.2 (Continued)
Vulcanizing Accelerators Found in Natural and Synthetic Rubbers

Thiazoles and Sulfenamides	Chemical Structure
2-Mercaptobenzothiazole (MBT) CAS# 149-30-4	
2,2-Dibenzothiazyl disulfide (MBTS) CAS# 120-78-5	
N-Cyclohexyl-2-benzothiazolesulfenamide (CBS) CAS# 95-33-0	
Morpholinylmercapto-benzothiazole (MOR or MMBT) CAS# 102-77-2	
2-Mercaptobenzimidazole CAS# 583-39-1	

Thioureas	Chemical Structure
1,3-Dibutylthiourea (DBTU) CAS# 109-46-6	$C_4H_9 - N - C - N - C_4H_9$ (H, H above; S below, double bond)
N,N-Diphenylthiourea (DPTU) CAS# 102-08-9	

Sulfurless Compounds	Chemical Structure
1,3-Diphenylguanidine (DPG) CAS# 102-06-7	
Dibenzoyl peroxide CAS# 94-36-0	$O = C - O - O - C = O$

TABLE 3.2 (Continued)
Vulcanizing Accelerators Found in Natural and Synthetic Rubbers

Sulfurless Compounds	Chemical Structure
Dicumyl peroxide CAS# 80-43-3	

compounds (e.g., isophthalates and acrylates), and metal oxides or other metal complexes (Table 3.2).[31,34,68] Examples of sulfur-independent accelerators are guanidines and aldehyde amines, with slow to moderate rates. These sulfurless accelerators often are used jointly with other sulfur-based or sulfur-independent curing chemicals. The behavior, utility, and efficiency of these agents and accelerators depends on the rubber elastomer and other compounding agents used.

The mechanisms of polymer cross-link formation differ for these sulfurless agents and accelerators.[34] For example, aliphatic and aromatic peroxides (e.g., tert-butyl and benzoyl peroxide, respectively) generate radicals within the polymer chains that form carbon cross-links across polymer chains. By comparison, difunctional compounds can donate and form cross-links that bridge polymer chains. Metal oxides (or other complexes of zinc, magnesium, and lead) react with groups on the polymer side chains as in the reaction of zinc oxide with the chlorinated side chains in neoprene.

2. Antidegradants

Antidegradants include antioxidants and antiozonants (Table 3.3). These are used to protect natural and synthetic rubber and thermoplastic elastomers from age- and oxidant-related deterioration, prolonging their useful life.[33] Exposure to oxygen, ozone, oxidizing chemicals, light, heat, or radiation results in the generation of free-radical species. These free radicals damage elastomers by attacking their chemical cross-links and polymeric backbone, leading to chain breaks, vulnerable new cross-links and additional reactive oxygen molecules.[31,33,68] Practically speaking, the physical properties of rubber polymer begin to deteriorate by becoming more brittle or less elastic. Unsaturated polymers such as polyisoprene (natural and synthetic), styrene-isoprene copolymers, and polybutadiene are more prone to oxidation than saturated polymers such as ethylene propylene.

Antioxidants resist oxidative damage by scavenging oxygen-based radicals.[33] The most widely used categories of antioxidants in rubber are secondary amines (e.g., alkyl amines and aromatic amines or quinolines), phenols (substituted, bisphenols, and aminophenols), and phosphites.[33,66,68] Of these different groups of antioxidants, the most commonly used are the secondary amines.[31]

Of the secondary amines, p-phenylenediamine derivatives are most frequently used in the rubber industry. They are generally very effective antioxidants; some can also serve a dual function as an antiozonant.[31] Unfortunately, they also impart

TABLE 3.3
Antidegradants (Antioxidants and/or Antiozonants) Found in Natural and Synthetic Rubbers

Phenylenediamines	Chemical Structure
N,N-Diphenyl-p-phenylenediamine (PPD) CAS# 74-31-7	
N-cyclohexyl-N-phenyl-p-phenylenediamine (CPPD) CAS# 101-87-1	
N-isopropyl-N-phenyl-p-phenylenediamine (IPPD) CAS# 101-72-4	

Phenols	Chemical Structure
Butylated hydroxytoluene (BHT) CAS# 128-37-0	
Butylated hydroxyanisole (BHA) CAS# 25013-16-5	
2,2–methylene-bis-(4 methyl-6-t-butylphenol) CAS# 119-47-1	
Polymeric 2,2,4-trimethyl-1,2-dihydroxyquinoline CAS# 26780-96-1	

color or stain the rubber product. Therefore they are used in the manufacture of dark-colored and dry rubber products such as tires, hoses, etc. By comparison, phenols — often referred to as hindered phenols — do not discolor, and include compounds such as styrenated phenol, butylated hydroxytoluene, and butylated hydroxyanisole. Phenol antioxidants are frequently used in the manufacture of light-colored rubber products, and can be found in some medical gloves and condoms.[31,33,66] As with other compounding agents, the choice of antioxidant depends on the rubber polymer, manufacturing process, and often the vulcanization agents and accelerators.

Similar to the mechanisms described above, ozone (O_3) in our environment attacks the unsaturated carbon bonds in rubber polymers. Once broken, these weakened areas can expose other unsaturated bonds and ultimately lead to material failure at stress points where the polymer stretches or folds.[69] Rubber polymers differ in their ozone resistance. Ozone-exposed (5 ppm O_3) polyisoprene, styrene-butadiene, nitrile, and polybutadiene develop surface cracking due to the presence of unsaturated carbon bonds in these polymers.[69] (Note that the EPA's Clean Air Act considers an ambient air level of 0.28 ppm ozone in the "extreme" category.) Other polymers such as polyisobutylene and neoprene are considered moderately ozone resistant, whereas ethylene propylene and polyvinyl chloride elastomers are very ozone resistant, again due to the differences in bond saturation.

Ozone-induced deterioration is preventable using surface coatings or chemical additives with the rubber polymer. A protective barrier can be formed by the use of specialized wax coatings that migrate to the surface during product manufacture.[31,69] However, these brittle surface coatings perform best on inflexible finished products. Alternatively, rubber polymers vulnerable to ozone damage can be blended with other more ozone-resistant polymers. For continuously flexed products, antiozonants are added during compounding.[31,69]

Antiozonants are similar to — and sometimes identical to — antioxidants. They include some secondary amines (e.g., p-phenylenediamines and naphthylamines), 2,2,4-trimethyl-1,2-dihydroxyquinoline, and alkyl-aryl derivatives (typically in neoprene rubbers). Other antiozonants include thiourea derivatives and certain dithiocarbamates, which function also as vulcanizing accelerators.[31] Overall, secondary amines are again the most common, particularly the p-phenylenediamine derivatives used in dark and dry rubber applications.[69] Alternative antiozonants are better for light-colored and thin-film articles such as gloves, condoms, catheters, and dental dams.

3. Pigments, Fragrances, and Flavorants

Providing color to the finished product, pigments include inorganic chemicals such as zinc oxide and lithopone (a barium and zinc mixture), as well as a number of organic dyes (e.g., Irgalite orange F2G).[34,70] Fragrances (also known as odorants) are sometimes required to hide an offensive odor associated with compounding, or with certain polymers. Fragrances can be added to complement fruit-based and spice-derived flavorants in toys, dental gloves, baby nipples, rubber dams, and condoms.

4. Processing Aids

These chemicals generally aid mixing, promote elasticity, improve viscosity, lubricate, and disperse the components of rubber mixtures without affecting the polymer's physical properties.[34] For example, during the compounding and mastication of dry rubber, plasticizers (also known as peptizers) are often added to chemically cap broken polymer chains. Chemical softeners such as petroleum products, oils, waxes, pine tar, and fatty acids may be added to improve viscosity for proper compounding. Processing aids may be specific to the application. For example, foam rubber requires the addition of blowing agents such as azo compounds and carbonates before it is mechanically whipped, molded, and vulcanized.

5. Releasing Agents and Lubricants

Dipped or molded products often require the use of release agents to facilitate stripping of the finished product. Residual amounts of release agents can end up on the exterior surface and be useful in preventing blocking (self-sticking) and bricking (sticking to others).[38] Mold-release agents can include powdered calcium carbonate and bioabsorbable cornstarch, or liquid formulations of silicone, waxes, amides, and fluoropolymers.[22,27,38] These agents are usually applied to the former or mold directly, or may be included in the rubber polymer. Again, selection depends on the rubber elastomer, solvents, manufacturing process, and temperatures involved.

Lubricants are commonly used in the manufacture of gloves to improve their donnability. Since the late 1970s, the American Society for Testing and Materials (ASTM) standards for medical grade gloves have stipulated that these lubricants meet U.S. Pharmacopoeia specifications for absorbable dusting powders.[38,71] The use of talcum powder, cotton flock, or Lycopodium spores is no longer permitted. Accepted powdered lubricants for medical grade gloves include cornstarch, oatstarch, casein, and other bioabsorbable powders.[71,72] For powder-free medical grade gloves, manufacturers may add surface coatings made of silicone, polyacrylates (e.g., hydrogels), polyurethane, polyols, or botanically derived polysaccharides (e.g., aloe vera).[22,73,74]

Other compounds can be found in releasing agents and surface coatings used on various types of gloves and rubber products in addition to those mentioned above. Examples include polyethylene and polypropylene, lipids and fatty acids, polyglycolic acid, sodium metaphosphate, magnesium carbonate, oxidized cellulose, and granular vinyl chloride polymer.[73,75-77] As described in the manufacturing section, these releasing agents and surface coatings are often applied as suspensions. The suspensions of lubricants and release agents can contain antimicrobials, stabilizers, and surfactants to minimize bacterial contamination and improve the application processes.

B. ALLERGENICITY OF RUBBER ADDITIVES

The potential allergenicity of a rubber product reflects the amount of processing chemical added and the chemical's sensitizing potential. Rubber allergenicity can be influenced by the degree of leaching, washing, and other harsh treatments likely to remove processing chemicals, as well as their solubility in water, solvents, and the specific rubber polymer. Harsh (e.g., solvent exposure) or wet-use conditions can also increase the availability of allergenic chemicals in elastomeric products.

Locating and interpreting chemical content information is not always easy. Compounding agents may not be detectable in the finished product, either due to leaching, degradation, or alteration during rubber manufacture.[78] Manufacturing formulations and processing methods may be proprietary.[56] Moreover, the multiple chemical, common, and brand names used for rubber compounding chemicals can be confusing. For example, the fungicide Thiram is identified by over 20 different trade names, and several common names, including thiuram and TMTD. This abbreviation stands for the IUPAC (International Union of Pure and Applied Chemistry) chemical name tetramethylthiuram disulfide, the vulcanizing accelerator. However, this chemical is also classified by the Environmental Protection Agency as an ethylene bisdithiocarbamate.[79]

Medical gloves, which fall under the purview of the Food and Drug Administration (FDA), should have demonstrated minimal potential for skin irritation and sensitization, based on animal or human studies.[80,81] Based on new Quality System regulations from the FDA the manufacturer should also have documentation on the chemicals added during and prior to manufacturing. Information submitted to the FDA prior to sale of the product in the U.S. should identify any color or fragrance additives, as well as the powder or lubricants used, but not the various compounding agents.[80] In practice, allergenicity to specific rubber compounding chemicals is sometimes more frequently assessed from reported changes in allergy prevalence data.

1. Vulcanization Agents and Accelerators

The prevalence of type IV allergies to vulcanization agents and accelerators in rubber products can equal or exceed that of type I allergies to NRL proteins.[82] In healthcare, where glove-related dermatoses are common, between 5 and 12% of tested workers may be allergic to thiurams and/or carbamates.[83–86] Other workers who regularly use rubber gloves such as factory workers, housekeeping staff, food handlers, food processors, hairdressers, and construction workers can also develop accelerator-based type IV allergies.[12,87–89] Of the common vulcanization accelerators and agents, thiuram sulfides and the structurally related carbamates lead in the frequency with which they elicit allergic reactions.[78,90] Allergies to the mercaptobenzothiazoles are much less prevalent.

These prevalence trends are generally supported by the limited residual chemical content data in the literature. In the early 1990s, 60% of the tested medical gloves contained thiurams.[91] This was particularly significant as the gloves were extracted with aqueous-based media, in which thiurams and carbamates are practically insoluble. The levels of thiurams reported were also significantly greater than mercaptobenzothiazole levels reported by Emmet et al. to have been extracted from gloves.[92] By comparison, 8 years later, less than 16% of tested gloves contained detectable levels of thiurams when extracted in acetone, an efficient solvent for these accelerators.[78] A subsequent study found no detectable thiurams when extracted in aqueous salt solutions.[93] Although comparisons between these studies are difficult due to dissimilar analytical methods, the quantities of glove thiurams appear to have decreased over the 10 year period.

Of the common accelerators, thiurams and carbamates exhibit significant allergenic potency. De Jong et al. reported that carbamates and thiurams comprised the top eight most allergenic accelerators, with diethyl dithiocarbamate displaying the greatest allergenic potency.[94] It is interesting to note that this latter accelerator is also one of the most frequently detected.[78] However, these differences may have little clinical meaning as most carbamate-allergic patients also react to thiurams, due to their structural similarity and potential oxidation-conversion of carbamates to thiurams.[95]

Allergic reactions to accelerators in rubber products may be aggravated by their presence in nonrubber consumer and industrial goods. For example, carbamates are found in many agricultural products such as herbicides, pesticides, fungicides, and slimicides.[96] Thiuram disulfides are widely used as a fungicide in agricultural industries.[96] They can also be found in some soaps, shampoos, and adhesives. Tetraethylthiuram disulfide is also a component of Antabuse®, a drug used in the treatment of alcoholism.

2. Antidegradants

Found in industrial belts, hoses, boots, and gloves, the phenylenediamine group of antioxidants and antiozonants can be allergenic.[96,97] The commonly used N-isopropyl-N-phenyl-p-phenylenediamine (IPPD) can be found in the "black rubber mix" component of patch test kits. In the 1990s the frequency of allergies to this group of chemicals was far less than that of thiurams and carbamates.[88]

Of the antiozonants, thioureas and dithiocarbamates are more likely than the hindered phenols to elicit allergic reactions, probably due to their more widespread use and greater allergenicity.[94] As discussed above, dithiocarbamates are one of the most commonly used chemical additives, and a significant source of accelerator-related type IV allergies.[93]

3. Other Additives

The presence of pigments, processing aids, fillers, and other compounds may be minimal in finished products. However, they can potentially cause both irritant and allergic reactions, albeit infrequently. For example, over 3% of patch-tested individuals were allergic to the retarder cyclohexyl thiophthalimide, as compared to over 6% who were allergic to thiurams.[98] Retarders (also known as scorch retarders) are used to prevent scorching of the rubber when dry rubber is heated and extruded or mixed.[67] It is not used in the production of thin-film latex products.

Thermoplastic elastomers may also have allergenic properties. Polyethylene has been reported to cause contact urticaria in a rare case.[99] Di(2-ethylhexyl) phthalate, a plasticizer used in PVC gloves, is the acknowledged source of contact urticaria in a few isolated case reports.[100,101] However, overall, several dialkyl phthalates have been found not to be sensitizing or irritating in a larger population.[102] Finally, the pigment Irgalite Orange F2G used in PVC gloves was found to be allergenic in one individual.[70]

4. Release Agents and Lubricants

Despite public misconceptions, allergic reactions to release agents, lubricants, and surface coatings are infrequently reported. The use of talcum powder and Lycopodium was associated with postsurgical complications from granulomas and adhesions, but apparently not allergies.[38,71] Casein powder has been reported as a potential source of allergic reactions for individuals already sensitized to cow's milk.[103] Reactions to surface coatings have not yet been reported. In the one allergic reaction to aloe found in the literature, symptoms only appeared after several years of oral and topical use.[104] Moreover, sensitivity to these compounds in surface coatings may be less likely given their limited quantity in finished products, and their less widespread use.

The most commonly used lubricant — cornstarch powder — is still regarded as a rare sensitizer. Although cases may be underreported, there are few documented allergic reactions to the cornstarch or maize protein in glove powder.[105,106] In contrast, cornstarch glove powder is a well-recognized carrier of NRL protein allergens, and plays a pivotal role in sensitization to NRL as well as symptom elicitation.[72,107] A recent study suggests that cornstarch may also function as an immunoadjuvant, potentiating an individual's immune response to NRL proteins.[108]

IV. CONCLUSIONS AND FUTURE DEVELOPMENTS

Continued changes in rubber processing and compounding agents should be expected. As noted above, the residual chemical content of gloves has changed: levels of elutable thiurams appear lower than a decade ago.[78,93] The changes in the prevalence of allergies to thiurams and carbamates suggest that glove manufacturers may be lowering accelerator chemical levels. Alternatively, glove manufactures may be substituting new and different chemical additives. Because these chemicals would be less common, theoretically fewer workers would be sensitized, thus reducing symptom elicitation. In practice, this approach is not always successful in the long term, as illustrated by the increasing frequency of shoe rubber allergy due to dithiodimorpholine as compared previously to mercaptobenzothiazole.[109] Ideally, rubber manufacturers would reduce residual chemical content to below sensitization levels by developing new chemical additives with low sensitization potential and processes that remove as much compounding agents as practical. New processes may also be developed that use high-energy radiation and do not require the addition of vulcanizing agents.

The development and improvement of rubber polymers can also be anticipated. Deproteinized rubber has been used in dry rubber commercial applications in the automotive industry, but not yet in thin-film dipped product manufacturing.[110] Deproteinized rubber can be made by the treatment of crude natural rubber latex with proteolytic enzymes such as alcalase, or papain, or by gamma radiation.[37] Deproteinization occurs prior to centrifugation and reportedly can remove a significant portion of antigenic proteins. However, the physical properties (e.g., tensile strength) of deproteinized latex rubber films may not yet be sufficient. Additional research is needed before these treatments can be widely applied.

Alternative commercial natural rubber sources may also be developed. During World War II, the Southwestern guayule shrub was harvested and used to produce natural rubber.[20,43] When *Hevea* rubber again became available after the war, this resource was abandoned, due principally to the comparatively low yields. However, the rise in type I allergies to natural rubber have encouraged research and development of this alternative natural rubber again.[111] Multiple plant species produce rubber, and several produce a significant *cis*-1,4-polyisoprene component.[43] In the future, alternative rubber systems may be derived from these more diverse plant species, or even bioengineered fermenters. However, these rubbers are still likely to contain many of the same compounding agents such as accelerators and antidegradants. New polymer-derived allergens may surface, such as the sesquiterpene cinnamic acid found naturally in guayule.[112]

Regulatory agencies and consumers have suggested improving the identification of potential chemical allergens such as thiurams and carbamates in all natural and synthetic rubber gloves. However, this requires standardization of analytical methods as well as establishing sensitization thresholds, for which data is still limited. In the interim, it is prudent to generally assume that vulcanized rubbers are highly likely to contain at least one of the common accelerators and antidegradants. Another useful assumption is that nonvulcanized elastomers are far less likely to contain these same chemicals. Regardless of the source material and manufacturing techniques, dermatologists, allergists, and workers must continue to educate themselves about the chemical content of rubber products.

REFERENCES

1. Ownby, D.R., A history of latex allergy, *J. Allergy Clin. Immunol.*, 110, S27, 2002.
2. Geelhoed, G.W., The pre-halstedian and post-halstedian history of the surgical rubber glove, *Surg. Gynecol. Obstet.*, 167, 350, 1988.
3. Downing, J.G., Dermatitis from rubber gloves, *N. Engl. J. Med.*, 208, 196, 1933.
4. Prosser-White, R., *The Dermatoergoses or Occupational Diseases of the Skin*, HK Lewis, London, 1934.
5. Bonnevie, P. and Marcussen, P.V., Rubber products as a widespread cause of eczema: Report of 80 cases, *Acta Derm. Venereol.*, 25, 163, 1945.
6. Rietschel, R.L. et al., Relationship of occupation to contact dermatitis: Evaluation in patients tested from 1998 to 2000, *Am. J. Contact Dermatitis*, 13, 170, 2002.
7. Larson, E., Prevalence and correlates of skin damage on the hands of nurses, *Heart & Lung*, 26, 404, 1997.
8. Tarlo, S.M. et al., Outcomes of a natural rubber latex control program in an Ontario teaching hospital, *J. Allergy Clin. Immunol.*, 108, 628, 2001.
9. Holness, D.L. and Mace, S.R., Results of evaluating health care workers with prick and patch testing, *Am. J. Contact Dermatitis*, 12, 88, 2001.
10. Beltrami, E.M. et al., Transmission of HIV and hepatitis C virus from a nursing home patient to a health care worker, *Am. J. Infect. Control*, 31, 168, 2003.
11. Kucenic, M.J. and Belsito, D.V., Occupational allergic contact dermatitis is more prevalent than irritant contact dermatitis: a 5-year study, *J. Am. Acad. Dermatol.*, 46, 695, 2002.

12. Bauer, A., Geier, J., and Elsner, P., Type IV allergy in the food processing industry: Sensitization profiles in bakers, cooks and butchers, *Contact Dermatitis,* 46, 228, 2002.

13. Emmett, E.A., Occupational Contact Dermatitis II: Risk Assessment and Prognosis, *Am. J. Contact Dermatitis,* 14, 21, 2003.

14. Hosler, D., Burkett, S.L., and Tarkanian, M.J., Prehistoric polymers: Rubber processing in ancient Mesoamerica, *Science,* 284, 1988, 1999.

15. Morton, M., Introduction to polymer science, in *Rubber Technology,* Morton, M., Ed., Van Nostrand Reinhold, New York, 1987, chap. 1.

16. Editor, The rise of the rubber industry (from the history of rubber), *Natuurrubber,* 21, 2, 2001.

17. Editor, The Growing Rubber Culture, *Natuurrubber,* 25, 1, 2002.

18. Subramaniam, A., Commercial elastomers: Natural rubber, in *The Vanderbilt Rubber Handbook,* Ohm, R.F., Ed., R.T. Vanderbilt Company, Inc., Norwalk, CT, 1990.

19. Editor, The rise of the industry, *Natuurrubber,* 26, 2, 2002.

20. Estilai, A. and Waines, J.G., Improved guayule germplasm for domestic production of natural rubber, in *Advances in New Crops,* J. Janick and J.E. Simon, Eds., Timber Press, Portland, OR, 1990.

21. Hibbs, J., Commercial elastomers: Styrene butadiene rubbers, in *The Vanderbilt Rubber Handbook,* Ohm, R.F., Ed., R.T. Vanderbilt Co., Inc., Norwalk, CT, 1990.

22. Yip, E. and Cacioli, P., The manufacture of gloves from natural rubber latex, *J. Allergy Clin. Immunol.,* 110, S3, 2002.

23. Subramaniam, A., The chemistry of natural rubber latex, *Immunol. Allergy Clin. North Am.,* 15, 1, 1995.

24. Archer, B.L., Barnard, D., and Cockbain, E.G., Structure, composition and biochemistry of Hevea latex, in *The Chemistry and Physics of Rubber-Like Substances,* Bateman, L., Ed., John Wiley & Sons, New York, 1963.

25. Mellstrom, G.A. and Boman, A.S., Gloves: Types, materials, and manufacturing, in *Protective Gloves for Occupational Use,* Mellstrom, G.A., Wahlberg, J.E. and Maibach, H.I., Eds., CRC Press, Boca Raton, FL, 1994, p. 3.

26. Truscott, W., Manufacturing methods sought to eliminate or reduce sensitivity to natural rubber products, in *Program and proceedings. International Latex Conference: Sensitivity to latex in medical devices,* Food and Drug Administration Center for Devices and Radiological Health, Baltimore, 1992.

27. Pendle, T.D. and Gorton, D.T., *Dipping with natural rubber latex,* Malaysian Rubber Producers' Research Association, Hertford, 1980, p. 1.

28. Subramaniam, A., Reduction of extractable protein content in latex products, in *Program and proceedings. International Latex Conference: Sensitivity to latex in medical devices,* Food and Drug Administration Center for Devices and Radiological Health, Baltimore, 1992.

29. Pendle, T. D. The production, composition and chemistry of natural latex concentrates, in *Program and proceedings. International Latex Conference: Sensitivity to latex in medical devices,* Food and Drug Administration Center for Devices and Radiological Health, Baltimore, 1992.

30. Subramaniam, A. et al., Extractable protein content of gloves from prevulcanized natural rubber latex, in *Latex Proteins and Glove Industry: A report of the proceedings of the International Rubber Technology Conference,* Kadir, A.A.S.A., Ed., Rubber Research Institute of Malaysia, Kuala Lumpur, Malaysia, 1994.

31. Greek, B.F., Rubber-processing chemicals, *Chem. Engineer. News,* 29, 1987.

32. Hamann, C.P. and Sullivan, K., Natural rubber latex hypersensitives, in *Cutaneous Allergy*, Charlesworth, E.N., Ed., Blackwell Publishing, London, 1996, pp. 155–208.

33. Layer, R.W., Introduction to rubber compounding, in *The Vanderbilt Rubber Handbook*, Ohm, R.F., Ed., R.T. Vanderbilt Co., Inc., Norwalk, CT, 1990.

34. Stephens, H.L., The compounding and vulcanization of rubber, in *Rubber Technology*, Morton, M., Ed., Van Nostrand Reinhold, New York, 1987, chap. 2.

35. Yatim, A.H.M., Effect of leaching on extractable protein content, in *Latex Proteins and Glove Industry: A report of the proceedings of the International Rubber Technology Conference*, Kadir, A.A.S.A., Ed., Rubber Research Institute of Malaysia, Kuala Lumpur, Malaysia, 1994.

36. Dalrymple, S.J. and Audley, B.G., Allergenic proteins in dipped products: Factors influencing extractable protein levels, *Rubber Develop.*, 45, 51, 1992.

37. Perrella, F.W. and Gaspari, A.A., Natural rubber latex protein reduction with an emphasis on enzyme treatment, *Methods*, 27, 77, 2002.

38. Truscott, W., Glove powder reduction and alternative approaches, *Methods*, 27, 69, 2002.

39. Aziz, N.A.A., Chlorination of gloves, in *Latex Proteins and Glove Industry: A report of the proceedings of the International Rubber Technology Conference*, Kadir, A.A.S.A., Ed., Rubber Research Institute of Malaysia, Kuala Lumpur, Malaysia, 1994.

40. Roberts, A.D. and Brackley, C.A., Surface treatments to reduce friction: Rubber glove applications, *Rubber Chem. Tech.*, 63, 722, 1990.

41. Flory, P.J., Rubber elasticity, in *Principles of Polymer Chemistry*, Cornell University Press, Ithaca, NY, 1953, chap. 1.

42. Holden, G., Thermoplastic elastomers, in *Rubber Technology*, Morton, M., Ed., Van Nostrand Reinhold, New York, 1987, chap. 16.

43. Mooibroek, H. and Cornish, K., Alternative sources of natural rubber, *Appl. Microbiol. Biotechnol.*, 53, 355, 2000.

44. Costa, G.E., Johnson, J.D., and Hamilton, R.G., Cross-reactivity studies of gutta-percha, gutta-balata and natural rubber latex (*Hevea brasiliensis*), *J. Endod.*, 29, 584, 2001.

45. Goodman, A., Schilder, H., and Aldrich, W., The thermomechanical properties of gutta-percha: II. The history and molecular chemistry of gutta-percha, *Oral Surg.*, 37, 954, 1974.

46. Hamann, C. et al., Cross-reactivity between gutta-percha and natural rubber latex: Assumptions vs. reality, *J. Am. Dent. Assoc.*, 133, 1357, 2002.

47. Siler, D.J., Hamilton, R.G., and Cornish, K., Absence of cross-reactivity of IgE antibodies from subjects allergic to *Hevea brasiliensis* latex with new source of natural rubber latex from guayule (*Parthenium argentatum*), *J. Allergy Clin. Immunol.*, 98, 895, 1996.

48. Seil, D.A. and Wolf, F.R., Nitrile and polyacrylic rubbers, in *Rubber Technology*, Morton, M., Ed., Van Norstrand Reinhold, New York, 2003, chap. 11.

49. Purdon, J.R., Nitrile elastomers, in *The Vanderbilt Rubber Handbook*, Ohm, R.F., Ed., R.T. Vanderbilt Co., Inc., Norwalk, CT, 1990.

50. Carothers, W.H. et al., Polymers and their derivatives. II. A new synthetic rubber: Chloroprene and its polymers, *J. Amer. Chem. Soc.*, 53, 4203, 1931.

51. Gelbert, C.H., *A selection guide for Neoprene latexes (Tech. Report-NL-020.1 [R1])*, Du Pont Company, Wilmington, DE, 1987, p. 1.

52. Gelbert, C.H., *Basic Compounding of Neoprene Latex (Technical Report)*, Du Pont Company, Wilmington, DE, 1986, p. 1.

53. Kane, R.P., The neoprenes, in *The Vanderbilt Rubber Handbook,* Ohm, R.F., Ed., R.T. Vanderbilt Co., Inc., Norwalk, CT, 1990.

54. Daniels, C.A. and Gardner, K.L., Rubber-related polymers, part 1: Poly(vinyl chloride), in *Rubber Technology,* Morton, M., Ed., Van Nostrand Reinhold, New York, 2003, chap. 20.

55. Lewis, R., Vinyl chloride and polyvinyl chloride, *Occup. Med.,* 14, 719, 1999.

56. Hamann, C.P. and Kick, S.A., Allergies associated with medical gloves: Manufacturing issues, *Dermatol. Clin.,* 12, 547, 1994.

57. Tickner, J.A. et al., Health risks posed by use of di-2-ethylhexyl phthalate (DEHP) in PVC medical devices: a critical review, *Am. J. Ind. Med.,* 39, 100, 2001.

58. Hill, S.S., Shaw, B.R., and Wu, A.H., Plasticizers, antioxidants, and other contaminants found in air delivered by PVC tubing used in respiratory therapy, *Biomed. Chromatogr.,* 17, 250, 2003.

59. Schollenberger, C.S., Polyurethane elastomers, in *Rubber Technology,* Morton, M., Ed., Van Nostrand Reinhold, New York, 1987, chap. 15.

60. O'Connor, G.E. and Rader, C.P., Thermoplastic elastomers, in *The Vanderbilt Rubber Handbook,* Ohm, R.F., Ed., R.T. Vanderbilt Co., Inc., Norwalk, CT, 1990.

61. Henderson, J.N., Styrene-butadiene rubbers, in *Rubber Technology,* Morton, M., Ed., Van Nostrand Reinhold, New York, 1987, p. 7.

62. Kuzma, L.J., Polybutadiene and polyisoprene rubbers, in *Rubber Technology,* Morton, M., Ed., Van Nostrand Reinhold, New York, 1987, chap. 8.

63. Carpino, J.C. and Macander, R.F., Silicone rubber, in *Rubber Technology,* Morton, M., Ed., Van Nostrand Reinhold, New York, 1987, chap. 13.

64. Easterbrook, E.K. and Allen, R.D., Ethylene-propylene rubber, in *Rubber Technology,* Morton, M., Ed., Van Nostrand Reinhold, New York, 1987, chap. 9.

65. DuPont de Nemours, E.I., Ethylene propylene rubbers, in *The Vanderbilt Rubber Handbook,* Ohm, R.F., Ed., R.T. Vanderbilt Co., Inc., Norwalk, CT, 1990.

66. Belsito, D.V., Rubber, in *Handbook of Occupational Dermatology,* Kanerva, L., et al., Eds., Springer-Verlag, Heidelberg, Germany, 2000, p. 87.

67. Wilson, W., Compounding materials, in *The Vanderbilt Rubber Handbook,* Ohm, R.F., Ed., R.T. Vanderbilt Co., Inc., Norwalk, CT, 1990.

68. Fishbein, L., Chemicals used in the rubber industry: an overview, *Scand. J. Work Environ. Health,* 9 (suppl. 2), 7, 1983.

69. Layer, R.W. and Lattimer, R.P., Protection of rubber against ozone, *Rubber Chem. Tech.,* 63, 426, 1990.

70. Kanerva, L., Jolanki, R., and Estlander, T., Organic pigment as a cause of plastic glove dermatitis, *Contact Dermatitis,* 13, 41, 1985.

71. FDA. Medical Glove Powder Report 1-21. DHHS, Rockville, MD, 1997.

72. Swanson, M.C. and Ramalingam, M., Starch and natural rubber allergen interaction in the production of latex gloves: A hand-held aerosol, *J. Allergy Clin. Immunol.,* 110, S15-S20, 2002.

73. Dunn, R.N., Surgical gloves and surface treatment of surgical gloves for avoiding starch peritonitis and the like, U.S. Patent Appl. 551111; U.S. Patent 4,540,407, 1985.

74. Chou, B.L., Aloe vera glove and manufacturing method, Shen Wei (USA) Inc., U.S. Patent Appl. 898632; U.S. Patent, 6,423,328, 2002.

75. Lentz, D.J. and Khan, M.A., Oxidized cellulose as a medical lubricant, Warner-Lambert Company, U.S. Patent Appl. 544665; U.S. Patent 4,668,224, 1983.

76. Joung, J.G. Surgeon's glove and talc free process for forming same, American Hospital Supply Corporation, U.S. Patent Appl. 061790; U.S. Patent 4,310,928, 1982.

77. Hassan, N.A. and Yuen, C.C. Powder-free medical gloves. Ansell Shah Alam Sdn Bhd., U.S. Patent Appl. 487108; U.S. Patent 6,378,137, 2002.
78. Knudsen, B.B. et al. Allergologically relevant rubber accelerators in single-use medical gloves, *Contact Dermatitis,* 43, 9, 2000.
79. U.S. Environmental Protection Agency, Ethylene bisdithiocarbamates (EBDCs); Notice of intent to cancel and conclusion of Special Review, *Federal Register,* 57, 7434, 1992.
80. FDA, *Medical glove guidance manual: draft document,* FDA CDRH, 1999, pp. 1.1–12.2.
81. FDA, Premarket Notification [510(k)] submissions for Testing for Skin Sensitization to Chemicals in Natural Rubber Products 1-8. DHHS, Rockville, MD, 1999.
82. Nettis, E. et al., Type I allergy to natural rubber latex and type IV allergy to rubber chemicals in health care workers with glove-related skin symptoms, *Clin. Exp. Allergy,* 32, 441, 2002.
83. Wrangsjo, K., Swartling, C., and Meding, B., Occupational dermatitis in dental personnel: contact dermatitis with special reference to (meth)acrylates in 174 patients, *Contact Dermatitis,* 45, 158, 2001.
84. Wallenhammar, L.M. et al., Contact allergy and hand eczema in Swedish dentists, *Contact Dermatitis,* 43, 192, 2000.
85. Schnuch, A. et al., Contact allergies in healthcare workers: Results from the IVDK, *Acta Derm. Venereol.,* 78, 358, 1998.
86. Gibbon, K.L. et al., Changing frequency of thiuram allergy in healthcare workers with hand dermatitis, *Br. J. Dermatol.,* 144, 347, 2001.
87. Conde-Salazar, L. et al., Contact dermatitis in hairdressers: Patch test results in 379 hairdressers (1980–1993), *Am. J. Contact Dermatitis,* 6, 19, 1995.
88. Conde-Salazar, L. et al., Type IV allergy to rubber additives: A 10-year study of 686 cases, *J. Am. Acad. Dermatol.,* 29, 176, 1993.
89. Conde-Salazar, L. et al., Occupational allergic contact dermatitis in construction workers, *Contact Dermatitis,* 33, 226, 1995.
90. Marks, J.G., Jr. et al., North American Contact Dermatitis Group patch-test results, 1996–1998, *Arch. Dermatol.,* 136, 272, 2000.
91. Knudsen, B.B. et al., Release of thiurams and carbamates from rubber gloves, *Contact Dermatitis,* 28, 63, 1993.
92. Emmett, E.A. et al., Skin elicitation threshold of ethylbutyl thiourea and mercaptobenzothiazole with relative leaching from sensitizing products, *Contact Dermatitis,* 30, 85, 1994.
93. Brehler, R., Rutter, A., and Kutting, B., Allergenicity of natural rubber latex gloves, *Contact Dermatitis,* 46, 65, 2002.
94. De Jong, W.H. et al., Ranking of allergenic potency of rubber chemicals in a modified local lymph node assay, *Toxicol. Sci.,* 66, 226, 2002.
95. Bergendorff, O. and Hansson, C., Spontaneous formation of thiuram disulfides in solutions of iron(III) dithiocarbamates, *J. Agric. Food Chem.,* 50, 1092, 2002.
96. Fisher, A.A., Rietschel, R.L., and Fowler, J.F., Jr., Allergy to Rubber, in *Fisher's Contact Dermatitis,* Rietschel, R.L. and Fowler, J.F., Jr., Eds., Lippincott, Williams, Wilkins, Philadelphia, 2000, chap. 31.
97. Estlander, T., Jolanki, R., and Kanerva, L., Disadvantages of gloves, in *Handbook of Occupational Dermatology,* Kanerva, L. et al., Eds., Springer-Verlag, Heidelberg, Germany, 2003, chap. 54.
98. Kanerva, L., Estlander, T., and Jolanki, R., Allergic patch test reactions caused by the rubber chemical cyclohexyl thiophthalimide, *Contact Dermatitis,* 34, 23, 1996.

99. Sugiura, K. et al., Contact urticaria due to polyethylene gloves, *Contact Dermatitis,* 46, 262, 2002.

100. Sugiura, K. et al., Di(2-ethylhexyl) phthalate (DOP) in the dotted polyvinyl-chloride grip of cotton gloves as a cause of contact urticaria syndrome, *Contact Dermatitis,* 43, 237, 2000.

101. Sugiura, K. et al., A case of contact urticaria syndrome due to di(2-ethylhexyl) phthalate (DOP) in work clothes, *Contact Dermatitis,* 46, 13, 2002.

102. Medeiros, A.M., Devlin, D.J., and Keller, L.H., Evaluation of skin sensitization response of dialkyl (C6-C13) phthalate esters, *Contact Dermatitis,* 41, 287, 1999.

103. Ylitalo, L. et al., Cow's milk casein, a hidden allergen in natural rubber latex gloves, *J. Allergy Clin. Immunol.,* 104, 177, 1999.

104. Morrow, D.M., Rapaport, M.J., and Strick, R.A., Hypersensitivity to aloe, *Arch. Dermatol.,* 116, 1064, 1980.

105. Guin, J.D. et al., Occupational protein contact dermatitis to cornstarch in a paper adhesive, *Am. J. Contact Dermatitis,* 10, 83, 1999.

106. Crippa, M. and Pasolini, G., Allergic reactions due to glove-lubricant-powder in health-care workers, *Int. Arch. Occup. Environ. Health,* 70, 399, 1997.

107. Tomazic, V.J. et al., Cornstarch powder on latex products is an allergen carrier, *J. Allergy Clin. Immunol.,* 93, 751, 1994.

108. Barbara, J. et al., Immunoadjuvant properties of glove cornstarch powder in latex-induced hypersensitivity, *Clin. Exp. Allergy,* 33, 106, 2003.

109. Belsito, D.V., Common shoe allergens undetected by commercial patch-testing kits: Dithiodimorpholine and isocyanates, *Am. J. Contact Dermatitis,* 12, 95, 2003.

110. van Baarle, B., Deproteinised natural rubber, *Natuurrubber,* 27, 1, 2002.

111. Wood, M., Desert shrub may help preserve wood, *Agric. Res. Mag.,* 4, 10, 2002.

112. Rodriguez, E., Reynolds, G.W., and Thompson, J.A., Potent contact allergen in the rubber plant guayule (*Parthenium argentatum*), *Science,* 21, 1444, 1981.

4 Natural Rubber Latex Allergy: Clinical Manifestations

Ignatius C. Chua, Alison J. Owen,
and Paul E. Williams

CONTENTS

I. Introduction 57
II. Systemic Manifestations of Allergy 58
    A. IgE Mediated Immediate Hypersensitivity Reactions 59
    B. Sensitization to NRL and Development of Symptoms 59
III. Patients with Spina Bifida 60
IV. Surgical and Medical Procedures 60
V. Fatal Anaphylaxis 61
VI. Occupational Exposure to NRL 61
VII. Everyday Exposure to NRL 62
VIII. Case History 62
IX. Conclusions 63
References 63

I. INTRODUCTION

Natural rubber latex (NRL) allergy was uncommon two decades ago,[1] but has become much more common over the past 12 years.[2] Severe symptoms of NRL allergy were first found to affect surgical patients with spina bifida[3] and patients undergoing barium enema,[4] but over the last 10 years systemic symptoms following latex exposure have been found in other populations such as healthcare and industrial workers. The prevalence of NRL allergy seemed to be increasing,[5] and it is considered to be a serious medical problem for a number of patients and healthcare workers (HCW).[6,7] Immunologists, occupational and other physicians are all seeing patients who have NRL allergy.[8,9] NRL allergy is a common cause of anaphylactic shock during surgical procedures,[10–12] and therefore it is important for hospital physicians, surgeons, and anesthetists to recognize the systemic manifestations of NRL allergy so as to be able to manage the situation appropriately.[13] Latex allergy may initially present with local symptoms only and develop more serious systemic manifestations later on. A fundamental understanding of the pathogenesis of latex allergy is essential in order to be able to diagnose and manage the condition.

II. SYSTEMIC MANIFESTATIONS OF ALLERGY

The systemic manifestations of life-threatening NRL allergy are IgE mediated. NRL allergy may best be visualized as a continuum of signs and symptoms. Unlike anaphylaxis caused by other allergens such as peanut, NRL causes anaphylaxis through more than one route. Hence the sequence of events in NRL anaphylaxis may not always conform to the classical paradigm of anaphylaxis. The clinical manifestations of anaphylactic reactions are related to the amount and location of histamine released,[14] which varies according to the level of sensitivity of the individual, and the site and extent of exposure.[15,16]

Most individuals who test positive for NRL allergy on skin-prick or *in vitro* blood testing are asymptomatic,[17] or have only mild skin symptoms of eczema and urticaria[18] on skin exposure. Initial symptoms and signs of NRL allergic reaction are often sensations of warmth, pruritus, and tingling,[19] usually occurring at the site of contact. Skin manifestations occur frequently[4] and are often described as "weals," "nettle rash," or "blotches."[18] Cutaneous effects are not life threatening and may progress from a flush to generalized urticaria or to angioedema over several hours.

Eye, mouth, and nasal symptoms are common features, especially in HCW exposed to NRL aeroallergen.[20,21] Eye symptoms include burning, running, or itching, mouth symptoms include itchy throat, tongue and roof of mouth, and nasal symptoms include sneezing, rhinorrhea, itching, and mucosal edema. A symptom score had been devised based on the above symptom complexes.[22] Neutrophil and eosinophil counts in nasal washings are significantly higher in NRL allergic subjects provoked nasally with NRL.[22]

Upper airway obstruction may occur because of edema of the larynx, epiglottis, or surrounding tissues. Bronchoconstriction and edema cause lower airway obstruction. Initial symptoms and signs of upper airway obstruction include hoarseness, dysphagia, a sense of fullness or constriction of the throat, and development of respiratory stridor. Lower respiratory tract manifestations include wheezing, coughing, chest tightness, and increasing shortness of breath. Both upper and lower respiratory tract manifestations may progress to asphyxia.[23]

The term *anaphylaxis* as used here refers to severe systemic manifestations involving clinically significant impairment of the upper airway, bronchoconstriction, or fall in blood pressure occurring as a result of IgE-mediated NRL allergy. Initially, individuals may have an overwhelming sense of impending doom and complain of faintness. Cardiovascular collapse is often rapid in onset, mostly occurring in anesthetized patients. In nonsedated individuals, the feelings of faintness and retrosternal pain may precede syncope. Myocardial infarction has not been a recognized phenomenon in NRL anaphylaxis.

Biphasic and sustained reactions (when symptoms and signs recur at a later stage as a result of the action of secondary mediators) are uncommon in NRL allergy. Late bronchoconstriction has been reported.[24]

Surprisingly abdominal pain, vomiting, diarrhea, and bowel mucosal edema have not been reported, even after intestinal surgery where latex surgical gloves are used.[23]

A. IgE Mediated Immediate Hypersensitivity Reactions

All current studies suggest that systemic manifestations of NRL allergy are wholly IgE mediated. Skin, nasal,[22] and bronchial challenge[25] with NRL proteins have reproduced identical symptoms in affected patients. Both the structures of NRL allergens and specific IgE antibodies to latex have been elucidated in both human and murine studies (see Chapter 2). Interestingly, different patterns of sero-recognition for specific proteins have been demonstrated between healthcare workers (Hev b 2, b 5, b 6.02)[26] and children with spina bifida (Hev b 1 and b 3),[27–29] possibly due to different routes of sensitization.

Control groups used in latex studies were less likely to have specific IgE antibodies to latex.[3,4] Strong positive reactions to NRL allergens on skin prick testing[23] and high serum NRL specific IgE levels both correlate with severity of symptoms.[30] Basophil degranulation[31] with release of histamine[3] and tryptase[32] by NRL allergens has been demonstrated.

B. Sensitization to NRL and Development of Symptoms

Initial exposures to NRL cause sensitization, symptoms being triggered after subsequent exposures to NRL.[33] The factors that determine whether an individual becomes sensitized are still poorly understood. These probably include genetic factors, regarding which there is limited knowledge at present, and the frequency and degree of exposure to latex. Dental students in their third year were found to have higher prevalence rates compared to first- and second-year students.[34] Similarly patients with spina bifida and children were more likely to be sensitized to latex after six or more surgical procedures.[35]

Routes of NRL exposure include skin contact,[4] inhalation,[21] and internal exposure during surgical procedures. Latex penetrates abrasions, eczematous skin, and vaginal and buccal mucous membranes to a greater extent than normal skin.[4] Sensitization with IgE production against latex has been described following NRL exposure subcutaneously, intrathecally, and topically. This occurs by stimulation of peripheral blood CD4+ T-cells to induce a TH2 cytokine profile (high IL-5/IFN γ ratio)[26] directed against NRL proteins.[37]

The concentration of soluble NRL proteins that HCW are exposed to varies greatly according to the individual product.[38] Latex allergens are readily adsorbed by cornstarch and thus it is conceivable that aerosolization of cornstarch may aid transport of NRL to the mucous membranes of the respiratory tract so as to enable sensitization.[21,39] Poor environmental ventilation results in increased aeroallergen concentration and thus symptoms upon exposure in sensitized individuals.[20] With regard to local symptoms on skin contact with gloves in NRL-sensitized individuals, the duration of exposure to gloves rather than the number of gloves worn dictate symptom manifestation.[20,21,34] Latex allergen levels in disposable rubber gloves from different manufacturers can vary by 3000-fold.[38]

Once sensitized, any level of exposure to NRL may result in severe allergic reactions,[6] with no safe level of exposure. Concentrations of NRL aeroallergens as low as $0.6ng/m^3$ have been shown to produce symptoms.[21] NRL aeroallergen concentrations in the work place are often 10 times this level.[25] There is a strong association between NRL allergy and atopy to common allergens in all groups studied.[17,20,40] This suggests that skin reactivity to NRL allergen is more likely to develop in individuals who have a propensity to develop IgE-mediated allergy to other, unrelated allergens.[41]

III. PATIENTS WITH SPINA BIFIDA

Patients with spina bifida have a 23% prevalence of NRL allergy.[35,42] They are 500 times more likely to have an anaphylactic reaction during surgery[43] than the normal population. This discrete group whose mean age is often less than 10 years[44,45] have usually had multiple operations and urinary catheterizations. There is no convincing evidence that patients with spina bifida who develop NRL allergy are genetically predisposed.[44-46] These patients have a heavy exposure to NRL via the urethral mucosa and other routes at an early age. There is much evidence that exposure to allergens at an early age is more likely to result in TH-2 differentiation of activated allergen-specific T-cells rather than TH-1 differentiation, thus favoring the generation of allergy.[44,45,47] The most important risk factor predisposing to NRL allergy is the number of surgical interventions (> 6).[35,43,46,48] Many patients who develop NRL allergy are atopic[35,43] and have previously had mild reactions to latex exposure.[3,43] The threshold for sensitization and the level of NRL exposure required to elicit clinical reactions seem to be lower in atopic than nonatopic individuals.[48] High total serum IgE concentration[43] and high serum levels of specific IgE against NRL (> 3.5kU/L)[42] are both significant risk factors for the occurrence of symptoms following NRL exposure.

Most reactions to NRL experienced by patients who have spina bifida are mild,[48] including urticaria, rhinoconjunctivitis, and angiedema.[42] However anaphylaxis during surgery can be life threatening. This may manifest as profound hypotension, tachycardia, bronchoconstriction, low arterial oxygen saturation, skin flushing, urticarial rash, and angiedema.[3,49,50] Anaphylaxis can rarely manifest with bradycardia.[10] Prompt treatment with epinephrine infusion, hydrocortisone, and plasma expanders may be required and may reverse anaphylaxis quickly.[3,23,31,32,50,53,56]

Even with careful NRL precautions, spina bifida children are prone to exposure to balloons, rubber boots, and household gloves at home and may develop symptoms ranging from contact urticaria to systemic reactions.[51]

IV. SURGICAL AND MEDICAL PROCEDURES

NRL is a common cause of anaphylactic reaction during surgery both in children and adults.[10,11] NRL proteins are found in anaesthetic equipment, ultrasound probe coverings,[8] surgical dressings, rubber cuffs, and latex catheter tips used during barium enemas.[32]

Intraoperative reactions to NRL can usually be distinguished from reactions to anaesthetic drugs as they tend to occur about one hour after the time of anaesthetic induction, usually during surgery.[12,32,52,53] In addition, they may follow repeated and intense handling of internal organs by surgeons' gloves as this favors the elution and absorption of water-soluble NRL proteins.[32,54] In nonselected children undergoing general surgery, anaphylaxis due to NRL allergy occurs in approximately 1 in 8000 operations.[10]

Individuals who have NRL-induced anaphylaxis have often had previous mild reactions to latex, angioedema during blowing of balloons, or urticaria with gloves.[11,23,31,32,54,56] Many individuals have had previous uncomplicated surgical procedures and this may be falsely reassuring.[32,54] Therefore all patients should be asked preoperatively about the possibility of NRL allergy,[32,55] and appropriate tests performed if indicated.[23]

V. FATAL ANAPHYLAXIS

Fatalities from latex anaphylaxis are rare with U.S. mortality figures between 1988 and 1993 documenting 15 deaths.[6,57] In the U.K. between 1992 and 1998 no deaths had been attributed to latex.[58] Two published reports of fatalities are summarized below.

The first fatality occurred in a 49-year-old woman with a history of atopic dermatitis, allergic rhinitis, and asthma. Minutes after commencing a barium enema procedure, she complained of itching and warmth over her upper extremities. Within minutes, she became breathless and started wheezing. She did not respond to albuterol inhaler, became cyanotic, and had a respiratory arrest with unsuccessful resuscitation. Postmortem showed severe mucous plugging, pulmonary edema, and emphysema.[59,60]

The second fatality occurred in a 28-year-old woman with known asthma, multiple allergies (nut, house dust mite, cat, and dog), and eczema from wearing gloves. Within 5 minutes of having hair extensions bonded with an adhesive containing latex, she had a burning sensation in her scalp. Despite removing woven hairs and taking chlorpheniramine, she developed generalized urticaria and facial edema. Her breathing became increasingly labored with no improvement after salbutamol treatment and she collapsed. Despite prompt intubation and epinephrine administration, she died. Autopsy revealed severe lip, tongue, and laryngeal edema. There was also mucus plugging of the bronchi with mucosal edema and mediastinal emphysema.[61]

Both women had had severe reactions within minutes of latex exposure through bowel mucosa and skin respectively, culminating in sudden severe bronchoconstriction and respiratory arrest. Epinephrine had been administered early but without benefit, and this lack of response has been described in anaphylaxis from other causes in the presence of asthma.[58]

VI. OCCUPATIONAL EXPOSURE TO NRL

HCW and workers in the rubber manufacturing industry have similar symptoms following NRL exposure. The prevalence of NRL allergy in both groups is 5 to

10%[1,8,20,62] and may be increasing.[8] Among HCW, doctors, nurses, and laboratory workers have the highest prevalence of NRL allergy.[20]

The most frequent symptoms in HCW are contact urticaria from latex gloves.[8,64] Symptoms may be present for many years before the correct diagnosis is made.[34,64] Anaphylaxis to NRL is uncommon, making up 0 to 7% of all reactions.[34,64] Work related asthma in HCW often occurs very soon after exposure, often with accompanying cough, facial redness, sneezing, and ocular itching but not generalized urticaria, angioedema, or tachycardia.[24,34,65] One study reported that 2.5% of HCW have occupational asthma due to NRL.[66]

As many as 15% of workers in glove manufacturing factories may have symptoms of NRL allergy.[67] Affected individuals often have prominent upper (77%) and lower respiratory symptoms (60%),[68] with cough, shortness of breath, chest tightness, and wheezing often occurring soon after commencing work.[68] Sneezing, rhinorrhea, and facial flushing may also occur.[40,63] The chest x-ray is usually normal.[68] Lung function tests often reveal diminished FEV_1 of $\geq 15\%$ from baseline values both at the workplace and during NRL challenging.[25,40,63,68] Some individuals may have a delayed bronchoconstrictor response some hours after challenge.[24,40,65] Chronic asthma may occur following occupational exposure to NRL,[65] and this has serious implications.

VII. EVERYDAY EXPOSURE TO NRL

Seroprevalence studies of the general population indicate that 6.5 to 8.2% of the population may have detectable IgE antibodies against NRL,[5,17] and nonwhite individuals were twice as likely to have latex specific IgE antibodies.[17] NRL is ubiquitously used in balloons, condoms, clothing, shoes, car tires, and many other household objects. Rubber balloons have been found to have a high NRL allergen load.[38] These products are used by a wide variety of people including hairdressers, police officers, painters, and food-service workers.[7,69] Latex condoms have been associated with local urticaria and rarely anaphylaxis.[23]

There have been few reports of NRL anaphylaxis occurring as a result of inadvertent NRL exposure occurring in public places in individuals not known to have NRL allergy. Case reports include anaphylaxis in children playing in ball pits[70] and adults exposed to NRL in food wrappings.[71] Food may be contaminated with NRL from food handling or food wrappings.[69] In this situation food allergy may be mistakenly suspected. Certain fruits such as avocado, kiwi, chestnut, and banana may cross-react with NRL proteins due to structural homology (see Chapter 13).[72] Many NRL allergic individuals (40%) have perioral itching, urticaria, angiedema, rhinitis, and asthma after eating or handling these fruits.[73,74] There have also been reports of anaphylaxis occurring in the same situation,[74] and so NRL allergic individuals should avoid these fruits.

VIII. CASE HISTORY

A woman aged 37 was referred by her family doctor to the allergy clinic with a history of angiedema and wheezing after eating avocado, bananas, or fish. She had swelling of the hands after wearing household gloves and swelling of the lips after blowing up balloons. She had looked after children with special needs for 16 years, and began to have eczema and dermatitis after wearing latex gloves 4 years earlier. A year later she had facial and tongue swelling, wheezing, and difficulty breathing after eating avocado, with these symptoms improving after taking Loratidine. She had been given a Medicalert Bracelet and an Epipen.

She had had eczema, asthma, and hayfever as a child and suffered long-standing rhinitis when visiting relatives who had cats, dogs, and horses. She had had gestational diabetes and pre-eclampsia during pregnancy 2 years earlier, with postpartum hypertension treated with lisinopril 10mg a day.

Skin prick tests gave a 4mm diameter weal to histamine, house dust mite, cat and dog epithelium, and mixed grass and mixed tree pollens, with a 12mm diameter weal to latex. The total serum IgE concentration was 1146 kU/l (normal < 81) and allergen-specific IgE antibodies were present against latex at 48 kU/l (normal < 0.35).

She was informed of the diagnosis of NRL allergy, and given relevant written information (see Chapter 22). Her Epipen administration technique was checked and she was counseled about avoidance of exposure to latex, avocado, banana, kiwi fruit, and chestnut. She continued to use Loratidine as required, and when seen in the clinic 12 months later she had had no further reactions.

IX. CONCLUSIONS

Systemic manifestations of NRL allergy are dependent on environmental factors and the biological characteristics of each individual's reactivity. Many health facilities and industrial factories have instigated measures to reduce NRL exposure and benefit is already apparent.[25] Anaphylaxis to NRL was initially recognized in patients who have spina bifida, later in HCW, and now in the general public. Even infrequent exposure to small amounts of NRL might cause sensitization. Hence, continued vigilance would seem to be in order, especially for any new biological agents introduced into our environment.

REFERENCES

1. Liss, G.M. and Sussman, G.L., Latex sensitisation: Occupational versus general population prevalence rates, *Am. J. Ind. Med.*, 35, 196, 1999.
2. Carous, B.L. et al., Natural rubber latex allergy after 12 years: Recommendations and perspectives, *J. Allergy Clin. Immunol.*, 109, 31, 2002.
3. Slater, J.E., Rubber anaphylaxis, *New Engl. J. Med.*, 320, 1126, 1989.
4. Axelsson, J.G.K., Johansson, S.G.O., and Wrangsjo, K., IgE mediated anaphylactoid reactions to rubber, *Allergy*, 42, 46, 1987.
5. Ownby, D.R. et al., The prevalence of anti-latex IgE antibodies in 1000 volunteer blood donors, *J. Allergy Clin. Immunol.*, 97, 1188, 1996.
6. Sussman, G.L. and Beezhold, D.H., Allergy to latex rubber, *Ann. Intern. Med.*, 122, 43, 1995.
7. Torasson, M. et al., Latex allergy in the workplace, *Toxicol. Sci.*, 58, 5, 2000.

8. Mitsuya, K., Comprehensive analysis of 28 patients with latex allergy and prevalence of latex sensitisation among hospital personnel, *J. Dermatol.*, 28, 405, 2001.

9. Tarlo, S.M. et al., Outcomes of a natural rubber latex control program in an Ontario teaching hospital, *J. Allergy Clin. Immunol.*, 108, 628, 2001.

10. Murrat, I., Anaphylactic reactions during paediatric anaesthesia: Results of the survey of the French Society of Paediatric Anaesthesists, *Paediatric Anaesthesists*, 3, 339, 1993.

11. Laxenaire, M.C. and Mertes, P.M., Anaphylaxis during anaesthesia: Results of a two-year survey in France, *Br. J. Anaesth.*, 87, 549, 2001.

12. Lieberman, P., Anaphylactic reactions during surgical and medical procedures, *J. Allergy Clin. Med.*, 110, S64, 2002.

13. Woods, J.A. et al., Natural rubber latex allergy: Spectrum, diagnostic approach and therapy, *J. Emer. Med.*, 15, 71, 1997.

14. Pearce, F.L., Biological effects of histamine: An overview, *Agents and Actions*, 33, 4, 1991.

15. Sitter, H. et al., Causality-based diagnosis of histamine-related cardiorespiratory disturbances in surgical patients, *Inflamm. Res.*, 45, S71, 1998.

16. Winberry, S.L. and Lieberman P.L., Histamine and antihistamines in anaphylaxis, *Clin. Allergy Immunol.*, 17, 287, 2002.

17. Grzybowski, M. et al., The prevalence of latex-specific IgE in patients presenting to an urban emergency department, *Ann. Emerg. Med.*, 40, 411, 2002.

18. Handfield-Jones, S.E., Latex allergy in health-care workers in an English district general hospital, *Br. J. Derm.*, 138, 273, 1998.

19. Scriven, R.J., Cirocco, W.C., and Golub, R.W., Latex allergy — report of an anaphylactic reaction, *Surgery*, 117, 350, 1995.

20. Liss, G.M., Latex allergy: Epidemiological study of 1351 hospital workers, *Occup. Environ. Med.*, 54, 335, 1997.

21. Baur, C., Chen, Z., and Allmers, H., Can a threshold limit value for natural rubber latex airborne allergens be defined? *J. Allergy Clin. Immunol*, 101, 24, 1998.

22. Palczynski, C. et al., Nasal provocation test in the diagnosis of natural rubber latex allergy, *Allergy*, 55, 34, 2000.

23. Sussman, G.L., Tarlo, S.M., and Dolovich, J., The spectrum of IgE-mediated responses to latex, *J. Am. Med. Assoc.*, 265, 2844, 1991.

24. Pisati, G. et al., Bronchial provocation testing in the diagnosis of occupational asthma due to latex surgical gloves, *Eur. Respir. J.*, 7, 332, 1994.

25. Hunt, L.W. et al., Management of occupational allergy to natural rubber latex in a medical center: the importance of quantitative allergen measurement and objective follow up, *J. Allergy Clin. Immunol.*, 110, S96, 2002.

26. Johnson, B.D. et al., Purified and recombinant latex proteins stimulate peripheral blood lymphocytes of latex allergic patients, *Int. Arch. Allergy Immunol.*, 120, 270, 1999.

27. Breiteneder, H. and Scheiner, O., Molecular and immunological characteristics of latex allergens, *Int. Arch. Allergy Immunol.*, 116, 83, 1998.

28. Alenius, H. et al., Latex allergy: Frequent occurrence of IgE antibodies to a cluster of 11 latex proteins in patients with spina bifida and histories of anaphylaxis, *J. Lab. Clin. Med.*, 123, 712, 1994.

29. Ylitalo, L. et al., IgE antibodies to prohevein, hevein, and rubber elongation factor in children with latex allergy, *J. Allergy Clin. Immunol.*, 102, 659, 1998.

30. Kim, K.T. and Ghassan, S.S., Relation of latex-specific IgE titer and symptoms in patients allergic to latex, *J. Allergy Clin. Immunol.*, 103, 7, 1999.

31. Leynadier, F., Pecquet, C., and Dry, J., Anaphylaxis to latex during surgery, *Anaesthesia*, 44, 547, 1989.
32. Volcheck, G.W. and Li, J.T.C., Elevated serum tryptase level in a case of intraoperative anaphylaxis caused by latex allergy, *Arch. Intern. Med.*, 154, 2243, 1994.
33. Poley, G.E. and Slater J.E., Latex allergy, *J. Allergy Clin. Immunol.*, 105, 1054, 2000.
34. Tarlo, S.M. et al., Latex sensitivity in dental students and staff: A cross-sectional study, *J. Allergy Clin. Immunol.*, 99, 396, 1997.
35. De Swert, L.F.A. et al., Determination of independent risk factors and comparative analysis of diagnostic methods for immediate type latex allergy in spina bifida patients, *Clin. Exp. Allergy*, 27, 1067, 1996.
36. Woolhiser, M.R., Munson, A.E., and Meade, B.J., Immunological responses of mice following administration of natural rubber latex proteins by different routes of exposure, *Toxicol. Sci.*, 55, 343, 2000.
37. de Silva, H.D. et al., Human T-cell epitopes of the latex allergen Hev b 5 in health care workers,. *J. Allergy Clin. Immunol.*, 105, 1017, 2000.
38. Yunginger, J.W. et al., Extractable latex allergens and proteins in disposable medical gloves and other rubber products, *J. Allergy Clin. Immunol.*, 93, 836, 1994.
39. Elliot, E.A., Latex allergy: The perspective from the surgical suite, *J. Allergy Clin. Immunol.*, 110, S117, 2002.
40. Pisati, G. et al., Environmental and clinical study of latex allergy in a textile factory, *J. Allergy Clin. Immunol.*, 101, 327, 1998.
41. Gautrin, D. et al., Specific IgE-dependent sensitisation, atopy, and bronchial hyperresponsiveness in apprentices starting exposure to protein-derived agents, *Am. J. Respir. Crit. Care Med.*, 155, 1841, 1997.
42. Bernardini, R. et al., Risk factors for latex allergy in patients with spina bifida and latex sensitisation, *Clin. Exp. Allergy*, 29, 681, 1999.
43. Kelly, J.K. et al., A cluster of anaphylactic reactions in children with spina bifida during general anesthesia: Epidemiologic features, risk factors, and latex hypersensitivity, *J. Allergy Clin. Immunol.*, 94, 53, 1994.
44. Konz, K.R. et al., Comparison of latex sensitivity among patients with neurologic defects, *J. Allergy Clin. Immunol.*, 95, 950, 1995.
45. Mertes, P.M. et al., Latex hypersensitivity in spinal cord injured adult patients, *Anaesth. Intensive Care*, 29, 393, 2001.
46. Porri, F. et al., Association between latex sensitisation and repeated latex exposure in children, *Anesthesiology*, 86, 599, 1997.
47. Capriles-Hulett A. et al., Very low frequency of latex and fruit allergy in patients with spina bifida from Venezuela, *Ann. Allergy Asthma Immunol.*, 75, 62, 1995.
48. Mazon, A. et al., Factors that influence the presence of symptoms caused by latex allergy in children with spina bifida, *J. Allergy Clin. Immunol.*, 99, 600, 1997.
49. Gold, M. et al., Intraoperative anaphylaxis: An association with latex sensitivity, *J. Allergy Clin. Immunol.*, 87, 662, 1991.
50. Moneret-Vautrin, D.A., Laxenaire, M.C., and Bavoux, F., Allergic shock to latex and ethylene oxide during surgery for spina bifida, *Anesthesiology*, 73, 556, 1990.
51. Ylitalo, L. et al., Natural rubber latex allergy in children: A follow-up study, *Clin. Exp. Allergy*, 30, 1611, 1999.
52. Moscicki, R.A. et al., Anaphylaxis during induction of general anesthesia: Subsequent evaluation and management, *J. Allergy Clin. Immunol.*, 86, 325, 1990.
53. Hodgson, C.A. and Andersen, B.D., Latex allergy: An unfamiliar cause of intraoperative cardiovascular collapse, *Anaesthesia*, 49, 507, 1994.

54. Gerber, A.C. et al., Severe intraoperative anaphylaxis to surgical gloves: Latex allergy, an unfamiliar condition, *Anesthesiology,* 71, 800, 1989.
55. Nguyen, D.H. et al., Intraoperative cardiovascular collapse secondary to latex allergy, *J. Urology,* 146, 571, 1991.
56. Turjanmaa, K. et al., Allergy to latex gloves: Unusual complication during delivery, *Br. Med. J.,* 297, 1029, 1988.
57. Neugut, A.I., Ghatak, A.T., and Miller, R.L., Anaphylaxis in the United States, *Arch. Intern. Med.,* 161, 15, 2001.
58. Pumphrey, R.S.H., Lessons for management of anaphylaxis from a study of fatal reactions, *Clin. Exp. Allergy,* 30, 1144, 2000.
59. Fecko, P.J., Simms, S.M., and Bakiri, N., Fatal hypersensitivity reaction during a barium enema, *Am. J. Roent.,* 153, 275, 1989.
60. Ownby, D.R. et al., Anaphylaxis associated with latex allergy during barium enema examinations, *Am. J. Roent.,* 156, 903, 1991.
61. Pumphrey, R.S.H., Duddridge, M., and Norton, J., Fatal latex allergy, *J. Allergy Clin. Immunol.,* 107, 558, 2001.
62. Allmers, H, et al., Reduction of latex aeroallergens and latex-specific IgE antibodies in sensitized worker after removal of powdered natural rubber latex gloves in a hospital, *J. Allergy Clin. Immunol.,* 102, 841, 1998.
63. Orfan, N.A. et al., Occupational asthma in a latex doll manufacturing plant, *J. Allergy Clin. Immunol.,* 94, 826, 1994.
64. Turjanmaa, K. et al., Long-term outcome of 160 adult patients with natural rubber latex allergy, *J. Allergy Clin. Immunol.,* 110, S70, 2002.
65. Brugnami, G. et al., Work related late asthmatic response induced by latex allergy, *J. Allergy Clin. Immunol.,* 96, 457, 1995.
66. Vandenplas, O. et al., Prevalence of occupational asthma due to latex among hospital personnel, *Am. J. Crit. Care Med.,* 151, 54, 1995.
67. Buyukozturk, S. et al., Latex allergy in a glove plant, *Allergy,* 55, 196, 2000.
68. Tarlo, S.M. et al., Occupational asthma caused by latex in a surgical glove manufacturing plant, *J. Allergy Clin. Immunol.,* 85, 626, 1990.
69. Pandolfo, J. and Franklin, W., Latex as a food allergen, *New Engl. J. Med.,* 341, 1858, 1999.
70. Fiocchi, A. et al., Severe anaphylaxis induced by latex as a contaminant of plastic balls in play pits, *J. Allergy Clin. Immunol.,* 108, 298, 2001.
71. Bernardini, R. et al., Anaphylaxis to latex after ingestion of a cream-filled doughnut contaminated with latex, *J. Allergy Clin. Immunol.,* 110, 534, 2002.
72. Breiteneder, H. and Ebner, C., Molecular and biochemical classification of plant derived food allergens, *J. Allergy Clin. Immunol.,* 106, 27, 2000.
73. Brehler, R. et al., "Latex-fruit syndrome": Frequency of cross reacting IgE antibodies, *Allergy,* 53, 404, 1997.
74. de Corres, L.H. et al., Sensitisation from chestnuts and bananas in patients with urticaria and anaphylaxis from contact with latex, *Ann. Allergy,* 70, 35, 1993.

5 Natural Rubber Latex Allergy and Allergens: *In Vitro* Testing

Vesna J. Tomazic-Jezic*

CONTENTS

I.   Introduction...67
II. Basis and Principles of Test Development..68
III. *In Vitro* Diagnosis of NRL Allergy...69
     A. Development of *In Vitro* Tests for NRL Sensitivity..........................69
     B. Performance of Commercial *In Vitro* Diagnostic Tests....................70
     C. Significance of *In Vitro* Tests in Diagnosing NRL Sensitivity 71
IV. Evaluating the Allergenic Potential of NRL Products..............................71
     A. Methods for Measurement of Total NRL Protein 72
     B. Methods for Quantification of Antigenic NRL Proteins....................73
     C. Quantification of NRL Allergens...74
         1. Measurement of the Individual NRL Allergens 75
         2. Relative Performance of Total Protein, Antigen, and
             Allergen Tests...76
V.   Future Trends and Goals 80
References...81

I. INTRODUCTION

When allergy to natural rubber latex (NRL) emerged as a significant health problem, we had minimal knowledge about the origin or reasons for its sudden increase or the identity of possible allergens. An effective strategy for addressing such a health issue required appropriate diagnosis and preventive measures. Because NRL contains a large number of proteins, any of which might be allergens, it was soon clear that the approach to the resolution of the problem would be quite complex. Progress in testing could not occur prior to acquiring sufficient knowledge about properties and structures of numerous unidentified allergenic proteins. Because of many potential

---

* Statements contained in this chapter are the opinions of the author and do not represent Department of Health and Human Services policy.

allergenic proteins in NRL, none of the existing methods could be used directly. There was a need to either modify the existing tests for the specific task or to develop new test methods.

This chapter describes the efforts to develop appropriate *in vitro* tests for the diagnosis of NRL allergy as well as for the evaluation of allergens in NRL products. The specific issues discussed include accuracy and standardization of the tests, and future development of *in vitro* testing.

II. BASIS AND PRINCIPLES OF TEST DEVELOPMENT

The approach to diagnosis of the NRL allergy is rather complex for several reasons. As in any IgE-mediated allergy, sensitization develops gradually through prolonged exposure to allergens. Depending on the sensitization level, the indicators and/or manifestations of the sensitivity may be different, ranging from subclinical signs (presence of the IgE antibodies in serum) to the serious clinical reactions, which in extreme cases could be life threatening. Consequently, evaluation of the afferent vs. the efferent indicators of allergy development, e.g., serum IgE antibody vs. skin testing and clinical manifestation, may produce inconsistent results. For example, individuals with limited exposure to NRL may have a measurable level of IgE antibodies in the blood shortly after the exposure, but without positive skin test response or any detectable clinical reactivity. On the other hand, a highly allergic individual, who is consciously avoiding additional exposure to NRL may have very low or undetectable level of IgE antibodies in the blood, but can positively respond to a skin test and manifest a clinical reaction to additional exposure.

A large number of epidemiological studies have been published in the last several years in the attempt to reveal the magnitude of the NRL allergy health hazard, and to identify individuals or groups at high risk of developing allergy (see Chapter 1).[1] These studies uniformly defined high-risk groups and described factors contributing to the development of allergy to NRL proteins, but at the same time revealed a great diversity in the estimate of prevalence among the groups evaluated. The reasons for the observed diversity appear to be the inconsistent evaluation methodology and variable criteria for defining true NRL allergy. While clinical scientists are still discussing optimal diagnostic criteria,[2] it has been widely accepted that an accurate diagnosis of NRL allergy can only be established by multiple parameters.[3-6] The starting point is frequently a clinical history followed by a confirmatory *in vitro* IgE antibody test and skin testing. In cases were a discrepancy occurs between an *in vitro* test and the skin test, additional testing, such as a wear (use) test or a provocation test with aeroallergen can be performed.[7,8] While each single test may produce unreliable results, with an equal chance to be a false positive or a false negative, the combination of several tests minimizes the chances that sensitized individuals may be missed or misdiagnosed.

In addition to the appropriate combination of diagnostic tests, the selection of the appropriate reagent and a uniform assay protocol are equally essential elements for a reliable diagnosis. Reagent selection is especially important in this case, as a large number of proteins may be allergenic. It was suggested that up to 60 proteins in NRL may be allergenic.[9,10] Several of the major NRL allergenic proteins have been defined in the last few years, but new ones are still being added to the existing list (see Chapter 2).[11,12] Through the years, investigators have used a variety of in-house preparations of NRL proteins, extracted either from medical gloves or from native or ammonia treated raw latex. In many cases, the allergen content or even the total amount of protein in those extracts was not characterized and the testing protocols were not uniform.

Analyses of extractable proteins from NRL products have shown that allergen content and amount can vary markedly between products. The individual allergens may not be present in the same proportion in different products or some may not be present at all. This factor, as well as differences in human genetic profiles, are the reasons for the observed difference in the sensitization patterns and the IgE antibody specificities among NRL allergic individuals.[13–15] These facts underscore the complexity and the importance of selecting the appropriate repertoire of proteins for an accurate diagnosis.

For prevention or minimizing further sensitization, it is instrumental to have a method of evaluating the sensitizing potential of NRL products. The variability of protein composition in NRL products has to be addressed in this case also. Several assays have been developed that measure either total NRL proteins, or all antigenic proteins, or all allergenic proteins. A potential standard test for specific NRL allergens has yet to be developed. However, with the increasing number of defined NRL allergenic proteins and the expanding knowledge about their properties and their significance in the overall sensitization, the task to develop a perfect allergen test seems reachable. To ensure accuracy of the allergenicity assessment, the test would have to include all proteins with an allergenic potential, and should have the capability to measure the relative amount of each allergen.

III. *IN VITRO* DIAGNOSIS OF NRL ALLERGY

A. DEVELOPMENT OF *IN VITRO* TESTS FOR NRL SENSITIVITY

In vitro tests are an important aspect of the diagnosis of IgE-mediated allergy. While the medical history is usually a starting point, the skin prick test has been considered the most reliable and the most direct indicator of a potential clinical reaction. However, *in vitro* tests are equally important, as they can detect initial exposure to allergens in a preclinical stage of the sensitization process, as well as be a valuable confirmatory test when the clinical signs of allergy are present. The *in vitro* tests that have been applied to diagnosis of NRL allergy include lymphocyte proliferation assay;[16–18] basophil histamine release assay;[19,20] and the tests for identification of IgE antibodies in the sera, such as immunoblots,[21] the RAST, and ELISA assays.[22–24] The tests, which require primary cultures of individual human blood cells, are valuable research tools, but have less potential to become routine diagnostic tests. The measurement of the serum level of NRL-specific IgE antibodies appeared more accessible as an assay that can be standardized and routinely used.

The main challenge with the test for measuring NRL-specific IgE antibodies was the selection of an appropriate source of NRL proteins. Because the relative quantities of individual NRL allergens are vastly different among various sources of raw latex and among extracts from finished products,[15,25,26] the IgE antibody response among sensitized individuals could be quite heterogeneous.[13–15,27–29] For that reason, the source of proteins for diagnosing NRL allergy should have the capacity to interact qualitatively and quantitatively with the complete spectrum of IgE specificities. Scientists have different opinions as to which of the NRL protein sources would be the most suitable. The proteins extracted from nonammoniated raw latex (NAL) are assumed to represent the most complete repertoire of individual proteins in a native form and as such this appears to be the best choice.[22,23] On the other hand, all NRL products that cause allergy are manufactured from ammoniated raw latex (AL). It was assumed that hydrolysis of the proteins by ammonia, as well as the manufacturing process itself may reveal or create some epitopes not present in native proteins.[27,28] The clinical studies designed to evaluate the performance of various sources of NRL proteins for skin testing[30] indicated that the NAL proteins displayed a comparable performance to proteins extracted from AL or proteins from glove extracts. Similar evaluation of NRL protein sources by serological assays also indicated a good agreement in their capability to identify human anti-NRL IgE antibodies.[22] LaGrutta et al., in a recent study of spina bifida children allergic to latex, demonstrated that NAL may have a greater diagnostic accuracy than AL.[31] These data encouraged use of nonammoniated protein extract as the most complete, uniform, and easily reproduced source of NRL proteins.

B. Performance of Commercial *In Vitro* Diagnostic Tests

Based on data from clinical studies, three commercial *in vitro* tests for measurement of human anti-NRL IgE antibodies have been developed and cleared by the FDA; AlaSTAT (Diagnostic Products Co. Los Angeles, CA), CAP System FEIA (Pharmacia, Peapack, NJ) and Hycor HYTECH (Hycor Biomedical, Garden Grove, CA). All three are similar type of tests and all use the NAL protein as a solid phase antigen. Several research laboratories evaluated their performance by measuring the levels of IgE antibodies in comparison with skin testing data and medical histories of sensitized individuals.[32,33] In relation to the skin test results, the CAP and the AlaSTAT tests showed about 97% specificity and 76 and 73% sensitivity, respectively. Ownby compared two IgE tests on groups of allergic and nonallergic individuals observing approximately 79 and 74% sensitivity and 90 and 92% specificity for CAP and AlaSTAT tests respectively.[34] These levels of sensitivity and specificity indicate that these tests, although a valuable diagnostic tool, may produce up to 25% false negative results and about 10% false positive results, respectively. The accuracy of the test was shown to be markedly reduced when the serum antibody levels are close to the cut-off point.[33]

The lower than expected accuracy level of these tests has been attributed, in part, to the possibility that not all major allergens are adequately presented in the NRL protein extracts.[35] On the other hand, cross-reactivity of NRL allergens with some common foods, such as avocado, banana, chestnut, and kiwi, can result in a false positive IgE test in individuals who have known food allergies without any indication of NRL allergy.[36–38] Also, the high percentage of fruit sensitivity among the NRL allergic individuals[6,39,40] confirms that the cross-reactivity with other allergens may affect the accuracy of the NRL allergy diagnosis (see Chapter 13).

C. Significance of *In Vitro* Tests in Diagnosing NRL Sensitivity

There is no doubt that serological testing is a valuable and important identifier of sensitivity to NRL allergens, but caution must be exercised when interpreting the data that has not been confirmed by another test. Due to the well-documented cross-reactivity of NRL proteins with some food allergens, a low titer of NRL-positive IgE cannot be considered a reliable indication of NRL sensitivity, without concomitant testing for food allergens and confirmatory testing for NRL sensitivity. This could be a likely explanation for some recent findings in which, based on the presence of NRL specific IgE in the sera, about 6% of the general population appeared sensitized to NRL,[41,42] while the earlier estimates of about 1% were based on multiple diagnostic parameters including clinical testing.[43]

In extensive discussions among researchers and clinicians, the general view is that multiple criteria are needed for an accurate diagnosis of NRL allergy.[2-4] A uniform agreement among different tests cannot always be expected as they evaluate different aspects of allergic responses. The skin test usually correlates well with the clinical symptoms,[44] however the skin test response may be competitively inhibited with a high level of IgE present in the serum.[45] Clinical reactions are usually the result of prolonged multiple exposures and relatively high level of sensitivity. Tarlo et al. demonstrated that up to three years of continuous exposure is needed for the manifestation of clinical symptoms of NRL allergy.[46] The complexity of an accurate diagnosis of NRL allergy was clearly shown in a study of NRL allergy prevalence among the employees of one U.S. hospital.[47] The analysis of the total IgE and anti-NRL IgE, when used as the sole criteria for the estimate of NRL sensitivity, indicated no difference in the prevalence of NRL sensitivity among the employees who regularly used NRL gloves and those whose work did not require glove use. However, when additional criteria, such as clinical manifestations of NRL allergy, were analyzed on the same test subjects, there was a clear difference between the two groups: the glove users had a significantly higher incidence of clinical reactions than non-users. Furthermore, the intensity and frequency of clinical reactions correlated with the number of gloves used daily.[47]

These findings clearly demonstrate that the serum IgE assay should be used as a confirmatory test in conjunction with clinical tests and medical history. In cases where anti-NRL IgE assay is the only parameter used to define sensitization, the number may overestimate the real prevalence of NRL allergy.[48,49] All individuals with positive IgE tests should have additional evaluation. This would be especially important when evaluating the sensitivity to NRL proteins in the general population.

IV. EVALUATING THE ALLERGENIC POTENTIAL OF NRL PRODUCTS

The safety of NRL glove users became a major concern as glove use and the prevalence of NRL allergy increased. For individuals who have already developed NRL allergy, a complete avoidance of the exposure was, and still is, the best protective measure. To prevent further user sensitization, it is imperative to reduce the level or possibly eliminate allergenic proteins from NRL products. At the time when the problem was identified in the early 1990s, this task was difficult to achieve because of the lack of an appropriate methodology for risk assessment and also due to very limited knowledge of the nature of NRL proteins. As we learned more about this heterogeneous group of proteins, it became clear that the existing methodology for general protein quantification is not appropriate for measuring multiple potential allergens on NRL products.

The essential factor in evaluation of the allergenic potency of NRL products is to ensure that the measurement includes all relevant proteins that may be responsible for allergy induction. Among the large family of NRL proteins, there are numerous allergenic ones, and without the capability of identifying specific allergenic proteins, the best and safest approach was to measure all proteins present in NRL. With the rationale that any number of NRL proteins may be allergenic when present in sufficient amounts, and via an appropriate route of exposure, it was assumed that the total level of protein should indicate proportionally the level of potential allergens.

A. Methods for Measurement of Total NRL Protein

Routinely used chemical methods for protein quantification were considered in efforts to develop a reliable and accurate *in vitro* method to quantify NRL allergens. Depending on the specific reaction mechanism, the protein assays have different propensities to react with particular amino acids and therefore may not quantify all proteins with the same accuracy. This may not be an issue in cases when a single protein is measured with an appropriate standard. On the contrary, when the measurement includes a mixture of a large number of proteins with unknown physical and chemical properties, significant inaccuracies may occur. In addition, protein extracts from raw NRL and those from finished NRL products may contain other non-proteinaceous substances that may interfere with the assays.

To determine if any of the existing methods for protein analysis may be adopted for measurement of NRL proteins, our laboratory evaluated three readily available protein assays and several potential reference proteins.[50,51] The total protein methods including the Coomassie-based Bradford assay,[52] the BCA (2,2′-bicinchoninic acid) assay,[53] and the Lowry assay[54] were evaluated in comparison with gravimetric and total nitrogen values.[55] The Lowry assay, with ovalbumin as a reference protein, demonstrated the best correlation and precision of the three methods.[50] The analysis of proteins in NRL glove extracts indicated that chemical additives, used in the manufacturing process and extracted with the soluble proteins, interfere with estimates of protein levels.[56] The original protocol was, therefore, modified and precipitation of proteins with trichloroacetic acid (TCA) and deoxycholic acid (DOC) has been added to remove interfering chemicals.[57] The third precipitation with phosphotungstic acid (PTA) was added to ensure precipitation of small protein molecules that may be lost in the supernatant.[58]

The Modified Lowry assay has been validated through the ASTM and became the ASTM standard (D5712) in 1995 and revised in 1999.[59] The ASTM D5712 was the first standardized and validated method for quantification of NRL proteins and represented a significant advance in the management of NRL allergy. Based on this standard, the FDA issued a recommendation that manufacturers may label the total protein level on the finished products to guide users in product selection.[60] The manufacturers used it as guidance in the efforts to improve their products, and frequent users of NRL products had the opportunity to select better products. Since the availability of the D5712 method, many manufacturers have successfully reduced the protein levels to such a degree that the assay has become insufficiently sensitive to accurately quantify the remaining proteins. However, measurements below the detection limit of the test were not an indicator of product safety. Beezhold et al. showed that glove extracts with protein level below the detection limit of the Modified Lowry assay may still induce positive skin reactions.[61] With wide use of the Modified Lowry assay, it has been observed that the precipitation of protein does not completely eliminate chemical interference. Furthermore, as a total protein method, it would include in the measurement some non-NRL proteins that may have been added during the manufacturing process. These factors are probably responsible for the generally poor correlation of the Modified Lowry method with the measurements of biologically active proteins, obtained by other nonstandardized methods.[62–64]

Another chemical method, HPLC amino acid analysis, has been recently validated for the quantification of NRL proteins and accepted as a nonmandatory appendix to the ASTM Modified Lowry standard D5712. It is a sensitive analytical method and may serve as a good reference for the total protein evaluation, but the need for expensive equipment and specific technical expertise may prove this method impractical for routine testing. The HPLC analysis requires complete hydrolysis of the protein to single amino acids. As a result, the analysis would include in the measurement all small peptides and single amino acids that may not have any relevance in NRL allergy induction.

B. Methods for Quantification of Antigenic NRL Proteins

The Modified Lowry method for total protein measurement has been, undoubtedly, a valuable tool for manufacturers and consumers of NRL products. However, as its lack of sensitivity and specificity became more evident, a new and better standard test was needed. The knowledge about specific NRL allergens, although markedly improved, was still not sufficient to develop a reliable specific allergen assay. To ensure that no important allergens are missed, the next logical step was to develop a test that would include measurement of all biologically relevant NRL proteins.

The first such test was the indirect ELISA assay, based on protein recognition by rabbit anti-NRL antibodies[65] with the assumption that rabbits produce IgG antibodies against all proteins capable of inducing immune response. This more sensitive test, available as a kit (LEAP, Guthrie Research Institute, Sayre, PA), has been used in addition to the Modified Lowry standard for several years. The assay consists of binding the NRL reference or test protein to the assay plate and reacting with the rabbit anti-NRL serum. The protein binding to the plate, however, may vary depending on the molecular weight of individual proteins and the overall protein concentration. With known variations in the amount and size distribution of proteins in the glove extracts, differences in the binding efficiency could affect the accuracy of the assay. In this case, there was no mechanism to validate either the amount or the type of proteins bound to the plates.

Another format of the ELISA test, the ELISA Inhibition assay, appeared to be a better alternative.[64,66,67] As in the LEAP assay, the measurement of antigenic protein levels is based on the capacity of rabbit anti-NRL IgG antibodies to react with the NRL protein in a test sample. However, this assay includes a two-step protocol; inhibition of rabbit anti-NRL serum with protein in test sample as an initial step, followed by the transfer of the inhibited serum into the assay plates precoated with the standard reference antigen. Remaining free rabbit antibodies react with antigen on the plate. Secondary enzyme-conjugated antirabbit IgG antibodies are used to visualize binding. The percent of serum inhibition reflects the level of protein in the test sample. This method measures all proteins capable of inducing IgG antibody response in rabbits and is, therefore, defined as an antigenic protein assay.[66,67] In contrast to the LEAP assay, this format eliminates the need to use the test sample as a solid phase protein. The ELISA Inhibition protocol has been validated through the ASTM and became the standard assay ASTM D6499.[68] The reference antigen in the D6499 assay is a pool of six AL extracts, each with a specifically defined origin, and known dose and time of ammonia exposure. The rabbit anti-NRL antiserum in this test is a pool of sera from 3 to 4 rabbits from two different laboratories, immunized with the same reference protein preparation. The inter- and intralaboratory reproducibility and sensitivity of the test are good, and with the well-defined source of NRL proteins and immunization protocol, reproducibility of standard reagents has been confirmed.

C. QUANTIFICATION OF NRL ALLERGENS

The methods developed to measure total protein and total antigen have been successfully used as indicators of the relative sensitizing potential of NRL products, but did not eliminate the need for a specific allergen assay. The identification of the individual allergens has progressed significantly, but the uncertainty regarding additional yet undefined allergens still remains. The two-dimensional electrophoresis of NRL extracts revealed about 60 proteins that react with human IgE antibodies,[9] and another study described 30 significant allergenic proteins in NRL.[10] Although some of those allergenic proteins may be isomers or cleaved fragments of the larger molecules, they may be important contributors to overall allergenicity of NRL proteins.

Because of the limited knowledge about the total number and identity of all allergenic NRL proteins, the only reliable measure of potential allergenicity was to measure all allergens. Two tests routinely used for detection of allergens, the RAST Inhibition and the ELISA Inhibition assay, have been applied to evaluate allergen content in NRL extracts.[22-24] Both tests are essentially the same, except for the endpoint identifier (radioactive isotope versus enzyme) and are comparably sensitive and reproducible. The format of the tests is very similar to the already described total antigen test D6499.[68] The detection of allergen in test samples is based on human serum IgE reaction with the proteins that lead to sensitization. Because of variations in IgE specificities among sensitized individuals, the pools of sera from a number of sensitized donors have been used. Most laboratories use NAL extracts

TABLE 5.1
Frequency of Responses to Major Allergens in NRL-Sensitized Individuals

Allergen	Percent of Positive Test Responses				
	Immunoblots	ELISA	ELISA	Skin Test	Skin Test
Hev b1	3	13–19	36		23
Hev b2	28	48–61		7	63
Hev b3	0	19	36	7	24
Hev b4	75	23–61			39
Hev b5	31		57	62	65
Hev b6.2		45	93	65	63
Hev b7b	61	23–45		41	63
Reference	Yeang (79)*	Kurup (78)	Palosuo (81)*	Yip (77)*	Bernstein (80)**

* Recombinant proteins.
** Native allergens.

as a reference and as a solid phase protein. These tests appear to be sufficiently sensitive and accurate in measuring allergen levels because the pool of a large number of immune sera should have the capacity to identify and quantify most if not all important allergenic proteins. Unfortunately, neither of these methods could be developed as a standard allergen assay because of the very limited availability of human sera and inability to reproduce the potency and specificity of serum pools.

1. Measurement of the Individual NRL Allergens

In parallel with the progress in identification of the major NRL allergens, researchers are initiating efforts to develop a specific allergen test that would not be based on human anti-NRL IgE and would have the potential to become a standard allergen test. There are presently thirteen major allergens identified and sequenced.[11,12] Recombinant proteins for several of those allergens have been produced,[12,69–76] and a number of monoclonal antibodies are now available. A limited number of published studies evaluating the relative importance of these allergens in sensitized individuals have been summarized in Table 5.1. NRL-sensitive individuals and their sera were screened for the frequency of reactions with native and recombinant allergenic proteins.[77–81] In the ELISA inhibition test, Kurup et al. showed that 53 to 100% of the human sera IgE react with allergens Hev b 1 to Hev b 7.[78] This study indicated that most of the healthcare workers respond to Hev b 2, Hev b 4, Hev b 5, Hev b 6.2, and Hev b 7b. Skin testing of NRL allergic individuals with single allergens confirmed the *in vitro* findings.[81] Yip et al. obtained somewhat different results, when a group of sensitized individuals with positive skin test to whole NAL extract, were retested with six individual major allergenic recombinant proteins.[77] Although positive to NAL protein extract, some of the subjects responded to only one of the six allergens and one individual did not respond to any of the six allergens tested. It is not clear if the lack of the response in this case resulted from the difference in the recognition of recombinant proteins versus native allergens, or these individuals were sensitized to some other allergenic proteins in NRL. On the other hand, most of the tested individuals responded to more than one allergen (Table 5.1). These studies indicate that five allergens, Hev b 2, Hev b 4, Hev b 5, Hev b 6.2, and Hev b 7b have been the most frequent sensitizers in adult healthcare workers.[77–81] In spina bifida children, however, the pattern of response is different and the major allergens appear to be Hev b 1 and Hev b 3.[78,82–85] Based on these limited but valuable data, it seems that an appropriate combination of a few allergens might be sufficient for the identification of serum positive individuals. As a serum IgE test is not considered a strictly quantitative test, inclusion of several major allergens may be a reliable identifier of anti-NRL antibodies in the serum. The true level of sensitivity could only be established in combination with other tests, including skin testing and clinical history.[2–6]

In contrast to the diagnostic approach, the measurement of allergenic protein content in NRL products, intended as a single risk assessment tool, requires a very precise and accurate quantitative test. In developing such a test it is, therefore, imperative to ensure its capacity to recognize all potential allergens and to properly measure the amount of each individual allergen. Because of the variations in the total protein content[86] and the relative levels of individual allergens among NRL products,[86,87] an excess of antibodies should exist for each allergen to ensure a complete inhibition. Several investigators attempted to develop a sandwich ELISA format test for the measurement of a single allergen, using allergen-specific mono-clonal antibodies.[88] The first test for quantification of four NRL allergens has been developed as a commercial kit (FITkit®, Biotech Co. Tampere, Finland). FITkit® includes four individual tests for Hev b 1, 3, 5 and 6.02. Ongoing studies evaluating performance and accuracy of this test will be discussed in Chapter 6.

We used the FITkit® to evaluate the levels and relative proportion of four major allergens in extracts from raw ammoniated and nonammoniated NRL as well as in extracts from finished NRL products. Analysis of four NAL protein extracts from various sources showed relatively uniform ratios of four allergens, with the highest proportion of Hev b 6.02 (Figure 5.1A). The allergen ratios in AL protein extracts, however, differed markedly from sample to sample (Figure 5.1B). The diversity in proportion of four allergens was even more evident among extracts from NRL gloves (Figure 5.2). This study indicates that both processing of raw NRL as well as the glove manufacturing process affect, not only the amount of total protein on the finished product, but also the relative amounts of individual allergens. Interestingly, the gloves with a low amount of total allergen tended to have relatively balanced levels of four allergens. In glove extracts with a high amount of total allergen, the higher level was mainly due to Hev b 5 and Hev b 6.02 allergens. As the relative levels of allergens in glove extracts may vary up to 100 times, each sample will have to be tested at multiple dilutions to ensure complete inhibition of each allergen.

2. Relative Performance of Total Protein, Antigen, and Allergen Tests

As the evaluation of NRL product allergenicity is progressing from the measurement of total proteins to the quantification of individual allergens, there is a persistent question of accuracy and relevance of these tests for the risk assessment and for the

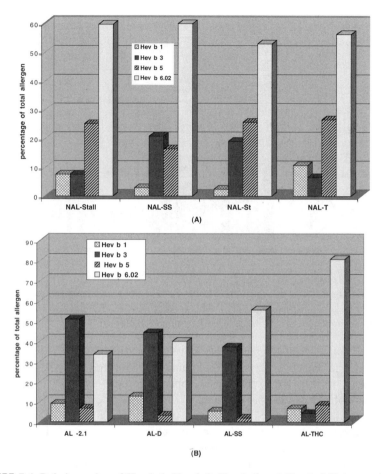

FIGURE 5.1 Relative ratios of Hev b 1, Hev b 3, Hev b 5, and Hev b 6.02 in samples of raw nonammoniated latex (NAL) protein extracts (A) and samples of ammoniated latex (AL) protein extracts (B). Value for each allergen represents percent of the sum of four allergens measured.

prevention of NRL allergy. With each of the methods developed so far, the general assumption was that both total protein and total antigenic protein represent a relative measure of allergen content. This assumption was based on the general understanding of the allergy development process and the nature of potentially allergenic proteins. Unfortunately, there is no established reference parameter or reference test, according to which all other tests could be evaluated.

In the diagnosis of NRL allergy, skin testing has been considered the gold standard. To some extent, it has also been used for the evaluation of specific allergens but ethical concerns limit wider use. However even with skin testing, a direct comparison of the existing data is complicated due to lack of uniform and standardized skin testing protocol and reference reagents. The two *in vitro* tests for total allergens, the RAST Inhibition, and the ELISA Inhibition, could be good candidates

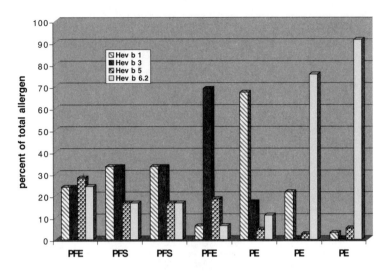

FIGURE 5.2 Relative ratios of Hev b 1, Hev b 3, Hev b 5, and Hev b 6.02 in protein extract samples from surgical and examination NRL gloves. Value for each allergen represents percent of the sum of four allergens measured. PFE — powder-free examination glove, PFS — powder-free surgical glove, PE — powdered examination glove.

for the validation of existing and newly developing tests, if a well-defined pool of human immune sera could be prepared. A number of such pools have been used by investigators, but there are no published comparative studies that evaluate uniformity of the sera pools or the data obtained.

Our laboratory conducted a number of studies to compare the performance of available tests for NRL proteins.[89] In a recent multicenter study, the ELISA Inhibition and the RAST Inhibition assays of glove extract proteins was performed, using different pools of human sera prepared from geographically and ethnically diverse populations of NRL allergic individuals.[90] The six sets of data generated in this study indicated a very good correlation between RAST and ELISA Inhibition tests without notable differences among various pools of immune sera. This observation suggests that these tests, with a representative pool of human anti-NRL IgE antibodies, could be a potentially reliable reference test. The concern here is availability of sufficient amount of immune sera in the light of the recent decrease in the prevalence of NRL allergy, with the use of improved NRL products.

To evaluate the performance of the total antigen assay ASTM D6499, we analyzed 15 glove extracts, comparing the data with several other tests, including total antigen LEAP test, two total protein assays including the HPLC amino acid analysis and the D5712 test, and the RAST Inhibition test for total NRL allergen content.[86] The D6499 correlated well with the LEAP assay. Less correlation was observed with the HPLC amino acid analysis, the D5712 assay, and with the RAST Inhibition test. In both total antigen tests, AL was the reference protein, while the allergen tests used NAL proteins. It is not clear if the data discrepancy between allergen and antigen tests was due to the difference in the protein source. NAL extract was shown to contain most of the proteins present in raw NRL and they remain in a native form,

TABLE 5.2
Significance of Antigen Source on the D6499 Assay Performance: Effects of NAL and AL Protein on the Correlation of Antigen Assay with Total Allergen Assay

Solid Phase Antigen	Reference Antigen	Rabbit Antiserum	D6499*	RAST Inhibition
NAL	NAL	Anti-AL	0.17	0.89
		Anti-NAL	0.16	0.95
NAL	AL	Anti-AL	0.11	0.98
		Anti-NAL	0.12	0.97
AL	AL	Anti-AL	0.84	0.43
		Anti-NAL	0.16	0.89
AL	NAL	Anti-AL	N/A	N/A
		Anti-NAL	0.30	0.99

Note: 15 surgical and examination gloves evaluated. Light gray area indicates standard D6499 conditions; dark gray area indicates the conditions assumed optimal.

* Our D6499 values compared to the mean value of seven sets of data from other laboratories testing the same glove samples.

while AL proteins are hydrolyzed to various degrees, depending on the ammonia level. Immunoblot analysis of the two extracts with rabbit anti-NRL sera showed that both, anti-AL and anti-NAL, sera recognize wider spectrum of proteins in the NAL than in the AL protein extract.[87]

The choice of AL or NAL as a reference protein in the various tests has been a controversial subject. Except for the LEAP and the D6499 assays, NAL has been used in most of the *in vitro* tests for both NRL allergy and NRL allergens, as well as in the commercial kits for human serum IgE detection. NAL has also been a source of proteins for the purification of allergens identified so far. A direct comparison of two reagents in skin testing showed equivocal responses at the same total protein level,[30] and somewhat better accuracy with NAL extract.[31]

To investigate the significance of the protein source in the performance of the D6499 test, we analyzed glove extracts, using either AL or NAL proteins as antigens, as well as using either anti-AL or anti-NAL rabbit sera (Table 5.2). For comparison, the same samples were simultaneously evaluated for allergen levels by the IgE ELISA Inhibition assay, using human anti-NRL IgE sera pool. When NAL proteins were used, an increased correlation between antigen and allergen values was obtained. The best correlation was observed when NAL was used as a coating antigen in the assay plates. This modification of the D6499 assay resulted in values closer to the allergenic protein measurements, and appeared to improve the accuracy of the assay. To confirm this finding, we evaluated a larger number of surgical and examination gloves comparing the standard D6499 with the modified protocol, replacing only AL protein with NAL protein as a solid phase antigen. The two sets

TABLE 5.3
Correlation of D6499 and Modified D6499 Test for NRL Antigen with the Tests for Total NRL Protein and Total Allergen Measurement

	D6499		M6499	
	Exp. 1*	Exp. 2*	Exp. 1*	Exp. 2*
D5712	0.41	0.08	0.53	0.73
AA		0.17		0.70
D6499	1.00	1.00	0.06	0.06
IgE ELISA*	0.01	0.09	0.75	0.96
IgE ELISA*	0.04	0.04	0.84	0.69
FITkit	0.01	0.07	0.77	0.90
M6499	0.06	0.06	1.00	1.00

* Data from two laboratories.
Note: Values represent correlation coefficients from two independent experiments on different glove extracts.

of data were compared to the IgE ELISA Inhibition assay (Table 5.3). This study confirmed our previous observation that changing the solid phase protein source from AL to NAL results in a better correlation of the D6499 test with the allergen assays. The ASTM is presently conducting validation studies to include this modification in the revision of the test. The revised method would provide a more accurate estimate of the allergen content in NRL products.

V. FUTURE TRENDS AND GOALS

When addressing future trends in the devleopment of *in vitro* methods, one should discuss the diagnostic tests separately from the tests for the quantitation of NRL allergens, as the purpose and requirements may be somewhat different.

Presently available *in vitro* diagnostic tests, although producing relatively reliable results, do not perform with 100% accuracy. The reasons are most likely due to uncertain reproducibility of protein composition in NRL extracts used in the tests, as well as the variability of human responses to individual allergens. Since the test performance is only as good as the allergen preparation used, the availability and use of pure recombinant allergens should improve allergy testing. However, because the sensitized individuals respond differently to single allergens, it would be difficult to determine an optimal combination and the relative amounts of individual allergens that would assure general accuracy of the test. The recombinant proteins will have to be highly purified and functionally identical to the native proteins. Limited published data indicate the possibility of differences in the allergenic specificity of recombinant and native NRL proteins,[77,80] which needs to be further investigated. From the observed response patterns among various high-risk groups, it may be necessary to develop more than one allergen test. It was suggested that several specific allergen test panels should be designed; one for spina bifida children, another for the adult population and the third for the individuals who also have food allergy.[11]

Accuracy of the test for quantification of allergens in NRL products is even more critical, as this would represent a direct and only measure of the potential risk for sensitization or allergic reaction. Therefore, such tests would have to be highly quantitative. They would have a capacity to detect not only the major allergenic proteins to which users become most frequently sensitized, but also any other protein in NRL that, under special circumstances, may have an allergenic potential. The number of major allergens already identified represents great progress, but we believe that more allergenic proteins will be identified in the future. As with the diagnostic tests, using a combination of individual recombinant allergens as the reference protein is a sound approach. However, for allergen quantitation test, there are even more questions that need to be resolved before a practical standard test can be developed. The most important question is how many and which allergens should be included in the test. It has been suggested that only a few proteins may be needed as "indicator allergens,"[91] but this may not ensure accuracy, considering great variations in the proportion of individual allergens in NRL products. Based on the most recent data,[77–81] it seems that four to seven major allergens may suffice, as those proteins represent a larger part of the total protein extractable from NRL products. If further studies confirm this to be true, the remaining issues to be resolved would be selection of the test format[92] and the most appropriate antibodies.

Current approaches to measure individual allergens using monoclonal antibodies are quite specific and accurate. However, the evaluation of each test sample separately for each of the major allergens would be impractical, time consuming and expensive. Several research laboratories through the ASTM auspices are discussing the feasibility of developing a single test using a combination of major allergens. This is a challenging task as it raises significant technical issues. One is determining the appropriate relative ratio of the individual allergens for the reference protein that would optimally reflect the most common ratio in the NRL product extracts. The other issue is related to selection of antibodies with one option to use polyclonal antibodies generated by immunization with the reference protein. Another option would be to use a mixture of monoclonal antibodies specific for each allergen in the test. The ratio of each antibody, in this case, would have to be determined based on the antibody affinity and the ratio of allergens in the reference proteins. More research and collaboration between investigators involved in allergen characterization and production of monoclonal antibodies is crucial for achieving this aim.

Future studies are likely to change the focus from identification of additional allergens to the identification of dominant allergenic epitopes, which would result in the production of a large number of monoclonal antibodies. This could shed a new light on the approach to *in vitro* testing.

REFERENCES

1. Turjanmaa, K. and Makinen-Kiljunen, S., Latex allergy: Prevalence, risk factors and cross-reactivity, *Methods,* 27, 10, 2002.

2. Turjanmaa, K., Diagnosis of latex allergy, *Allergy,* 56, 810, 2001.
3. Kelly, K.J. et al., The diagnosis of natural rubber latex allergy, *J. Allergy Clin. Immunol.,* 93, 813, 1994.
4. Tilles, S.A., Occupational latex allergy: Controversies in diagnosis and prognosis, *Ann. Allergy Asthma Immunol.,* 83, 640, 1999.
5. Tarlo, S.M., Natural rubber latex allergy and asthma, *Curr. Opinion Pulmon. Med.,* 7, 27, 2001.
6. Nettis, E. et al., Latex hypersensitivity: Personal data and review of the literature. *Immunopharm. Immunotoxicol.,* 24, 315, 2002.
7. Hamilton, R.G. and Atkinson, N.F., Validation of latex glove provocation procedure in latex-allergic subjects, *Ann. Allergy Asthma Immunol.,* 79, 266, 1997.
8. Kurtz, K.M. et al., Hooded exposure chamber (HEC) for particulate latex allergen challenge, *J. Allergy Clin. Immunol.,* 99, 638, 1997 (abstract).
9. Posch, A. et al., Characterization and identification of latex allergens by two-dimensional electrophoresis and protein micro sequencing, *J. Allergy Clin. Immunol.,* 99, 385, 1997.
10. Wagner, S. et al., Natural rubber latex contains more than 30 significant allergens, *J. Allergy Clin. Immunol.,* 107, s117, 2001.
11. Breiteneder, H. and Scheiner, O., Molecular and immunological characteristics of latex allergens, *Int. Arch. Allergy Immunol.,* 116, 83, 1998.
12. Yeang, H.Y. et al., Allergenic proteins of natural rubber latex, *Methods,* 27, 32, 2002.
13. Sussman, G.L., Tarlo, S., and Dolovich, J., The spectrum of IgE-mediated responses to latex, *J. Am. Med. Assoc.,* 265, 2844, 1991.
14. Beezhold, D.H. et al., Identification of a 46-kD latex protein allergen in health care workers, *Clin. Exp. Immunol.,* 98, 408, 1994.
15. Tomazic, V.J., Withrow, T.J., and Hamilton, R.G., Characterization of the allergen(s) in latex protein extracts, *J. Allergy Clin. Immunol.,* 96, 635, 1995.
16. Murali, P.S. et al., Investigations into cellular immune responses in latex allergy, *J. Lab. Clin. Med.,* 124, 638, 1994.
17. Raulf-Heimshoth, M. et al., Lymphocyte response of latex-sensitized patients to purified allergen Hev b 1, *J. Allergy Clin. Immunol.,* 98, 640, 1996.
18. Johnson, B.D. et al., Purified and recombinant latex proteins stimulate peripheral blood lymphocytes of latex allergic patients, *Int. Arch. Allergy,* 120, 270, 1999.
19. Crockard, A.D. and Ennis, M., Basophil histamine release tests in the diagnosis of allergy and asthma, *Clin. Exp. Allergy,* 31, 345, 2001.
20. Ebo, D.G. et al., Validation of two-color flow cytometry assay detecting *in vitro* basophile activation for the diagnosis of IgE-mediated natural rubber latex allergy, *Allergy,* 57, 706, 2002.
21. Gruber, C. et al., Is there a role for immunoblots in the diagnosis of latex allergy? Intermethod comparison of *in vitro* and *in vivo* IgE assay in spina bifida patients, *Allergy,* 55, 476, 2000.
22. Hamilton, R.G. et al., Serologic methods in the laboratory diagnosis of latex rubber allergy: Study of non-ammoniated, ammoniated latex, and glove (end product) extracts as allergen reagent sources, *J. Lab. Clin. Med.,* 123(4), 594, 1994.
23. Turjanmaa, K. et al., Latex allergy diagnosis: *In vivo* and *in vitro* standardization of a natural rubber latex extract, *Allergy,* 52, 41, 1997.
24. Palosuo, T., Alenius, H., and Turjanmaa, K., Quantitation of latex allergens, *Methods,* 27, 52, 2002.
25. Lu, L. et al., Comparison of latex antigens from surgical gloves, ammoniated and non-ammoniated latex: Effect of ammonia treatment on natural rubber latex proteins, *J. Lab. Clin. Med.,* 126(2), 161, 1995.

26. Yunginger, J.W. et al., Extractable latex allergens and proteins in disposable medical gloves and other rubber products, *J. Allergy Clin. Immunol.*, 93, 836, 1994.

27. Asakava, A., Hsieh, L.-S., and Lin, Y., Serum reactivities to latex proteins (*Hevea brasiliensis*), *J. Allergy Clin. Immunol.*, 95, 1196, 1995.

28. Asakava, A., Hsieh, L.-S., and Lin, Y., Comparison of latex specific IgE binding among non-ammoniated latex, ammoniated latex and latex glove allergenic extracts by ELISA and immunoblot inhibition, *J. Allergy Clin. Immunol.*, 97, 1116, 1996.

29. Kurup, V.P. and Fink, J.N., The spectrum of immunologic sensitization in latex allergy, *Allergy*, 56, 2, 2001.

30. Hamilton, R.G. and Adkinson, N.F., Natural rubber latex skin testing reagents: Safety and diagnostic accuracy of non-ammoniated latex, ammoniated latex, and latex rubber glove extracts, *J. Allergy Clin. Immunol.*, 98, 872, 1996.

31. LaGrutta, S. et al., Comparison of ammoniated and non-ammoniated extracts in children with latex allergy, *Allergy*, 58, 814, 2003.

32. Hamilton, R.G., Biagini, R.E., and Krieg, E.F., Diagnostic performance of FDA-cleared serological assays for natural rubber latex specific IgE antibody, *J. Allergy Clin. Immunol.*, 103, 925, 1999.

33. Biagini, R.E. et al., Receiver operating characteristics analyses of Food and Drug Administration cleared serological assays for natural rubber latex-specific IgE antibody, *Clin. Diag. Lab. Immunol.*, 8, 1145, 2001.

34. Ownby, D.R., Magera, B., and Williams, B., A blinded, multi-center evaluation of two commercial *in vitro* tests for latex-specific IgE antibodies, *Ann. Allergy Asthma Immunol.*, 84, 193, 2000.

35. Hamilton, R.G. et al., Latex-specific IgE assay sensitivity enhanced using Hev b5 enriched latex allergosorbent. *J. Allergy Clin. Immunol.*, 111, s172, 2003 (abstract).

36. Diez-Gomez, M.L. et al., Fruit-pollen-latex cross-reactivity: Implication of profilin (Bet v 2), *Allergy*, 54, 951, 1999.

37. Moller, M. et al., Determination and characterization of cross-reacting allergens in latex, avocado, banana and kiwi fruit, *Allergy*, 53, 289, 1998.

38. Blanco, C., Latex-fruit syndrome, *Curr. Allergy Asthma Rep.*, 3, 47, 2003.

39. Brehler, R. et al., Latex-fruit syndrome: Frequency of cross-reacting IgE antibodies, *Allergy*, 52, 404, 1997.

40. Kim, K.T. and Hussain, H., Prevalence of food allergy in 137 latex-allergic patients, *Allergy Asthma Proc.*, 20, 95, 1999.

41. Ownby, D.R. et al., The prevalence of anti-latex IgE antibodies in 1000 volunteer blood donors, *J. Allergy Clin. Immunol.*, 97, 1188, 1996.

42. Lebenbom-Mansour, M.H. et al., The incidence of latex sensitivity in ambulatory surgical patients: A correlation of historical factors with positive serum immunoglobulin E levels, *Anesth. Analg.*, 85, 44, 1997.

43. Liss, G.M. and Sussman, G.L., Latex sensitization: Occupational versus general population prevalence rates, *Am. J. Ind. Med.*, 35, 196, 1999.

44. Hadjiliadis, D., Banks, D.E., and Tarlo, S.M., The relationship between latex skin prick test responses and clinical allergic responses, *J. Allergy Clin. Immunol.*, 97, 1202, 1996.

45. Witteman, A.M. et al., The relationship between RAST and skin test results in patients with asthma or rhinitis: A quantitative study with purified major allergens, *J. Allergy Clin. Immunol.*, 97, 16, 1996.

46. Tarlo, S.M., Sussman, G.L., and Holness, D.L., Latex sensitivity in dental students and staff: A cross-sectional study, *J. Allergy Clin. Immunol.*, 99, 396, 1997.

47. Page, E.H. et al., Natural Rubber latex: Glove use, sensitization and airborne and latent dust concentration at the Denver Hospital, *J. O. E. M.*, 42, 613, 2000.

48. Yeang, H.Y., Prevalence of latex allergy may be vastly overestimated when determined by *in vitro* assays, *Ann. Allergy Asthma Immunol.*, 84, 628, 2000.
49. Pridgeon, C. et al., Assessment of latex allergy in a healthcare population: Are the available tests valid?, *Clin. Exp. Allergy*, 30, 1444, 2000.
50. Tomazic-Jezic, V.J. et al., Quantitation of natural rubber latex proteins: Evaluation of various protein measurement methods, *Toxicol. Methods*, 9, 153, 1999.
51. Lucas, A.D. and Tomazic-Jezic, V.J., Modification of the Lowry method for analysis of soluble latex proteins, *Toxicol. Methods*, 10, 165, 2000.
52. Compton, S.J. and Jones, C.G., Mechanism of dye response and interference in the Bradford protein assay, *Anal. Biochem.*, 151, 369, 1985.
53. Smith, P.K., Measurement of protein using bicinchoninic acid, *Anal. Biochem.*, 150, 76, 1985.
54. Peterson, G.L., Review of the folin phenol protein quantitation method of Lowry, Rosenbrough, Farr and Randall, *Anal. Biochem.*, 100, 201, 1979.
55. Koch, F.S. and McMeekin, T.L., A new direct nesslerization micro Kjeldahl method and a modification of the Nessler-Folin reagent for ammonia, *J. Am. Chem. Soc.*, 46, 2066, 1924.
56. Chen, S.F., Teoh, S.C., and Porter, M., A false-positive result with the ASTM D5712-95 test method for protein given by the common vulcanization accelerator, *J. Allergy Clin. Immunol.*, 100, 713, 1997.
57. Siler, D.J. and Cornish, K., Measurement of protein in natural latex rubber particle suspensions, *Anal. Biochem.*, 229, 278, 1995.
58. Yusof, F. and Yeang, H.Y., Quantitation of proteins from natural rubber latex gloves, *J. Natl. Rubber Res. Inst.*, 7, 206, 1992.
59. ASTM D 5712-99, Standard test method for the analysis of aqueous extractable protein in natural rubber and its products using the Modified Lowry method, in *Annual Book of ASTM Standards*, Conshohocken, PA, 1999.
60. FDA guidance for protein level labeling, *Guidance for medical glove: A workshop manual*, U.S. Department of Health and Human Services, FDA96-4257, 6, 1996.
61. Beezhold, D.H. et al., Correlation of protein levels with skin prick test reactions in patients allergic to latex, *J. Allergy Clin. Immunol.*, 98, 1097, 1996.
62. Beezhold, D.H. et al., Measurement of natural rubber proteins in latex glove extracts: Comparison of the methods, *Ann. Allergy Asthma Immunol.*, 76, 520, 1996.
63. Baur, X. et al., Protein and allergen content of various natural latex articles, *Allergy*, 52, 661, 1997.
64. Chabane, H. et al., Competitive immunoassay for antigenic latex protein measurement: Rabbit antiserum-based assay compared to Modified Lowry and human IgE-inhibition methods, *Invest. Allergol. Clin. Immunol.*, 9, 372, 1999.
65. Beezhold, D.H., LEAP: Latex ELISA for antigenic proteins, *Guthrie J.*, 61, 77, 1992.
66. Tomazic-Jezic, V.J., Woolhiser, M.R., and Beezhold, D.H., ELISA inhibition assay for the quantitation of antigenic protein in natural rubber latex, *J. Immunoassay Immunochem.*, 23, 261, 2002.
67. Beezhold, D.H., Kostyal, D.A., and Tomazic-Jezic, V.J., Measurement of latex proteins and assessment of latex protein exposure, *Methods*, 27, 46, 2002.
68. ASTM D 6499-00, Standard test method for the immunological measurement of antigenic protein in natural rubber and its products, in *Annual Book of ASTM Standards*, ASTM, Conshohocken, PA, 2000.
69. Hye, M.L. and Cheung, K.Y., Beta-1,3-glucanase is highly-expressed in lacifers of *Hevea brasiliensis*, *Plant Mol. Biol.* 29, 397, 1995.

70. Akasawa, A. et al., A novel acidic allergen, Hev b 5, in latex: Purification, cloning and characterization, *J. Biol. Chem.*, 271, 25389, 1996.
71. Chen, Z. et al., Purification and characterization of rubber elongation factor from *Hevea Brasiliensis* (Hev b 1) that acts as a major allergen in latex allergic patients with spina bifida, *Allergy*, 52, 79, 1997.
72. Chen, Z. et al., Identification of hevein (Hev b 6.02) in Hevea latex as a major cross-reacting allergen with avocado fruit in patients with latex allergy, *J. Allergy Clin. Immunol.*, 102, 476, 1998.
73. Kostyal, D.A. et al., Cloning and characterization of a latex allergen (Hev b 7): Homology to patatin, a plant PLA2, *Clin. Exp. Immunol.*, 112, 355, 1998.
74. Yeang, H.Y. et al., Amino acid sequence similarity of Hev b3 to two previously reported 27- and 23-kDa latex proteins allergenic to spina bifida patients, *Allergy*, 53, 513, 1998.
75. Slater, J.E. et al., Identification, cloning and sequence of a major allergen (Hev b5) from natural rubber latex (*Hevea brasiliensis*), *J. Biol. Chem.*, 271, 25394, 1996.
76. DeSilva, H.D. et al., Human T-cell epitopes of the latex allergen Hev-b 5 in health care workers, *J. Allergy Clin. Immunol.*, 105, 1017, 2000.
77. Yip, L. et al., Skin prick test reactivity to recombinant latex allergens, *Int. Arch. Allergy Immunol.*, 121, 292, 2000.
78. Kurup, V.P. et al., Detection of immunoglobulin antibodies in the sera of patients using purified latex allergens, *Clin. Exp. Allergy*, 30, 359, 2000.
79. Yeang, H.Y. et al., Hev b 2 and Hev b 3 content in natural rubber latex and latex gloves, *J. Allergy Clin. Immunol.*, 107, s118, 2001 (abstract).
80. Bernstein, D.I. et al., In vivo sensitization to purified *Hevea brasiliensis* proteins in health care workers sensitized to natural rubber latex, *J. Allergy Clin. Immunol.*, 111, 610, 2003.
81. Palosuo, T. et al., Recombinant allergen-based ELISA for the simultaneous detection of IgE to clinically relevant latex allergens, *J. Allergy Clin. Immunol.*, 111, s172, 2003 (abstract).
82. Alenius, H. et al. IgE reactivity to 14-kD and 27-kD natural rubber proteins in latex-allergic children with spina bifida and other congenital anomalies, *Int. Arch. Allergy Immunol.*, 102, 61, 1993.
83. Lu, L-J. et al., Characterization of a major latex allergen associated with hypersensitivity in spina bifida patients, *J. Immunol.*, 155, 2721, 1995.
84. Alenius, H. et al., Purification and partial amino acid sequencing of a 27-kD natural rubber allergen recognized by latex-allergic children with spina bifida, *Int. Arch. Allergy Immunol.*, 106, 258, 1995.
85. Yeang, H.Y. et al., The 14.6 kD (ref, Hev b1) and 24kD (Hev b3) rubber particle proteins are recognized by IgE from spina bifida patients with latex allergy, *J. Allergy Clin. Immunol.*, 98, 628, 1996.
86. Tomazic-Jezic, V.J. and Lucas, A.D., Evaluation of antigens in the ELISA inhibition assay for natural rubber latex proteins, *The Toxicologist*, 54, 125, 2000.
87. Tomazic-Jezic, V.J. and Truscott, W., Identification of antigenic and allergenic natural rubber latex proteins by immunobloting, *J. Immunoassay Immunochem.*, 23, 369, 2002.
88. Raulf-Heimsoth, M. et al., Development of a monoclonal antibody-based sandwich ELISA for detection of the latex allergen Hev b 1, *Int. Arch. Allergy Immunol.*, 123, 236, 2000.
89. Tomazic-Jezic, V.J. et al., The ASTM Semi-annual Meeting, June 2003 (minutes).

90. Tomazic-Jezic, V.J. et al., Performance of methods for the measurement of natural rubber latex (NRL) protein, antigen and allergen, *J. Allergy Clin. Immunol.*, Jan 2004, in press.
91. Hamilton, R.G., Aria, S.A.M., and Yeang, H.Y., Quantification of Hev b1/Hev b6 levels in prospective latex allergen reference preparations by immunoenzymetric assays, *J. Allergy Clin. Immunol.*, 105, s82, 2000 (abstract).
92. Bacarese-Hamilton, T. et al., Detection of allergen-specific IgE on microarrays by use of signal amplification techniques, *Clin. Chem.*, 48, 1367, 2002.

6 New Developments in Measuring Allergens in Natural Rubber Latex Products

Katja Frisk, Tytti Kärkkäinen, Hely Reinikka-Railo, and Timo Palosuo

CONTENTS

I.   Introduction 87
II. NRL Allergens in the Source Material and in Manufactured
     Products 88
III. Methods for Measuring Natural Rubber Latex Allergens 89
     A. Qualitative Methods 89
        1. IgE-Immunoblotting Analysis (Western Blotting) 89
        2. IgE-Immunoblotting after Isoelectric Focusing and
           Electrophoresis (Two-Dimensional Immunoblotting) 90
     B. Semiquantitative Methods 90
        1. Skin Prick Testing in Voluntary Latex-Allergic Subjects 90
        2. RAST Inhibition and IgE-ELISA Inhibition Assay 90
     C. Quantitative Methods 91
        1. Capture Enzyme Immunoassays (EIA) for NRL Allergen
           Quantification 91
IV. Conclusions 94
References 95

I. INTRODUCTION

Immediate allergic reactions to natural rubber latex (NRL) proteins have been recognized for almost 20 years as an important medical and occupational health problem. An important source of sensitization has been considered to be proteins or peptides eluting from protective NRL gloves.[1] Minimizing allergen concentration in latex gloves to prevent sensitization and the development of clinical allergy to NRL is acknowledged to be of mutual interest for rubber manufacturers and regulatory health authorities.

For several years, there has been an increasing need for accurate measurement of the allergenic potential of NRL goods but the availability of specific methods has been scanty. In several studies, the amount of extractable total protein has correlated relatively well with the true allergen content of NRL gloves measured by skin prick test (SPT) or human IgE-based immunological inhibition assays.[2-5] A well-known shortcoming of the total protein methods is, however, that they measure also non-allergenic proteins that are likely to be irrelevant in NRL allergy. It is commonly believed that allergen-specific assays would provide much more accurate and reliable information. Yet, there is still incomplete knowledge on the wide spectrum of NRL allergens and on their overall significance, which has made it difficult to decide which of the numerous allergens present in the NRL source material should be measured to obtain sufficient and clinically useful information about the allergenic potential of a given NRL product.

Specific semiquantitative methods based on human IgE-containing reagents, such as RAST inhibition, have been available for several years mostly in research laboratories but these methods suffer from the paucity of human sera containing clinically relevant latex-specific IgE antibodies. In addition, the methods are difficult to standardize. The principle that an ideal test for assessing allergenic potential of NRL products should be based on specific allergen quantification assays has recently been adopted and endorsed by both European[6,7] and U.S.[8] standardization organizations.

In recent years, substantial progress has been made in the characterization and purification of NRL allergens and in the development of specific and quantitative assays for individual latex allergen quantification.[9,10] The new assays are usually based on the capture-enzyme immunoassays (EIA) principle and on the use of monoclonal antibodies and purified or recombinant allergens. These assays are specific and can be properly standardized, and are of sufficient sensitivity and reproducibility. In this chapter, new developments in methods for NRL allergen measurement are reviewed with emphasis on specific allergen quantification. The methods for total protein and antigenic latex proteins were dealt with in Chapter 5.

II. NRL ALLERGENS IN THE SOURCE MATERIAL AND IN MANUFACTURED PRODUCTS

Of the some 250 different proteins or polypeptides demonstrated in the liquid latex of the rubber tree, *Hevea brasiliensis*, about one fourth have been shown to bind with IgE and represent allergens.[11,12] The NRL source material is a typical mixture of plant kingdom proteins reflecting in fact the stress response of the rubber tree to wounding (the tapping procedure). Several of these proteins are defense proteins that have been well-preserved during evolution. Obviously, the structural homologies shared with these proteins provide the molecular basis for many if not all of the very common allergen cross-reactions toward various plant proteins seen in NRL allergic patients. All the important allergens probably are present in the liquid NRL but it should also be taken into account that, according to the current state of knowledge, the great majority of proteins and polypeptides present in the NRL source material are likely to be irrelevant in the assessment of allergenic properties of manufactured NRL products. The WHO/IUIS Allergen Nomenclature Committee (October 2003) lists 13 NRL allergens characterized at the molecular level (www.allergen.org), most of which have been cloned and produced by recombinant DNA techniques. Up-to-date knowledge of these allergens was dealt with in Chapter 2.

A relatively limited number of allergens have so far been unequivocally demonstrated in manufactured NRL products. Allergens or their biologically relevant fragments must retain their IgE binding properties during the harsh rubber manufacturing processes to be detectable in manufactured products as genuine rubber product-specific proteins or peptides. Consensus exist that these peptides are responsible for the sensitization processes in allergy to rubber products. The current literature supports the contention that at least Hev b 1, Hev b 3, Hev b 5 and Hev b 6.02, and/or fragments or polymers of them expressing IgE-binding epitopes, can be present in manufactured products.[13–18] Other allergens possibly detectable in gloves or other NRL products may include Hev b 2.[19] Whether additional allergens, such as Hev b 7 and Hev b 13, also belong to the so-called rubber product-specific allergens, still awaits to be elucidated. A new problem in assessing the role of relevant allergens in rubber products is that some of the seemingly important allergens appear to be difficult to purify to absolute homogeneity and/or to produce as biologically active IgE binding molecules by recombinant DNA technology. At present, the possibility occurs that small but biologically significant amounts of the major and most abundant NRL allergen in the source material, i.e., hevein (Hev b 6.02), copurify with other proteins when standard protein chemistry and chromatographic methods are applied.[20] The specificity of the immunoassays designed for allergen detection is of course dependent on the purity of the immunizing preparations.

III. METHODS FOR MEASURING NATURAL RUBBER LATEX ALLERGENS

A. QUALITATIVE METHODS

Numerous studies, mainly in the early 1990s, based on immunoelectrophoretic methods and/or immunoblotting have described and tentatively characterized a large variety of NRL proteins binding IgE from sera of NRL-allergic patients. However, it is agreed that these methods carry marked limitations and are suitable neither for reliable identification nor for quantification of allergens.[11]

1. IgE-Immunoblotting Analysis (Western Blotting)

The Western blot procedure assesses the molecular weight distribution of proteins by first separating the proteins on sodium-dodecyl-sulphate–polyacrylamide-gel electrophoresis (SDS-PAGE)[21] and then transferring (blotting) them onto nitrocellulose membrane. The NRL allergens can be demonstrated using human sera with IgE antibodies to latex allergens. The standard SDS-PAGE is one of the most widely used analytical tools in protein chemistry, but it must be noted that in the standard reducing conditions the proteins are denatured and conformational epitopes may be destroyed. In addition, in the standard assays, small molecular weight peptides such as hevein, the most important NRL allergen, easily escape detection.

2. IgE-Immunoblotting after Isoelectric Focusing and Electrophoresis (Two-Dimensional Immunoblotting)

In two-dimensional immunoblotting, proteins are first separated by isoelectric focusing. In the second dimension, the proteins are separated according to their size in SDS-PAGE.[22] The transfer to nitrocellulose and the following steps are identical to those used in one-dimensional immunoblotting. The method has proved to be useful and informative in characterizing individual proteins in mixtures containing large numbers of unknown proteins,[11,12] but it is technically demanding and only suitable for use in research laboratories.

B. Semiquantitative Methods

1. Skin Prick Testing in Voluntary Latex-Allergic Subjects

Allergenicity of NRL extracts can be assessed in a semiquantitative manner by skin prick testing (SPT) in NRL-allergic patients since the size of the reaction is dependent on and directly proportional to the quantity of the allergens to which the patient has IgE class antibodies.[2] From the biological point of view, SPT would make an ideal test to assess clinically relevant allergenicity, but due to factors such as ethical constraints, this approach cannot be routinely used as a test for monitoring allergen contents in NRL gloves.

2. RAST Inhibition and IgE-ELISA Inhibition Assay

Two types of assays are available both based on the same (inhibition) principle, RAST inhibition (RAST, radioallergosorbent test), and ELISA inhibition (ELISA, enzyme linked immunosorbent assay). The critical reagent is the pooled human serum containing IgE antibodies to relevant NRL allergens.

RAST inhibition[22] has been used to evaluate latex allergens in various medical and consumer products that are made of NRL.[3,4,24] In the assay procedure, optimal amount of NRL allergens are bound to activated paper discs. Unknown samples and the standard are incubated with pooled high-titered IgE sera from individuals with confirmed latex allergy. When the IgE antibody binds to the soluble allergen, it is completely or partly prevented from binding to the solid phase allergen. After incubation, an immobilized paper disc is added and the free IgE antibodies are bound to the allergens on the disc. Specific binding is then measured using a radio-labeled anti-IgE and a gamma counter. The amount of inhibition is proportional to the quantity of soluble allergens in the extract.

In allergen specific IgE-ELISA inhibition assay,[4] NRL proteins are first immobilized to microtiter wells. Either native (nonammoniated) NRL or ammoniated NRL can be used as a coating reagent and a standard. We have assigned an arbitrary concentration of 100,000 allergen units (AU) per 1 ml for the standard nonammoniated NRL preparation with a total protein concentration of 10 mg/ml. After blocking the unbound sites on the polystyrene wells with 1% human serum albumin and washes, serial dilutions of glove extracts and standard NRL preparation dilutions are incubated with an optimally diluted IgE serum pool containing characterized high-titered sera from NRL-allergic adults and children with spina bifida. These mixtures are then transferred to the microtiter wells, where the remaining free IgE is bound to the immobilized NRL proteins and detected by biotinylated goat anti-human IgE and streptavidin-conjugated alkaline phosphatase. Substrate, p-nitrophenylphosphate, is added and the developed color read at 405 nm. The dilutions of glove extracts are analysed for their inhibitory capacity and the results calculated from the standard curve formed by the results obtained with serial dilutions of the standard NRL preparation. The decrease in binding of IgE from the serum pool to the solid-phase antigens (allergens) is directly proportional to the concentration of allergens in the extract tested.[4]

RAST inhibition and IgE-ELISA inhibition belong to the first allergen-specific methods that have provided reliable semiquantitative information on allergen contents of NRL gloves.[3,4,25] Highly significant correlation (r = 0.94–0.96) have emerged between the results of RAST inhibition and ELISA inhibition and the results of SPT, the gold standard for diagnosing latex allergy.[4] These human IgE-based methods have, however, well-known shortcomings. There is already a shortage of human sera with desired IgE antibodies to NRL allergens and such antibodies or serum pools are difficult if not impossible to standardize. A noticeable shortcoming is also the lack of standardized allergens. Likewise, a specific problem is the particular scarcity of human sera containing IgE antibodies to the hydrophobic rubber particle-associated allergens Hev b 1 and Hev b 3, characteristic of spina bifida–associated NRL allergy in children.

C.   QUANTITATIVE METHODS

1.   Capture Enzyme Immunoassays (EIA) for NRL Allergen Quantification

a.   Background

The progress in characterizing new NRL allergens and evaluating their significance as well as in producing allergens with recombinant DNA technology and monoclonal antibodies has prompted several research groups to study and develop new methods for reliable demonstration and quantification of NRL allergens in manufactured products. We advocated the idea that an optimal assay should be designed to detect only those NRL proteins that have been shown to be present in manufactured products, i.e., rubber product-specific allergens. It is emphasised that the knowledge of the number and significance of such rubber product-specific allergens is based on the published literature and the picture may change when further studies are performed. At any rate, this principle would limit the desired allergens to a reasonable number and it would easily allow testing the performance of the new assays in relation to human IgE-based methods.

TABLE 6.1
Performance Characteristics of the FITkit® Capture EIA

		Hev b 1	Hev b 3	Hev b 5	Hev b 6.02
Detection limit		1.2 µg/l	2.3 µg/l	0.5 µg/l	0.1 µg/l
Repeatability (N=16)	Low	5.6%	5.3%	4.4%	4.6%
	Medium	4.6%	3.4%	2.5%	4.1%
	High	2.8%	4.6%	5.1%	5.8%
Reproducibility (N=5)	Low	6.8%	6.9%	5.2%	5.6%
	Medium	5.6%	6.0%	2.6%	4.3%
	High	4.6%	7.6%	5.4%	6.9%
Recovery%		73–115	87–124	81–101	94–116
Linearity%		96–132	85–124	105–120	92–110

Only four NRL allergens, i.e., Hev b 1, Hev b 3, Hev b 5, and Hev b 6.02, have so far been unequivocally demonstrated to be present in extracts of NRL gloves.[13,15,16,17,26] The two most important allergens relevant for healthcare workers and children with no history of surgery are Hev b 5 and Hev b 6.02 (hevein).[15,17,27] Hev b 1 and Hev b 3 are the two most important latex allergens for patients with spina bifida.[28] Given this information, allergen-specific capture enzyme immunoassays (EIA) to quantify these four clinically relevant NRL allergens were developed in collaboration with a Finnish biotechnology company, (FITBiotech Ltd, Tampere, Finland) which resulted in the launching of assay kits (FITkit®), in December 2001.

b.   Description of Capture EIA Methods

The capture EIAs use specific monoclonal antibodies against the four allergens and either purified allergens or proteins produced by recombinant DNA technology as standards. The microtiter wells are coated in each test with one specific monoclonal antibody that binds the desired allergen from the sample. After incubation, unbound material is removed by washing the wells. In the second incubation, horseradish peroxidase (HRP)-labeled allergen-specific monoclonal antibody binds to allergen molecules bound on the microtiter plate in the first incubation. After washing, substrate for HRP is added. The absorbance at 414 nm is measured after stopping the reaction. The intensity of the color produced is directly proportional to the allergen concentration of the sample. According to the manufacturer's information (FITkit® insert leaflets, www.fitbiotech.com), the limit of detection for the 4 allergens range from 0.1 µg/l (Hev b 6.02) to 2.3 µg/l (Hev b 3). Repeatability ranges from 2.8 to 5.8%, and reproducibility from 2.6 to 7.6% (Table 6.1).

c.   Performance of Capture EIAs in Comparison with IgE-Based
*   Allergen Assays*

The important question with regard to the applicability of FITkit® and similar capture EIAs is whether the information provided would be useful for glove-using persons in the process of selecting adequate gloves. These specific allergen tests have now been used in several series of gloves in Finland and elsewhere to evaluate their performance in assessing allergenicity in comparison to specific human IgE-based assays. The best verification of the allergenic potential of a given extract would be reflected in its reactivity in the skin of a large number of NRL-allergic patients. In a study of 22 NRL gloves, highly significant correlation emerged when the sum quantity of these 4 allergens was related to results from human IgE based assays.[10] Correlation was remarkably high with regard to SPT in 20 NRL allergic volunteers (r = 0.95) and IgE-ELISA inhibition (r = 0.90) but not with total protein measured with the Modified Lowry method (r = –0.11). In another series of 58 NRL gloves reported in the same communication,[10] the correlation between the sum of the four allergens measured by the FITkit® and total allergen activity by IgE-ELISA inhibition was 0.84. It thus appears that the sum of the four allergens reflects the total allergenic potential of the glove extracts in a biologically meaningful manner. Extended studies with a large number of gloves are, of course, needed to further evaluate this, but it can now be speculated whether additional allergens in the assay framework would significantly affect the outcome.

To obtain information on the role of the individual allergens and to investigate whether these tests would enable estimating limits that could serve as tentative guidelines for glove users and regulatory authorities, we investigated the performance of FITkit® in assessing allergen content of 230 gloves. The gloves had been collected during national market surveys, organized by the National Agency of Medicines, Finland, between 1995 and 2003. The gloves had been blindly coded and tested earlier with human IgE-based ELISA inhibition. There were 109 gloves (47% of all gloves tested) with a low total allergen content (< 5 AU/ml) and, as can be seen in Figure 6.1, such gloves seldom contained measurable amounts of any of the four allergens (with the exception of Hev b 6.02). In the remaining 121 gloves with allergen content more than 5 AU/ml, the proportion of gloves with measurable quantities of any of the four allergens increased in relation to the total allergen content. This was most readily seen with regard to the amount of Hev b 6.02. These observations confirm the earlier contention that Hev b 6.02 and Hev b 5 are the most common and most abundant allergens demonstrable in NRL gloves.[18]

Current evidence reveals that the correlation between the total allergen activity by human IgE assays and the sum of four allergens measured by the FITkit® is highest in highly allergenic gloves (r about 0.95). Highly allergenic NRL products are thus readily picked up by the assay. In more recent years, when the proportion of highly allergenic gloves on the market has been on a steady decrease, slightly lower correlation coefficients (r = 0.78–0.84) have been observed. At present, there is not enough data to suggest any safety limits for gloves in general, either for individual allergens, or for their sum. We have previously suggested a limit for low allergen content for gloves at the level of 10 AU/ml.[4] In light of present studies with capture EIA, these values may need to be reassessed. It can be noted though, that the earlier mentioned level 1 µg/g [10] specifies gloves with high allergenicity to which almost all latex-allergic patients showed SPT reactivity. On the other hand, our preliminary analyses suggest that gloves in which the sum of the four allergens is less than 0.1–0.2 µg/g, have also very low allergen content measured by human IgE based-allergen methods. For glove users, these figures could serve as an interim

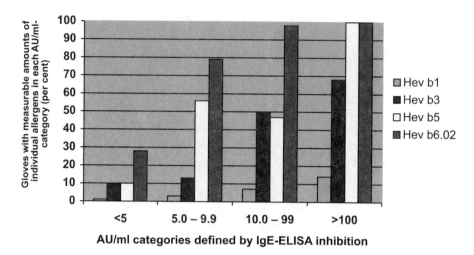

FIGURE 6.1 Occurrence in 230 NRL gloves of measurable amounts of four NRL allergens (Hev b 1, Hev b 3, Hev b 5, and Hev b 6.02) in relation to total allergen activity measured by IgE-ELISA inhibition. The columns represent percentages of gloves with measurable amounts of the four allergens in relation to the total amount of gloves in each AU/ml category. The study series consisted of 109 (47%) gloves in the < 5 AU/ml category, 39 (17%) in the 5–9.9 category, 60 (26%) in the 10–99 category and 22 (10%) gloves in the > 100 AU/ml category. As can be seen, all gloves in the highest total allergen category contained Hev b 5 and Hev b 6.02. The gloves were analysed in connection with the Finnish national market surveys during 1995–2003.

rough estimate for their glove selection policy. Further studies are needed to set up more exact recommendations.

IV. CONCLUSIONS

Minimizing allergen concentration in NRL goods to prevent sensitization to NRL and thereby the development of clinical allergy is acknowledged as important for both rubber manufacturers and regulatory health authorities. Measuring total protein cannot be deemed as a satisfactory regulatory measure to control allergen content. Specific methods based on human IgE-containing reagents, such as RAST inhibition, have been available for many years in certain laboratories for demonstrating NRL allergens in rubber products but the methods lack standardization and suffer from the lack of optimal reagents. Capture EIA assays for specific quantification of clinically relevant NRL allergens overcome several of the significant limitations of previous methods by using characterized and highly purified allergens, and specific monoclonal antibodies, against four NRL allergens known to be present in NRL products such as rubber gloves. The assays have excellent specificity, irrespective of presence of any other proteins or chemical substances derived from the manu-facturing process of NRL products, and high sensitivity capable of measuring rele-vant allergen in the range of nanograms/ml. The methods are convenient to perform and the results can be obtained in a short assay time (< 2 hours).

Currently, commercial tests for measuring four individual NRL allergens by capture-EIA-based assays using monoclonal antibodies and purified or recombinant allergens (FITkit®, FIT Biotech, Tampere, Finland) have become available. Kits for measuring these four allergens in NRL products are available but reagents and other laboratory equipment required to carry out the tests can also be purchased separately. Should additional allergens be discovered to be specific for rubber products (not only the rubber tree proteins) and lead to improvement of the performance of the existing assays, new kits to measure other proteins can be developed with ease. The new method has the advantage that the assessment of biologically meaningful threshold levels for safety purposes is becoming possible to evaluate. This could eventually lead to specific guidelines for the rubber industry and regulatory health authorities.

REFERENCES

1. Turjanmaa, K. et al., Natural rubber latex allergy, *Allergy,* 51, 593, 1966.
2. Turjanmaa, K. et al., Rubber contact urticaria: Allergenic properties of 19 brands of latex gloves, *Contact Dermatitis,* 19, 362, 1988.
3. Yunginger, J.W. et al., Extractable latex allergens and proteins in disposable medical gloves and other rubber products, *J. Allergy Clin. Immunol.,* 93, 836, 1994.
4. Palosuo, T. et al., Measurement of natural rubber latex allergen levels in medical gloves by allergen-specific IgE-ELISA inhibition, RAST inhibition, and skin prick test, *Allergy,* 53, 59, 1998.
5. Yip, E. et al., Allergic responses and levels of extractable proteins in NR latex gloves and dry rubber products, *J. Nat. Rubber Res.,* 9, 79, 1994.
6. CEN/STAR Document N 409 — Endorsement by star of research proposal on immunological test to measure allergens in natural rubber latex (document CEN/TC 205 N 1187), European Committee for Standardisation, Brussels, 2002.
7. Scientific committee on medicinal products and medical devices, Opinion on natural rubber latex allergy, European Commission, http://europa.eu.int/comm/foods/fs/sc/scmp/out31_en.pdf, 2000.
8. Hamilton, R.G. and Palosuo, T., Minutes of the ASTM meeting on immunoenzymetric assay (IEMA) task group (D11.40.08), Denver, CO, 2003.
9. Turjanmaa, K. et al., Recent developments in latex allergy, *Curr. Opin. Allergy Clin. Immunol.,* 2, 407, 2002.
10. Palosuo, T., Alenius, H., and Turjanmaa, K., Quantitation of latex allergens, *Methods,* 27, 52, 2002.
11. Alenius, H. et al., Latex allergy: Frequent occurrence of IgE antibodies to a cluster of 11 latex proteins in patients with spina bifida and histories of anaphylaxis, *J. Lab. Clin. Med.,* 123, 712, 1994.
12. Posch, A. et al., Characterization and identification of latex allergens by two-dimensional electrophoresis and protein micro sequencing, *J. Allergy Clin. Immunol.,* 99, 385, 1997.
13. Czuppon, A.B. et al., The rubber elongation factor of rubber trees (*Hevea brasiliensis*) is the major allergen in latex, *J. Allergy Clin. Immunol.,* 92, 690, 1993.
14. Lu, L-J. et al., Characterization of a major latex allergen associated with hypersensitivity in spina bifida patients, *J. Immunol.,* 155, 2721, 1995.
15. Alenius, H. et al., The main IgE-binding epitope of a major latex allergen, prohevein, is present in its N-terminal 43-amino acid fragment, hevein, *J. Immunol.,* 156, 1618, 1996.

16. Akasawa, A. et al., A novel acidic allergen, Hev b 5, in latex: Purification, cloning and characterization, *J. Biol. Chem.*, 271, 25389, 1996.
17. Sutherland, M.F. et al., Specific monoclonal antibodies and human immunoglobulin E show that Hev b 5 is an abundant allergen in high protein powdered latex gloves, *Clin. Exp. Allergy*, 32, 583, 2002.
18. Palosuo, T. et al., The major latex allergens Hev b 6.02 (hevein) and Hev b 5 are regularly detected in medical gloves with moderate or high allergen content, *J. Allergy Clin. Immunol.*, 107, S321, 2001 (abstract).
19. Yeang, H.Y. et al., Hev b 2 and Hev b 3 content in natural rubber latex and latex gloves, *J. Allergy Clin. Immunol.*, 107, S118, 2001 (abstract).
20. Palosuo, T. et al., Prevalence of IgE antibodies to extensively purified Hev b 13 and Hev b 2 in natural rubber latex (NRL) allergic patients, *J. Allergy Clin. Immunol.*, 113, 577, 2004 (abstract).
21. Laemmli, U.K., Cleavage of structural proteins during the assembly of the head of bacteriophage T4, *Nature*, 77, 680, 1970.
22. O'Farrell, P.H., High-resolution two-dimensional electrophoresis of proteins, *J. Biol. Chem.*, 250, 4007, 1975.
23. Yman, L., Ponterius, G., and Brandt, R., RAST-based allergen assay methods, *Dev. Biol. Stand.*, 29, 151, 1975.
24. Crippa, M. et al., Prevention of latex allergy among health care workers: Evaluation of the extractable latex protein content in different types of medical gloves, *Am. J. Ind. Med.*, 44, 24, 2003.
25. Baur, X. et al., Protein and allergen content of various natural latex articles, *Allergy*, 52, 661, 1997.
26. Ylitalo, L. et al., IgE antibodies to prohevein, hevein, and rubber elongation factor in children with latex allergy, *J. Allergy Clin. Immunol.*, 102, 659, 1998.
27. Alenius, H. et al., IgE reactivity to 14-kD and 27-kD natural rubber proteins in latex-allergic children with spina bifida and other congenital anomalies, *Int. Arch. Allergy Immunol.*, 102, 61, 1993.
28. Yeang, H.Y. et al., The 14.6 kD rubber elongation factor (Hev b 1) and 24 kD (Hev b 3) rubber particle proteins are recognized by IgE from patients with spina bifida and latex allergy, *J. Allergy Clin. Immunol.*, 98, 628, 1996.

7 Contact Urticaria: Clinical Manifestations

Sarah H. Wakelin

CONTENTS

I. Introduction 97
II. Classification 98
   A. Nonimmunological Contact Urticaria 98
   B. Immunological Contact Urticaria 98
   C. Contact Urticaria with Undetermined Mechanisms 100
III. Clinical Features of NRL Contact Urticaria 100
IV. Conclusions 103
References 103

I. INTRODUCTION

Contact urticaria is a localized wheal and flare reaction following external contact of a substance with the skin and or mucous membranes. It usually appears within 10 to 30 min and clears completely within hours, without residual signs of irritation. The term was introduced by Fisher in 1973,[1] but this phenomenon had been recognized for many years. For example, urticarial reactions to nettles and hairy caterpillars were reported during the last century,[2] and contact urticants such as aromatic oils and balsams have been used therapeutically for many years to induce cutaneous erythema (rubifacients) and as counterirritants.[3]

Contact urticaria is not uncommon, and a large and expanding list of substances, ranging from simple chemicals to macromolecules, have been reported as causes. Because symptoms are usually transient and mild, they are often overlooked and epidemiological studies of many of its causes are lacking. Natural rubber latex (NRL) has undoubtedly emerged as the most important cause of contact urticaria in modern society. NRL is not new to our environments and has been used in many household, industrial, and medical items for over a century. However, the increased occurrence of a range of adverse reactions to NRL arose as a consequence of the exponential increase in use of disposable powdered latex gloves following the institution of universal precautions for protection against HIV infection and viral hepatitis in 1987.[4] The effect of the recent "epidemic" of NRL allergy among healthcare workers in particular, has been wide-ranging, with medical, occupational, legal, and financial implications. This has fueled research in the fields of epidemiology and allergy, making NRL the most thoroughly studied agent among substances that can cause contact urticaria.

II. CLASSIFICATION

The mechanisms underlying contact urticaria are broadly classified as nonimmunological irritant and immunological or allergic. A third category exists for reactions with mixed features or undetermined pathomechanisms.

A. NONIMMUNOLOGICAL CONTACT URTICARIA

Substances which cause nonimmunological contact urticaria (NICU) are encountered frequently in our environment as preservatives or fragrances and flavorings in cosmetics, toiletries, topical medicaments, and food. Examples include sorbic acid, benzoic acid, and cinnamaldehyde. At concentrations in common use, they have been shown to elicit contact reactions. For example, contact urticaria affected 18 of 20 school children who applied a salad dressing containing sorbic acid and benzoic acid to their faces.[5] Many household, industrial, and laboratory chemicals and insecticides can also cause NICU. Substances which cause NICU produce a reaction without any previous sensitization in most or almost all exposed persons,[6] and it has been assumed that NICU is the commonest form of contact urticaria. The pathogenesis of NICU is not clearly understood, and different urticariogens may act by different mechanisms. However, it appears to involve the release of vasogenic mediators such as prostaglandins without involvement of immunological processes. NICU reactions are inhibited by prior treatment with topical or oral nonsteroidal anti-inflammatory drugs,[7,8] but are unaffected by antihistamines, suggesting that histamine is not the main mediator.[6]

NICU reactions remain localized to the sites of contact without any systemic effect and are invariably mild. There is a problem in defining what constitutes the mildest form of reaction, as only macular erythema or in some cases pruritus alone may be manifestations of contact urticaria without obvious whealing. Kligman has argued that "sub-urticogenic" reactions are underreported, underrecognized forms of contact urticaria, and has shown that by diluting classical urticariogens the immediate response can be limited to erythema or even pruritus alone.[9] However, simple erythema of the skin appearing within minutes of contact with the eliciting substance cannot be regarded as contact urticaria unless at least some subjects get urticarial reactions at the application site.[10]

B. IMMUNOLOGICAL CONTACT URTICARIA

Immunological (allergic) contact urticaria (ICU) is a form of immediate-type/type I hypersensitivity, and involves interaction of allergen and allergen-specific IgE in a sensitized individual. People with atopy are predisposed to develop ICU due to their propensity to develop IgE antibodies. This is the mechanism underlying contact urticaria and other systemic immediate reactions to NRL, specifically its proteinaceous components.[11] IgG4 antibodies have been detected in parallel with IgE antibodies against NRL proteins, and it has been speculated that they may also play a role in the pathogenesis of latex allergy.[12]

Sensitization to immediate-type allergens can occur via the skin, mucous membranes or via other organs such as the respiratory or gastrointestinal tract. The primary route of exposure to NRL via which individuals become sensitized is not always clear. Body sweat inside latex gloves may make latex proteins soluble, and the solublized proteins could then be absorbed through the skin, sensitizing the wearer to the foreign protein. In addition, surface proteins are present on gloves, which transfer immediately onto a moist skin membrane.[13] In healthcare workers, the use of glove powder that generates aerosolised allergens has been linked with increased latex allergy,[14] and it has been suggested that latex exposure through the respiratory tract may play an important role in the induction of immediate-type sensitization.[15] Animal studies have confirmed that it is possible to induce dermal hypersensitivity by bronchial exposure to NRL.[16] Conversely, it has been shown that dermal exposure to NRL can induce NRL-specific IgE and lead to airway hyperreactivity.[17]

Following skin or mucosal exposure in a sensitized individual, a variable amount of allergen penetrates through the epithelium, then binds and cross-links allergen-specific IgE attached via high affinity receptors on to the membranes of mast cells, causing degranulation and release of histamine and other vasoactive substances (Figure 7.1). Other inflammatory mediators such as arachidonic acid metabolites (prostaglandins and leukotrienes), kinins, and cytokines, including eosinophil chemotactic factor and neutrophil chemotactic factor, are also released and may

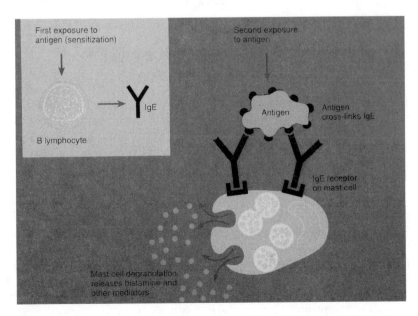

FIGURE 7.1 (See color insert following pg. 112). Schematic diagram of immediate-type allergic reaction.

influence the clinical response. Histamine and kallikrein-generating factors cause vasodilation, increased vascular permeability, and smooth muscle contraction of airways, which depending on the severity of response, may manifest clinically as urticaria, bronchospasm, hypotension, and anaphylactic shock. Thus, the consequences of ICU are potentially far more serious than for NICU, as urticarial reactions may not remain localized to the area of contact, and angioedema, or involvement of internal organs such as the respiratory or gastrointestinal tract may ensue, culminating in anaphylactic shock, and death. Such a potential for multisystem involvement has been highlighted by the term "contact urticaria syndrome" introduced by Maibach and Johnson in 1975.[18]

Although natural rubber latex is the commonest occupational cause of ICU, other vegetable and animal proteins can cause similar reactions in those who come into regular contact with them, such as food handlers, agricultural workers, and veterinary workers. In addition a wide range of metals, medicaments, inorganic, and organic chemicals have been reported as causes. Many of these are listed by Amin and Maibach.[19]

C. CONTACT URTICARIA WITH UNDETERMINED MECHANISMS

A third category exists for substances which elicit mixed features of NICU and ICU, or where the mechanism remains unestablished. The bleaching agent ammonium persulphate is a classic example and may produce both localized and generalized reactions and even vascular collapse.[20] Although the clinical picture resembles an IgE-mediated reaction, antibodies against ammonium persulphate have not been identified.

III. CLINICAL FEATURES OF NRL CONTACT URTICARIA

NRL was first described as a cause of contact urticaria in 1979 by Nutter.[21] She briefly reported a housewife who developed contact urticaria to household rubber gloves. A report of contact urticaria to surgical gloves by Fröström followed shortly in 1980.[22] Systemic allergic reactions including anaphylaxis were reported later.[23] The underlying mechanism of IgE-mediated type I hypersensitivity was proposed by Kopman and Hanuksela, Frosch and coworkers, and Turjanmaa et al. [24–26]

The clinical presentations of NRL hypersensitivity fall into the categories denoted the "contact urticaria syndrome" by Maibach and Johnson in 1975.[18] These comprise localized urticaria (stage 1); generalized urticaria and angioedema (stage 2); asthma, rhinoconjunctivitis, and other extracutaneous symptoms (stage 3); and anaphylaxis (stage 4) (Table 7.1).[20] The nature of symptoms on exposure of a sensitized individual depends on the route of exposure.[27] The allergen dose and exposed individual's degree of hypersensitivity are important factors in determining the severity of symptoms and progression to systemic features. Clinical manifestations of hypersensitivity reactions to NRL can, therefore, be variable because they reflect the dose of bioavailable allergen and route of exposure, as well as the individual's inherent level of hypersensitivity.

TABLE 7.1
The Contact Urticaria Syndrome

Stage 1:	Localized urticaria
	Nonspecific symptoms (itching, tingling, burning)
	Dermatitis (eczema)
Stage 2:	Generalized urticaria
Stage 3:	Extracutaneous involvement (rhinoconjunctivitis, bronchospasm, orolaryngeal, gastrointestinal)
Stage 4:	Anaphylactic shock

Source: From Von Krogh, G. and Maibach, H.I., 1981. With permission.[20]

Hands most frequently come into contact with NRL in the form of household or disposable gloves, and cutaneous reactions (localized contact urticaria) are the most common presentation in latex allergic patients.[28,29] Serious allergic reactions following glove wearing are rare as the intact epidermis provides a good barrier against the penetration of protein allergens. Penetration through mucosal surfaces is greater and much more rapid leading to a larger dose of allergen, and higher risk of systemic symptoms. Serious allergic reactions are therefore most frequently associated with an abraded mucosa.[30]

The external layer or stratum corneum is paper thin and provides the main barrier function of the epidermis. When intact, it is a highly effective barrier against protein penetration but when damaged or inflamed, as in chronic hand dermatitis, penetration is enhanced which allows greater allergen exposure.[31] The epidermis may be damaged or compromised by several different mechanisms (Table 7.2). *In vitro* penetration models using surgical samples of human skin and hairless guinea pig skin have demonstrated that less than 1% of latex proteins penetrate through intact skin, whilst up to 23% of applied proteins passed through abraded skin within 24 hr of exposure.[32] The presence of hand dermatitis had been identified as a risk factor for sensitization to NRL,[33] as well as increasing the likelihood of developing symptoms on subsequent exposure to NRL. Excessive glove use may increase skin hydration and cause irritation, which combined with frequent hand washing, may also cause further skin damage. The role of barrier creams and emollients is controversial, as they have

TABLE 7.2
Causes of Reduced Stratum Corneum Barrier Integrity in Normal Skin

Preexisting dermatitis	e.g., irritant, allergic
Physical damage	e.g., burned, shaved, wounded
Chemical damage	e.g., detergents and other penetration enhancers
Increased hydration	e.g., excessive hand washing
Occluded skin	e.g., wearing of gloves

Source: From Smith-Pease, C.K. and Basketter, D.A., 2002. With permission.[31]

been shown to favor skin uptake of allergens from gloves rather than decrease this as intended (see Chapter 17).[34]

Contact urticaria to gloves presents clinically with itching, redness, and wheal formation, particularly on the dorsum of the hands and fingers, and around the wrists.[35] Symptoms are less common on the palmar aspects where the stratum corneum is thicker. After donning NRL gloves, symptoms usually appear within a few to 30 minutes and disappear spontaneously within 1 to 2 hours of their removal.[36] Symptoms increase as a direct function of the time-usage of NRL gloves, and have been found to be more prevalent in operating room staff who wear gloves for prolonged periods compared to other health workers.[37]

The clinical presentation is often complicated and confused by the presence of coexisting hand dermatitis, as sufferers are frequently atopic, and may have chronic endogenous hand dermatitis. NRL allergy may also be preceded or accompanied by delayed type (type IV) hypersensitivity to rubber chemicals,[38,39] which requires evaluation by patch testing (see Chapter 11). If a person who has NRL hypersensitivity is touched by another person wearing NRL gloves, e.g., nursing or dental personnel, they may also develop symptoms. Contact urticaria by definition, begins at the place of contact, so the person being examined may develop swelling and edema at whatever body site has been touched, for example, the vulva and vagina following gynacological examination or the lips and tongue following dental treatment. Cornstarch glove powder enhances the sensitizing capacity of NRL gloves and also allows airborne dissemination of allergens. Aerosolized powder containing NRL proteins has resulted in rhinoconjunctivitis, asthma, and in severe cases, bronchospasm and anaphylaxis (see Chapter 4). In a German study of 70 patients with NRL allergy, all (100%) had contact urticaria, 51% rhinitis, 44% conjunctivitis, 31% dyspnea, 24% systemic symptoms, and 6% severe systemic symptoms during surgery.[29]

Contact urticaria manifesting as mucosal swelling and irritation may also follow exposure to other items made of NRL, especially condoms[40] and balloons. Items made from dry rubber latex may also, less frequently, cause symptoms. The list of reported causes is wide and ranges from rubber face masks, infusion sets, sticking plasters, tourniquets, urinary catheters, and pacifiers to rubber shoes and sports racquet handles.[41] Another unsuspected source of NRL exposure resulting in severe symptoms was from the mat in playground ball pits.[42] NRL may also be used as an adhesive, and in this form has caused immediate-type hypersensitivity symptoms including anaphylaxis from obscure sources such as sweet wrappers and hair extensions.[43,44]

Late phase type I reactions typically occur 6 to 12 hours after antigenic challenge and cause burning, induration, and inflammatory cell infiltration. The clinical significance of late phase in NRL reactions remains unclear, and they appear to be uncommon in practice. In addition, NRL may be a cause of so-called protein contact dermatitis which presents with inflammation and eczematous vesicles within 20 minutes of contact. The term was originally introduced by Hjorth and Roed-Petersen to describe an allergic or nonallergic eczematous reaction to proteinaceous materials amongst food handlers.[45] It is important to specifically ask patients who present with chronic hand dermatitis about immediate symptoms on contact with NRL gloves in order to avoid overlooking an immediate-type allergy.

IV. CONCLUSIONS

Contact urticaria needs to be distinguished from simple irritant symptoms or *glove itch* which is frequent among healthcare workers who wear gloves for prolonged periods, especially if there is any associated hand dermatitis. Awareness of the potential problem of NRL allergy is now achieving a higher profile amongst nursing staff and other healthcare workers, and may be a potential source of anxiety. Many studies investigating glove symptoms have reported that nonimmunological glove irritation is much commoner than genuine type I allergy to latex protein.[46,47] It is very important that patients with ambiguous symptoms are formally investigated to determine whether they have NRL allergy or not.

NRL glove urticaria also needs to be differentiated from symptomatic dermographism, a form of physical urticaria. This may also present with whealing on wearing tight gloves, but sufferers usually have symptoms at other body sites, unrelated to latex exposure, and will react similarly on wearing tight gloves made out of materials other than NRL.

REFERENCES

1. Fisher, A.A., *Contact Dermatitis,* 2nd Ed., Lea & Febiger, Philadelphia, 1973, p. 283.
2. Lesser, E., Lehrbuch der Haut und Teschlechtskrankheiten fur studirende und arzte, Verlag von FCW Vogel, Leipzig, 1894, Capitel, Urticaria, p. 134.
3. Burdick, A.E. and Mathias, T., The contact urticaria syndrome, *Dermatol. Clin.,* 3, 71, 1985.
4. Sussman, G.L., Beezhold, D.H., and Liss, G., Latex allergy: Historical perspectives, *Methods,* 27, 3, 2002.
5. Clemmenson, O. and Hjorth, N., Perioral contact urticaria from sorbic acid and benzoic acid in a salad dressing, *Contact Dermatitis,* 8, 1, 1982.
6. Lahti, A., Non-immunologic contact urticaria, *Acta Dermatovener (Stockholm),* S60, 3, 1980.
7. Lahti, A. et al., Acetylsalicylic acid inhibits non-immunologic contact urticaria, *Contact Dermatitis,* 16, 133, 1987.
8. Johannson, J. and Lahti, A., Topical non-steroidal anti-inflammatory drugs inhibit non-immunologic immediate contact reactions, *Contact Dermatitis,* 19, 161, 1988.
9. Kligman, A.M., The spectrum of contact urticaria: Wheals, erythema and pruritus, *Dermatol. Clin.,* 8, 57, 1990.
10. Lahti, A., Non-immunologic contact urticaria, In *The Contact Urticaria Syndrome,* Amin. S., Lahti, A., and Maibach, H.I., Eds., CRC Press, Boca Raton, 1997, p. 5.
11. Turjanmaa, K. et al., Allergens in latex surgical gloves and glove powder. *Lancet,* 336, 1588, 1990.
12. Alenius, H. et al., Detection of IgG4 and IgE antibodies to rubber proteins by immunoblotting in latex allergy, *Allergy Proc.,* 13, 75, 1992.

13. Beezhold, D., Kostyal, D.A., and Wiseman, J., The transfer of protein allergens from latex gloves, *AORN Journal,* 59, 605, 1994.

14. Brehler, R. et al., Glove powder — A risk factor for the development of latex allergy? *Eur. J. Surg.,* 163, 23, 1997.

15. Baur, X., Chen, Z., and Allmers, H., Can a threshold limit value for natural rubber latex airborne allergens be defined? *J. All. Clin. Immunol.,* 101, 24, 1998.

16. Reijula, K.E. et al., Latex-induced dermal and pulmonary hypersensitivity in rabbits, *J. All. Clin. Immunol.,* 94, 891, 1994.

17. Howell, M.D., Weissman, D.N., and Meade, B.J., Latex sensitisation by dermal exposure can lead to airway hyperreactivity, *Int. Arch. All. Immunol.,* 128, 204, 2002.

18. Maibach, H.I. and Johnson, H.L., Contact urticaria syndrome: Contact urticaria to diethyltoluamide (immediate type hypersensitivity), *Arch. Dermatol.,* 111, 726, 1975.

19. Amin, S. and Maibach, H.I., Immunologic contact urticaria definition, in *The Contact Urticaria Syndrome,* Amin, S., Lahti, A., Maibach, H.I., Eds., CRC Press, Boca Raton, 1997.

20. Von Krogh, G. and Maibach, H.I., The contact urticaria syndrome — An updated review, *J. Am. Acad. Dermatol.,* 5, 328, 1981.

21. Nutter, A.F., Contact urticaria to rubber, *Br. J. Dermatol.,* 101, 597, 1979.

22. Fröström, L., Contact urticaria from latex surgical gloves, *Contact Dermatitis,* 6, 33, 1980.

23. Slater, J., Rubber anaphylaxis, *N. Engl. J. Med.,* 320, 626, 1989.

24. Kopman, A. and Hannuksela, M., Contact urticaria to rubber, *Duodecim,* 99, 221, 1983.

25. Frosch, P.J. et al., Contact urticaria to rubber gloves is IgE mediated, *Contact Dermatitis,* 14, 241, 1986.

26. Turjanmaa, K. et al., Severe IgE-mediated allergy to surgical gloves, *Allergy,* 139, 39, 1989 (abstract).

27. Warshaw, E.M., Latex allergy, *J. Am. Acad. Dermatol.,* 39, 1, 1998.

28. Mahler, V. et al., Prevention of latex allergy by selection of low-allergen gloves, *Clin. Exp. All.,* 30, 509, 2000.

29. Jaeger, D. et al., Latex specific proteins causing immediate type cutaneous, nasal, bronchial and systemic reactions, *J. All. Clin. Immunol.,* 89, 759, 1992.

30. Tomazic, V.J. et al., Latex associated allergies and anaphylactic reactions, *Clin. Immunol.,* 64, 89, 1992.

31. Smith-Pease, C.K. and Basketter, D.A., Skin as a route of exposure to protein allergens, *Clin. Exp. Dermatol.,* 27, 296, 2002.

32. Hayes, B.B. et al., Evaluation of percutaneous penetration of natural rubber latex proteins, *Toxocol. Sci.,* 56, 262, 2000.

33. Boxer, M., Hand dermatitis: A risk factor for latex hypersensitivity, *J. All. Clin. Immunol.,* 98, 855, 1996.

34. Baur, X. et al., Results of wearing test with two different latex gloves with and without the use of skin-protection cream, *Allergy,* 53, 441, 1998.

35. Turjanmaa, K., Latex glove contact urticaria, Thesis, *Acta Universitatis Tamperensis,* Ser A, vol 254, University of Tampere, 1988.

36. Turjanmaa, K., Allergy to natural rubber latex: a growing problem, *Ann. Med.,* 26, 297, 1994.

37. Larese Filon, F. et al., Latex symptoms and sensitisation in health care workers, *Int. Arch. Occup. Environ. Health,* 74, 219, 2001.

38. Kleinhans, D., Contact urticaria to rubber gloves, *Contact Dermatitis,* 10, 124, 1984.

39. Van Ketel, W.G., Contact Urticaria from rubber gloves after dermatitis from thiruams, *Contact Dermatitis,* 11, 323, 1984.
40. Fisher, A.A., Condom conundrums: Part II, *Cutis,* 48, 433, 1991.
41. Hamann, C.P., Natural rubber latex protein sensitivity in review, *Am. J. Contact Dermatitis,* 4, 4, 1993.
42. Fiocchi, A. et al., Severe anaphylaxis induced by latex as a contaminant of plastic balls in play pits, *J. All. Clin. Immunol.,* 108, 298, 2001.
43. Meirion Hughes, T., Natural rubber latex allergy to adhesive in chocolate bar wrappers, *Contact Dermatitis,* 44, 46, 2001.
44. Wakelin, S.H., Contact anaphylaxis from natural rubber latex used as an adhesive for hair extensions, *Br. J. Dermatol.,* 146, 340, 2002.
45. Hjorth, N. and Roed-Pedersen, J., Occupational protein contact dermatitis in food handlers, *Contact Dermatitis,* 2, 28, 1976.
46. Nettis, E. et al., Type I allergy to natural rubber latex and type IV allergy to rubber chemicals in health care workers with glove-related symptoms, *Clin. Exp. All.,* 32, 441, 2002.
47. Chowdhury, M.M.U. and Statham, B.N., Natural rubber latex allergy in a health-care population in Wales, *Br. J. Dermatol.,* 148, 737, 2003.

8 Contact Urticaria Syndrome: Predictive Testing

Antti I. Lauerma and Howard I. Maibach

CONTENTS

I. Introduction 107
II. Immunologic Contact Urticaria (ICU) 108
    A. Mechanisms 108
    B. Respiratory Chemical Allergy as an Animal Model for ICU 108
    C. Contact Chemical Allergy as an Animal Model for ICU 109
    D. Protein Allergy as an Animal Model for ICU 109
III. Nonimmunologic Contact Urticaria 110
    A. Mechanisms 110
    B. Animal Models for NICU 110
IV. Predictive Testing: Perspectives 110
    A. Predictive Testing for Agents Causing ICU or NICU 110
    B. Predictive Testing for Medicaments for ICU or NICU 111
V. Conclusions 111
References 111

I. INTRODUCTION

Contact urticaria is a skin disease of increasing importance. The usefulness of products made from natural rubber latex has caused an increase in allergic (immunologic) contact urticaria, often causing work-related disability. Other forms of contact urticaria continue to be common. The symptoms experienced in contact urticaria range from local tingling to systemic anaphylaxis. A common factor in urticaria is release of inflammatory mediators, such as histamine, from cutaneous mast cells, which causes pruritus and swelling of the skin tissue.

Immunologic contact urticaria (ICU) and nonimmunologic contact urticaria (NICU) are two different forms of contact urticaria. They are separate in their mechanisms and etiology, while similarities in their clinical pictures may be seen. The most important distinguishing factor is the role of immunologic memory in these diseases. ICU occurs only in patients sensitized previously to the causative agent, whereas NICU does not require immunologic memory and can occur in any person. Due to these differences, the diagnostic procedures in patients are different.

An increasing number of new substances, especially chemicals, are being used in skin care and as medication. Therefore, contact urticaria to new substances is a constant threat. To avoid these problems, predictive tests to exclude the possibility that new products cause contact urticaria, are needed. Additionally, as ICU and NICU are common skin problems, medications are also needed. To develop new treatments for contact urticarias, models of NICU and ICU for predictive testing would be highly desirable. As *in vitro* models for ICU and NICU are not available, this chapter will concentrate on *in vivo* models, i.e., animal models.

II. IMMUNOLOGIC CONTACT URTICARIA (ICU)

A. Mechanisms

Immunologic contact urticaria is caused by molecules, entering the body through skin, which are perceived as foreign. It is mediated through IgE antibodies identifying the molecule. The responsible molecule has to penetrate epidermis before it is able to attach to IgE bound on mast cell surfaces in the dermis. The responsible molecules have to have sufficient size and contain amino acid structures to be able to bind to IgE. Therefore the most usual molecules causing ICU are proteins or large molecule size polypeptides. Smaller peptides or chemicals have to bind to a carrier protein to be able to trigger immune response. After the responsible protein, polypeptide, or hapten-carrier-complex binds to the IgE on mast cell, the cell releases inflammatory mediators, such as histamine, which cause itch, inflammation, and swelling in the skin. The swelling is seen as edema, the principal feature of urticaria.[1]

B. Respiratory Chemical Allergy as an Animal Model for ICU

Asthma-like symptoms in persons that have been exposed to anhydrides, including trimellitic anhydride (TMA) is well studied.[2] The immunologic reactions in lungs of experimental animals and patients feature anaphylactic (type I), complement mediated (type II), antibody complex mediated (type III), and cell mediated (type IV) reactions. Nonimmunologic (irritant) reactions may also participate,[3] possibly due to degradation of trimellitic anhydride to trimellitic acid.

TMA causes skin reactivity if sensitization is done through skin.[4] The skin reactions appear in two phases (immediate and delayed) implying that both type I and type IV reactions are involved.[1,4]

Experimental animals can be sensitized through airways[5] or skin. Cutaneous sensitization can be done intradermally (guinea pigs)[3] or topically (mice).[4] Intradermal sensitization of guinea pigs can be done with TMA 30% in corn oil at 0.1ml dose. The guinea pigs can be used for challenges 3 to 4 weeks after the injection. When mice, such as BALB/C mice that are widely used in allergy research, are sensitized with TMA, topical application can be utilized. The first dose has been 100 μl TMA at 500 mg/mL. To enhance development of anti-TMA-IgE-antibodies, a second sensitization has been performed with 50 μl TMA at 250 mg/ml at the same site. The animals have been used for elicitation 1 week after the second sensitization.

In mice that are sensitized to TMA, an immediate-type reaction is seen at 1 hour after dosing and a second delayed-type swelling reaction is seen at 24 hours. A dose-dependent swelling is also seen in nonsensitized animals,[1] which can be caused by trimellitic acid, a hydrolization product of TMA.[6] Such reactions could possibly be a form of nonimmunologic contact urticaria (NICU).

Mice sensitized to topical TMA can be used for study of topical drugs. In one study, an antihistamine suppressed early, a glucocorticosteroid suppressed both early and delayed, and a nonsteroidal anti-inflammatory drug enhanced early skin reaction, in line with the clinical findings seen in patients in practice when these medications have been given in atopic IgE-mediated diseases.[1]

Haptens other than TMA that are capable of inducing respiratory allergy, such as diphenyl-methane-4,4-diisocyanate (MDI) and phthalic anhydride, could possibly also be used to establish an animal model for ICU.

C. CONTACT CHEMICAL ALLERGY AS AN ANIMAL MODEL FOR ICU

When mice are repeatedly sensitized with strong contact allergen dinitrofluoroben-zene (DNFB), an immediate-type reaction kinetic emerges at the expense of the more typical delayed-type response to this contact allergen. Such reaction kinetic shift coincided with an increase of the number of mast cells in the skin area used for sensitization and elicitation. Antigen-specific IgE was also seen, and the reactions were dependent on presence of mast cells in mice.[7]

D. PROTEIN ALLERGY AS AN ANIMAL MODEL FOR ICU

Rabbits sensitized through airways or through skin with natural rubber latex show wheal-and-flare responses when prick tested.[8] Therefore it could be that such animals can be used as an animal model for ICU to study the pathogenesis and possible medications for treatment. However, it has not been studied whether open application could be sufficient for ICU in this model as the rate of cutaneous penetration of natural rubber latex proteins has not been established. Also mice exposed to NRL have elevated IgE levels and eosinophilia. Other proteins, such as ovalbumin, that are able to cause type I IgE-mediated reactions,[9] should be studied to see if they could be used in a similar manner.

Recently, a murine animal model for atopic dermatitis has been developed. It is based on sensitization to ovalbumin in repeated epicutaneous applications, sup-plemented by tape-strippings. This model has been shown to be useful in screening possible strategies for treating eczema.[9,10] It has also been utilized to study latex allergy in the form of protein contact dermatitis.[11] The model has not yet been used to try to induce contact urticaria in sensitized mice for study of possible medicaments and/or screening against possible contact urticants, but is promising for such purposes.

III. NONIMMUNOLOGIC CONTACT URTICARIA

A. Mechanisms

Nonimmunologic immediate contact reactions range from erythema to urticaria and occur in individuals that have not necessarily been previously exposed to them and who are also not sensitized to them. It is likely that nonimmunologic contact urticaria reactions are more common than immunologic contact urticaria reactions. The reactions arise most likely from the causative agent's ability to induce release of histamine and/or leukotrienes from skin tissue, therefore being pharmacological in nature. The agents causing NICU are numerous and include, among others, benzoic acid, sorbic acid, cinnamic aldehyde, and nicotinic acid esters. Provocative skin tests for NICU include the rub test and open test. The kinetics of NICU reactions are somewhat slower than those of ICU, i.e., the peak being at 45 to 60 minutes instead of 15 to 20 minutes.[12]

B. Animal Models for NICU

Animal models have been searched in the hope to find a suitable screening method for compounds causing NICU.[13] The different agents causing NICU often have varied mechanisms and therefore an *in vivo* end point, i.e., thickness of ear, has been utilized.

Guinea pigs are more sensitive to NICU than mice and rats, and therefore guinea pigs have been used in most studies.[14] Substances studied are applied openly on guinea pig ear lobe, and edema is quantified with a micrometer. The reactions are seen at their maximum approximately 50 minutes after the application; the largest swellings are two-fold. NICU model can also be used to study pharmacological agents for treatments.[15]

IV. PREDICTIVE TESTING: PERSPECTIVES

A. Predictive Testing for Agents Causing ICU or NICU

At present there is no standardized method for predicting the contact urticaria potential of substances. This is surprising, as contact urticaria can cause problems, comparable in severity and management difficulty to allergic or irritant contact dermatitis, and occasionally much worse (anaphylaxis). Work-related disabilities due to contact urticaria are on the rise as atopic predisposition becomes more common both in industrialized and developing countries.

For immunologic contact dermatitis it seems that only strong sensitizers (such as TMA) are able to sensitize and cause IgE-mediated contact urticaria when animals are sensitized with single or double applications. For less potent sensitizers, including possibly proteins, the model should probably include multiple sensitizations and skin manipulation in the form of tape-stripping. Alternatively, use of adjuvants, such as aluminium hydroxide (AlOH) or Freund's Complete Adjuvant (FCA), may be needed. Adjuvant use would, however, compromise the reliability of positive results if controls are not planned in an appropriate manner.

Agents causing nonimmunologic contact urticaria could seem easier to screen, with the guinea pig ear model being the most useful for this purpose at present. However, large-scale studies are still missing.

B. Predictive Testing for Medicaments for ICU or NICU

This chapter describes animal models for both NICU[13] and chemical-induced ICU.[1] These models have been successfully implemented for the study of topical medications against these forms of contact urticaria. However, the models do need further research to become standardized. Furthermore, a model for protein-induced ICU is missing, although the model for latex-induced respiratory allergy[8] and ovalbumin-induced atopic dermatitis[9] could be pursued for feasibility to study ICU.

V. CONCLUSIONS

It seems that mice sensitized to TMA and possibly also other respiratory chemical allergens may be used as animal models for ICU. For NICU the guinea pig ear lobe method may be most useful. These models need more refinement and standardization. Alternative methods may include *in vitro* mast cell cultures with specific IgE obtained from patients for ICU. For NICU, several tissue culture systems should be tried. If *in vitro* methods are used, also percutaneous absorption of the responsible agents should be studied, as it is the prerequisite for both ICU and NICU.

The work for developing predictive testing for contact urticaria is only beginning. However, due to the increase of atopic disposition worldwide, it is work that certainly needs to be done.

REFERENCES

1. Lauerma, A.I., Fenn, B., and Maibach, H.I., Trimellitic anhydride-sensitive mouse as an animal model for contact urticaria, *J. Appl. Toxicol.,* 17, 357, 1997.
2. Zeiss, C.R. et al., Trimellitic anhydride-induced airway syndromes: Clinical and immunologic studies, *J. Allergy Clin. Immunol.,* 60, 96, 1977.
3. Hayes, J.P. et al., Bronchial hyperreactivity after inhalation of trimellitic anhydride dust in guinea pigs after intradermal sensitization to the free hapten, *Am. Rev. Respir. Dis.,* 146, 1311, 1992.
4. Dearman, R.J. et al., Differential ability of occupational chemical contact and respiratory allergens to cause immediate and delayed dermal hypersensitivity reactions in mice, *Int. Arch. Allergy Immunol.,* 97, 315, 1992.
5. Obata, H. et al., Guinea pig model of immunologic asthma induced by inhalation of trimellitic anhydride, *Am. Rev. Respir. Dis.,* 146, 1553, 1992.
6. Patterson, R., Zeiss, C.R., and Pruzansky, J.J., Immunology and immunopathology of trimellitic anhydride pulmonary reactions, *J. Allergy Clin. Immunol.,* 70, 19, 1982.
7. Natsuaki, M. et al., Immediate contact hypersensitivity induced by repeated hapten challenge in mice, *Contact Dermatitis,* 43, 267, 2000.
8. Reijula, K.E. et al., Latex-induced dermal and pulmonary hypersensitivity in rabbits, *J. Allergy Clin. Immunol.,* 94, 891, 1994.

9. Spergel, J.M. et al., Epicutaneous sensitization with protein antigen induces localized allergic dermatitis and hyperresponsiveness to methacholine after single exposure to aerosolized antigen in mice, *J. Clin. Invest.,* 101, 1614, 1998.
10. Homey, B. et al., CCL27-CCR10 interactions regulate T cell-mediated skin inflammation, *Nat. Med.,* 8, 157, 2002.
11. Lehto, M. et al., Epicutaneous natural rubber latex sensitization induces T helper 2-type dermatitis and strong prohevein-specific IgE response, *J. Invest. Dermatol.,* 120, 633, 2003.
12. Gollhausen, R. and Kligman, A.M., Human assay for identifying substances which induce non-allergic contact urticaria: The NICU-test, *Contact Dermatitis,* 13, 98, 1985.
13. Lahti, A. and Maibach, H.I., An animal model for nonimmunologic contact urticaria, *Toxicol. Appl. Pharmacol.,* 76, 219, 1984.
14. Lahti, A. and Maibach, H.I., Species specificity of nonimmunologic contact urticaria: Guinea pig, rat, and mouse, *J. Am. Acad. Dermatol.,* 13, 66, 1985.
15. Lahti, A. et al., Pharmacological studies on nonimmunologic contact urticaria in guinea pigs, *Arch. Dermatol. Res.,* 279, 44, 1986.

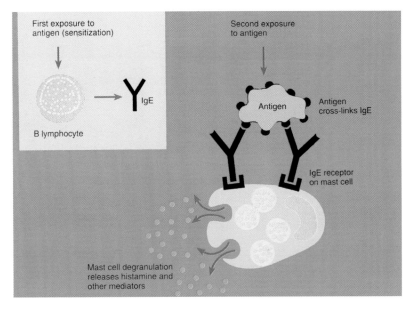

COLOR FIGURE 7.1 Schematic diagram of immediate-type allergic reaction.

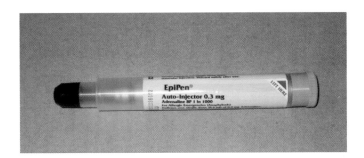

COLOR FIGURE 22.2 Epipen device. (Photo courtesy of ALK-Abelló, U.K.)

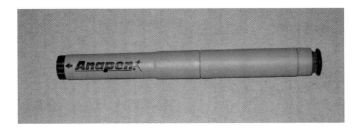

COLOR FIGURE 22.3 Anapen device. (Photo courtesy of Celltech Pharmaceuticals Ltd., U.K.)

9 Contact Urticaria Syndrome: Prognosis

Sarah H. Wakelin

CONTENTS

I. Introduction 113
II. Follow-up Studies of Adults with Occupational NRL Allergy 113
III. Primary Prevention 115
IV. Patients with Spina Bifida 116
V. Conclusions 117
References 117

I. INTRODUCTION

Allergy to natural rubber latex (NRL) is an important occupational problem in healthcare workers and other glove-wearing occupations. Most recent studies have concentrated on the clinical and immunological aspects of NRL allergy, and there is still relatively little information on the long-term outcome of NRL allergy in large patient populations. This is not surprising, since it is a relatively new clinical problem. From an occupational perspective, the most important issues are whether the condition improves with NRL avoidance in order to preserve employment for the latex sensitive worker; and secondly, what measures are effective in the primary prevention of NRL allergy. The outcome of NRL allergy is also important for the affected individual, as those with severe allergy are at risk of potentially fatal reactions on repeated exposure.

II. FOLLOW-UP STUDIES OF ADULTS WITH OCCUPATIONAL NRL ALLERGY

The first follow-up study on the occupational prognosis of the NRL-sensitized workers was published by Wrangjo of Sweden in 1994.[1] Twenty-five of 27 NRL-allergic medical, dental, and laboratory workers were reexamined an average of 7 years after diagnosis. Five had changed occupation and 5 had changed tasks within their occupation because of NRL allergy. Fifteen of 19 still in the same job (79%) reported work-related allergic symptoms. The dominating symptoms were glove-related contact urticaria with rhinitis or periorbital reactions and asthma. The majority of patients reported that their reactions increased in severity, and incidental exposure to NRL was difficult to avoid both at work and at home. This report highlighted that latex-allergic healthcare and laboratory workers did not easily get rid of their work-related allergic symptoms simply by avoiding latex themselves. It is notable that only in a few cases had there been a reduction or total change to nonpowder or nonlatex gloves by workmates to reduce indirect allergen exposure.

Similarly in 1996, a shorter follow-up questionnaire study from the United States of 41 patients with NRL allergy reported that the majority continued to have symptoms at work. A third had lost work time because of significant and sometimes incapacitating symptoms, and the number reporting systemic symptoms increased, including 5 individuals who suffered from anaphylaxis.[2] It has been shown that even if NRL-allergic healthcare workers avoid direct contact with NRL gloves, they remain at risk of suffering respiratory symptoms as long as powdered gloves are used in the workplace.[3]

The high rate of continued symptoms evident in these studies indicated the need to develop a safer environment for NRL-sensitized individuals. Legislation regarding standards for glove manufacture was therefore introduced in order to reduce latex exposure in the medical environment (see Chapter 19). In the U.K., the 1998 directive from the Medical Devices Agency effectively banned the use of glove powder in hospital. This directive also defined an upper limit for the extractable NRL protein content of examination gloves.[4] Similar strategies were advocated in North America by the American Academy of Allergy Asthma and Immunology.

Subsequent to the introduction of these policies, a report in the year 2000 of 20 NRL-sensitized anaesthetists found that 14 of 16 (88%) individuals, with an initially positive serological test (RAST), showed a reduction in latex specific IgE 10 to 15 months after the hospital had replaced all NRL examination gloves with nitrile and vinyl alternatives.[5] All twelve subjects who were symptomatic (8 with mild, localized glove symptoms, and 4 with ocular, respiratory, and cardiovascular symptoms) became and remained symptom free during the follow-up period. Another study by Allmers et al. showed a decrease in latex-specific IgE antibodies in healthcare workers with NRL allergy who avoided all latex products when, at the same time, powdered latex gloves were eliminated from the workplace.[6]

The importance of eliminating glove powder for severely allergic individuals is illustrated by the report by Tarlo et al. of a laboratory worker who had occupational NRL sensitization and repeated episodes of anaphylaxis. Her allergic symptoms only cleared when coworkers changed to powder-free gloves. Analysis of airborne latex allergen levels showed that levels were below the level of detection in a laboratory using powder-free NRL gloves, but were detectable and variable with powdered gloves.[3] Tilles reported a dental hygienist with NRL allergy who developed work-related symptoms culminating in repeated anaphylaxis with airborne exposure to NRL glove powder, and suggested that her sensitivity increased due to continued aerosolized exposure.[7] Early identification is also a key issue in the secondary prevention of latex allergy as appropriate allergen avoidance may halt progression of symptoms.

The largest published follow-up study of NRL allergy, was conducted by Turjanmaa and coworkers in 1995–1996.[8] This involved 160 adults (71 healthcare workers and 89 nonhealthcare workers) with NRL-allergy who were reexamined a median of 3 years after diagnosis. Hospital workers had been routinely using low-allergenic gloves for over 5 years, but these were normally powdered. On follow up, none of the healthcare workers had retired or changed work because of NRL allergy and there was a significant fall in the prevalence of hand eczema from 54 to 38%. It is of interest that most (61) of the hospital workers in this study had continued to use low allergen NRL gloves rather than nonlatex alternatives, which contrasts with current recommendations. The study did not specify any ongoing work-related symptoms, but several individuals had symptoms from nonoccupational NRL exposure including contact urticaria or irritation from dentists' gloves, rubber bands and undergarments, balloons, condoms, and other items. Two of the nonhealthcare workers, both men working in a rubber band factory, had to stop working because of persistent respiratory symptoms. The authors concluded that the outcome amongst NRL-allergic healthcare workers and nonhealthcare workers was generally good. The study also implies that for those working in production of NRL-containing items, where exposure cannot be avoided, a change in occupation may become necessary.

It is possible that the prognosis for patients with lower respiratory symptoms may be different from those presenting with contact urticaria. A small study of 19 patients diagnosed with occupational asthma due to NRL, found although most had changed their tasks or jobs, only 16% were free of symptoms without treatment, suggesting a poor prognosis.[9] However, another study of NRL occupational asthma, using different measures of outcome, reported that symptoms improved with reduced exposure as well as complete avoidance. The authors suggested that reducing exposure was a reasonably safe measure and had fewer socioeconomic consequences.[10] A U.S. study of 67 NRL-allergic healthcare workers found that work-related skin, respiratory, and systemic symptoms resolved in 44 of 49 (90%) NRL allergic healthcare workers who switched to non-NRL gloves whilst remaining in their current job. These data suggest a generally good outcome. However, 4 of 24 workers (17%) with work-related asthma were compelled to change employment to NRL-safe workplaces, resulting in a loss of annual income.[11]

We still do not understand clearly how direct skin exposure to latex affects the progression of allergic symptoms from localized urticaria to anaphylaxis. Therefore, sensitized healthcare workers should be advised against wearing latex gloves even if they have been shown to be of low allergenicity by *in vitro* and *in vivo* methods.[12]

III. PRIMARY PREVENTION

Exposure to allergen is clearly important for the development of IgE sensitization and subsequent allergic symptoms. However, there is little quantitative data that documents the relationship between dose and response for occupational allergens in humans, and it has therefore not been possible to establish threshold exposure limits for most allergens. Glove powder plays a key role in eliciting symptoms in those sensitized to NRL, but there is a lack of information on the effectiveness of using powder-free low protein gloves as a primary prevention strategy. However, one study has shown that no new cases of latex sensitivity were observed among hospital staff where only powder-free gloves were used during a 1-year follow-up period.[6] Similarly, in 1075 skin prick-negative healthcare workers followed over a 1-year period, a 1% incidence of clinically relevant symptomatic latex allergy was observed in a subgroup wearing powdered latex gloves, whereas there was only a nonsymptomatic conversion in the SPT in 2 individuals wearing nonpowdered gloves of low protein content.[13]

Prophylactic selection of low protein, nonpowdered gloves was found to be associated with an absence of NRL sensitization in a study of 189 dental students.[14] These students were not tested prior to glove use, so this study did not give conclusive evidence that use of powdered gloves was responsible for sensitization. Data from the German statutory accident insurance company for healthcare workers showed steady decline in the incidence of suspected occupational NRL allergy cases after 1998 when use of nonpowdered low protein gloves became mandatory, which adds further support to this intervention.[15]

Not all studies have confirmed that changing gloves has a primary protective effect. A prospective study among Canadian healthcare workers found no difference in the rate of new positive skin prick tests after 2 years, among 208 subjects using powdered gloves compared with 227 using nonpowdered latex alternatives.[13] However, the authors subsequently retested the converters in the nonpowder intervention group and found them to be latex skin prick negative, and only those working with powdered gloves had symptoms.[16]

IV. PATIENTS WITH SPINA BIFIDA

It has been apparent since the early 1990s that children with spina bifida are at increased risk of NRL allergy and may suffer severe allergic reactions due to mucosal and intraoperative NRL exposure.[17] The risk of intraoperative anaphylaxis in this group has been estimated to be increased 500 fold.[18] Follow up studies of this group in a hospital setting have shown that systemic reactions can be avoided if operations are performed in an allergen-free environment.[19] A time-dependent (but not significant) decrease in mean latex-specific IgE of patients with spina bifida has been reported when surgery is subsequently performed in a NRL-free environment.[20]

However, a study by Ylitalo of 24 children who were sensitized to NRL and followed up a few years after diagnosis found that avoidance of NRL in the home environment was difficult.[21] Although these patients were carefully and comprehensively advised, the great majority reported further NRL exposure at follow-up. In this group, no decrease in skin prick reactivity or RAST to latex allergens was observed over a follow up period of 2.8 years. Mazon et al. even observed a 5:1 ratio of increased to decreased rates of NRL hypersensitivity in a 2 year follow-up study of children with spina bifida who were advised about medical prophylaxis and home prophylaxis.[22] This illustrates the progressive nature of latex sensitization in these patients, which again may be due to difficulty in complying with avoidance advice.

A larger follow-up study by Reider et al. over a 5-year period from 1995–2000 reported the outcome of 100 children with shunted hydrocephalus with or without additional spina bifida.[23] All children and/or their parents were given detailed avoidance advice for latex exposure, although only those who knew they were sensitized tended to follow these recommendations. Reevaluation of the 30 children with initially positive latex specific IgE, showed a fall in RAST-class in 20, no change in 7, and an increase in 3 individuals, suggesting that secondary prevention had been effective. Patients were questioned about the avoidance measures they had followed and medical prophylaxis appeared to be more important than home prophylaxis.

There is little data on the primary prevention of NRL allergy in spina bifida, but a recently published study carried out in children treated in a latex-free environment from birth showed a fall in prevalence of latex sensitization from 4/15 (26.7%) to 1/22 (4.5%) over 6 years.[24]

V. CONCLUSIONS

Recent legislation regarding glove quality and banning of powder has played a critical role in protection of healthcare workers against NRL allergy, and there is emerging evidence to support its effectiveness in both primary and secondary prevention of NRL allergy. Additional prospective data are needed, but it appears that the prognosis for occupational NRL allergy is good provided that proper latex avoidance is undertaken. Studies in children with spina bifida provide examples of non-occupational exposure. The importance of strict latex avoidance both in a hospital setting and at home has emerged. Continued and more widespread awareness of NRL allergy is needed in order to improve primary prevention and readily identify and protect those already sensitized.

REFERENCES

1. Wrangsjo, K., Latex allergy in medical, dental and laboratory personnel — a follow up study, *Am. J. Contact Dermatitis,* 5, 194, 1994.
2. Taylor, J.S. and Praditsuwan, P., Latex allergy: Review of 44 cases including outcome and frequent association with allergic hand eczema, *Arch. Dermatol.,* 132, 265, 1996.
3. Tarlo, M. et al., Control of airborne latex by use of powder-free gloves, *J. Allergy Clin. Immunol.,* 93, 985, 1994.
4. Medical Devices Agency Safety Notice (SN9825): Latex medical gloves (surgeons' and examination), powdered latex medical gloves (surgeons' and examination), July 1988.
5. Hamilton, R.G. and Brown, R.H., Impact of personal avoidance practices on health care workers sensitised to natural rubber latex, *J. Allergy Clin. Immunol.,* 105, 839, 2000.
6. Allmers, H. et al., Reduction of latex aeroallergens and latex specific IgE antibodies in sensitised workers after removal of powdered natural rubber latex gloves in a hospital, *J. Allergy Clin. Immunol.,* 102, 841, 1998.
7. Tilles, S.A., Occupational latex allergy: Controversies in diagnosis and prognosis, *Ann. Allergy Asthma Immunol.,* 83, 640, 1999.
8. Turjanmaa, K. et al., Long-term outcome of 160 adult patients with natural rubber latex allergy, *J. Allergy Clin. Immunol.,* 110(S2), S70, 2002.
9. Acero, S. et al., Occupational asthma from natural rubber latex: Specific inhalation challenge test and evolution, *J. Invest. Allergol. Clin. Immunol.,* 13, 155, 2003.
10. Vandenplas, O. et al., Occupational asthma caused by natural rubber latex: Outcome according to cessation or reduction of exposure, *J. Allergy Clin. Immunol.,* 109, 125, 2002.

11. Bernstien, D.I. et al., Clinical and occupational outcomes in health care workers with natural rubber latex allergy, *Ann. Allergy Asthma Immunol.,* 90, 209, 2003.

12. Smedley, J., Occupational latex allergy: The magnitude of the problem and its prevention, *Clin. Exp. Allergy,* 30, 458, 2000.

13. Sussman, G.L. et al., Incidence of latex sensitisation among latex glove users, *J. Allergy Clin. Immunol.,* 101, 171, 1998.

14. Levy, D.A. et al., Powder-free protein poor natural rubber latex gloves and latex sensitisation, *J. Am. Med. Assoc.,* 281, 988, 1999.

15. Allmers, H., Schmengler, J., and Skudlik, C., Primary prevention of natural rubber latex allergy in the German health care system through education and intervention, *J. Allergy Clin. Immunol.,* 110, 318, 2002.

16. Sussman, G.L., Liss, G.M., and Wasserman, S., Update on the Hamilton, Ontario latex sensitisation study, *J. Allergy Clin. Immunol.,* 102, 333, 1998.

17. Kelly, K.J. et al., A cluster of anaphylactic reactions in children with spina bifida during general anaesthesia: Epidemiologic features, risk factors and latex hypersensitivity, *J. Allergy Clin. Immunol.,* 94, 53, 1994.

18. Tosi, L.L. et al., Latex allergy in spina bifida patients: Prevalence and surgical implications, *J. Pediatr. Orthop.,* 13, 709, 1993.

19. Cremer, R. et al., Longitudinal study on latex sensitisation in children with spina bifida, *Pediatr. Allergy Immunol.,* 9, 40, 1998.

20. Niggemann, B. et al., Latex allergy in spina bifida: At the turning point? *J. Allergy Clin. Immunol.,* 106, 1201, 2000.

21. Ylitalo, L. et al., Natural rubber latex allergy in children: A follow up study, *Clin. Exp. Allergy,* 30, 1611, 2000.

22. Mazon, A. et al., Latex sensitisation in children with spina bifida: Follow up comparative study after two years, *Ann. Allergy Asthma Immunol.,* 84, 207, 2000.

23. Reider, N. et al., Outcome of a latex avoidance program in a high-risk population for latex allergy: A five-year follow up study, *Clin. Exp. Allergy,* 32, 708, 2002.

24. Nieto, A et al., Efficacy of latex avoidance for primary prevention of latex sensitisation in children with spina bifida, *J. Paediatr.,* 140, 370, 2002.

10 Allergic Contact Dermatitis: Clinical Manifestations

Natalie M. Stone

CONTENTS

I.   Introduction 119
II. Sites Involved 120
III. Eczematous Variants 121
IV. Rubber Purpura 121
V.   Rubber Depigmentation 121
VI. Unusual Delayed-Type Reactions 122
VII. Allergic Contact Dermatitis to Natural Rubber Latex 122
References 123

I. INTRODUCTION

Natural rubber latex products are composed of polymerized isoprene protein and chemical additives such as accelerators and antioxidants, added during the manufacture of rubber products.[1] Allergic contact dermatitis (ACD) to rubber classically occurs to the low molecular weight chemical additives, such as thiurams and thiazoles, and not to the high molecular weight isoprene protein.[2] ACD to rubber additives is a problem for consumers of rubber products as well as an occupational problem for rubber industry workers.

Occupational and nonoccupational allergic contact dermatitis to rubber is increasing in incidence due to an increased worldwide use of rubber products. Contact with rubber additives is also increasing due to the use of these compounds in nonrubber items such as paints and insecticides.[1–3]

Delayed-type hypersensitivity reactions have been reported to occur to natural rubber latex, in the absence of reactions to the rubber additives. It is not yet known if this is a common problem or the exact allergen involved. Type IV allergy to natural latex remains a controversial subject.[4–6]

ACD to rubber usually presents with localized areas of dermatitis where there has been direct contact with rubber and sometimes more generalized eczematous

0-8493-1670-7/05/$0.00+$1.50

TABLE 10.1
Site and Cause of Rubber Allergy

Site	Rubber Containing Item	Allergen
Eyelids[3]	Eyelash curler	Phenyl beta naphthylamine
Thigh[3]	Garter	MBT, thiuram
Palm[3]	Squash ball	IPPD
Penis[3]	Condom	MBT, carbamates
Face[3]	Balloons	Thiurams
Ears[9]	Ear plugs	MBT, thiurams
Wrist[10]	Keyboard rest	Thioureas

eruptions. Unusual presentations of ACD to rubber additives can also occur, such as purpura[7] and leukoderma.[8]

II. SITES INVOLVED

ACD to rubber additives classically presents with an eczematous rash at the site of contact with a rubber item (Table 10.1). Processed rubber items release small amounts of chemical additives over time, known as *blooming*. This is enhanced when rubber is moist and warm due to direct skin contact, such as when wearing rubber gloves. Patients allergic to their rubber gloves may present with dermatitis over the dorsum of the hand, with a band at the wrist due to contact with the glove cuff. Hand eczema is the most common site of involvement in patients presenting with a type IV rubber allergy. Other common presentations include lower leg eczema due to rubber containing bandages and foot dermatitis due to shoes or boots containing rubber. Fingertip dermatitis is recognized to occur in bank clerks due to the use of rubber fingerstalls.[1] Unusual site specific presentations include the inner ear due to rubber earplugs,[9] unilateral leg dermatitis due to a rubber containing leg brace,[10] eyelid dermatitis due to rubber-containing eyelash curlers,[3] and wrist dermatitis due to use of a rubber wrist support when typing on a keyboard.[10]

The eyelids have been described as an ectopic site of rubber allergy. Jordan reported the cases of several healthcare workers presenting with eyelid dermatitis, in the absence of hand dermatitis, who had developed allergy to the accelerator in their rubber gloves.[11] He suggested that accelerators leached into glove donning powder would remain in contact with the eyelid but would be washed off the hands after removal of the gloves. Calnan similarly reported a patient allergic to thiurams and carba mix who presented with eyelid and penile edema, in the absence of hand eczema, after laying a rubber-backed carpet.[12] The hands may transfer chemicals to sensitive sites such as the eyelid where the skin is thin and allergens penetrate more easily.

A specific localized presentation occurs with the bleached rubber syndrome.[13] An eczematous rash develops under rubber-elastic areas of clothing if it has been washed with laundry bleach. Patch testing is negative for the usual rubber additives but positive for the item of clothing. The allergen is dibenzylcarbamyl chloride which is produced when sodium hypochlorite in the laundry bleach interacts with the accelerator, zinc dibenzyldithiocarbamate.

III. ECZEMATOUS VARIANTS

Conde-Salazar has reported pompholyx-type eczema occurring predominantly on the dorsolateral aspects of the dominant hand of workers who frequently use rubber bands.[14] The allergens involved were thiurams and thiazoles.

Hyperkeratotic eczema is recognized to occur particularly with allergic contact dermatitis to the amine antioxidant n-isopropyl-n-phenyl-paraphenylenediamine (IPPD).[15] IPPD is an allergen present in most black or grey rubber, and allergy can present with hyperkeratotic eczema on the hands of mechanics handling black rubber tires or on the feet of patients wearing black rubber-soled shoes. Conde-Salazar has named this condition "black rubber hands and feet."[14] The differential diagnosis of hyperkeratosis of the hands includes endogenous hand dermatitis and psoriasis.

Positive patch tests to rubber chemicals and improvement of the rash on avoiding rubber can help with the diagnosis. IPPD hand eczema can however be persistent, despite allergen avoidance.

Widespread, generalized, eczematous rashes, simulating atopic eczema, can occur due to type IV allergy to rubber additives. This may be caused by several body sites being in contact with rubber, indirect manual transfer of the allergen by the patient, or the use of rubber gloves to apply creams.[16] An airborne pattern of allergic contact dermatitis to rubber additives has been reported,[17] and the possibility of a generalized rash caused by systemic contact dermatitis to rubber chemicals leaching into foods from rubber containers has been hypothesized.[18]

IV. RUBBER PURPURA

Purpura secondary to delayed-type rubber allergy was first described by Fisher in 1974. He used the term "PPPP syndrome" to describe pruritus, petecheiae, and purpura produced by contact with IPPD.[7] Several cases of purpura have since been reported to occur due to contact with items such as rubber boots, a rubber diving suit, and a rubber knee support.[19–21] Other rubber additives have been implicated, including mercaptobenzothiazole and thiurams.[22] The positive patch test reaction may be purpuric.[23]

V. RUBBER DEPIGMENTATION

Hydroquinone and its derivatives are used as rubber antioxidants and stabilizers, as well as therapeutically as skin lightening agents for conditions such as chloasma and post-inflammatory hyperpigmentation. Oliver et al. first described occupational depigmentation caused by rubber gloves containing the monobenzyl ether of hydroquinone.[8] The monobenzyl ether of hydroquinone is a potent depigmenting agent and also a recognized potent allergen.[24] It has been recognized to cause depigmentation even at sites distant to contact. Patients classically present with a confetti-type hypopigmentation over the dorsum of the hands due to wearing rubber gloves. This presentation is now rare as hydroquinone-type compounds are less frequently used in the rubber industry, but they are still used in the photographic industry.[1] A case of peri-orbital depigmentation due to use of rubber swimming goggles has been reported.[25]

VI. UNUSUAL DELAYED-TYPE REACTIONS

Lichenoid-type pigmented contact dermatitis has been reported in patients occupationally exposed to IPPD from rubber tires.[26] Clinically the eruption can mimic classical lichen planus in distribution and morphology, however the clue to diagnosis lies in the rash clearing when the patient is away from work. Pustular reactions to rubber chemicals have also been reported, one presenting as plantar pustulosis in a patient allergic to mercaptobenzothiazole[27] and one allergic to hexafluorosilicate used to manufacture foam rubber.[28] Erythema multiforme-type rashes have also been described occurring due to contact with rubber gloves and a rubber watch strap.[29, 30]

VII. ALLERGIC CONTACT DERMATITIS TO NATURAL RUBBER LATEX

It has been suspected for many years that delayed-type allergy to latex protein may exist, with several patients being described with allergic reactions to their gloves but no reactions to known rubber additives. It is much more recently that type I hypersensitivity reactions have been recognized to occur to latex protein.[31] Wyss et al. reported the first case of a patient with allergic contact dermatitis to natural latex, in the absence of a type I reaction to latex or a type IV reaction to known rubber additives.[32] Many further cases of positive patch test reactions to latex protein have since been reported, some in combination with and some without contact urticaria to latex.[33–35]

The largest series of delayed hypersensitivity reactions to latex was a multicenter study reported by Sommer et al. in 2002.[36] They used latex preserved solely in ammonia to patch test 2738 consecutive patients from 5 patch testing centers. Twenty-seven (1%) had a positive patch test reaction to latex, interpreted as allergic, of which 14 also had a positive specific IgE test or prick test to latex. Four patients had a positive patch test to latex which was thought to be of current relevance, in the confirmed absence of a type I allergy to latex. These patients presented with eczema at different sites (Table 10.2). Seven reactions to latex were interpreted as irritant.

In a previous study, Wilkinson and Burd tested an at-risk population of 117 patients with hand eczema and history of glove use.[37] They found an increased prevalence of delayed-type reactions to latex, with 7 patients (6%) having a positive patch test reaction to latex preserved in ammonia, of which 3 did not have a type I allergy to latex. Gottlober et al. similarly tested 167 at-risk patients with hand eczema and history of rubber contact.[35] They report 4 patients with an allergic patch test reaction to latex, of whom 3 did not have a type I allergy to latex protein.

TABLE 10.2
Patients with a Relevant Allergic Patch Test to Latex, with a Negative Prick Test to Latex

Sex	Age	Site	Occupation	NRL Prick Test	NRL Patch Test	Patch Test Relevance
F	26	Hands	Hairdresser	Negative	Positive	CR
M	20	Face, neck	Student	Negative	Positive	CR
M	50	Hands, face	Plumber	Negative	Positive	CR
M	71	Legs	Pensioner	Negative	Positive	CR

Source: From Sommer, S. et al., 2002. With permission.[36]

Positive patch and prick test reactions to latex seem to be strongly associated.[38] This may be interpreted as representing a protein contact dermatitis to latex protein, as opposed to separate type I and type IV allergies to the protein.[39] Positive patch test reactions to pure latex, in the absence of a type I reaction, are less common, but do occur. It seems to be most relevant to patients with hand eczema and a history of rubber contact. Allergic contact dermatitis to natural latex should be considered as a potential diagnosis in patients with a history of rubber intolerance.

REFERENCES

1. Belsito, D.V., Rubber, in *Handbook of Occupational Dermatology*, Kanerva L., Elsner P., Wahlberg J.E. and Maibach H.I., Eds., Springer-Verlag, Berlin, Heidelberg, 2000, chap. 87, p. 701.
2. Conde-Salazar, L. et al., Type IV allergy to rubber additives: A 10 year study of 686 cases, *J. Am. Acad. Dermatol.*, 176, 29, 1993.
3. Cronin, E., Rubber, in *Contact Dermatitis*, Cronin, E., Ed., Churchill Livingstone, Edinburgh, 1980, p. 714.
4. Wilkinson, S.M. and Beck, M.H., Allergic contact dermatitis from latex rubber, *Br. J. Dermatol.*, 134, 910, 1996.
5. Shaffrali, F.C.G. and Gawkroger, D.J., Allergic contact dermatitis from natural rubber latex without immediate sensitivity, *Contact Dermatitis*, 40, 325, 1999.
6. Wilkinson, S.M. and Burd, R., Latex: A cause of allergic contact eczema in users of natural rubber gloves, *J. Am. Acad. Dermatol.*, 38, 36, 1998.
7. Fisher, A.A., Allergic petechial and purpuric rubber dermatitis: The PPPP syndrome, *Cutis*, 14, 25, 1974.
8. Oliver, E.A., Schwartz, L., and Warren, L.H., Occupational leukoderma: Preliminary report, *J. Am. Med. Assoc.*, 113, 927, 1939.
9. Deguchi, M. and Tagami, H., Contact dermatitis of the ear due to a rubber earplug, *Dermatology*, 193, 251, 1996.
10. McClewsky, P.E. and Swerlic, R.A., Clinical review: Thioureas and allergic contact dermatitis, *Cutis*, 68, 387, 2001.
11. Jordan, W.P., 24 and 48 hour patch tests, *Contact Dermatitis*, 6, 151, 1980.

12. Calnan, C.D., Rubber sensitivity presenting as eyelid oedema, *Contact Dermatitis,* 1, 124, 1975.
13. Jordan, W.P. and Bourlas, M.C., Allergic contact dermatitis to underwear elastic, chemically transformed by laundry bleach, *Arch. Dermatol.,* 111, 593, 1975.
14. Conde-Salazar, L., Rubber Dermatitis: Clinical forms, *Contact Dermatitis,* 8, 49, 1990.
15. Conde-Salazar, L. and Gomez Urcuyo, F.J., Sensibilidad a aminas antioxidants: Revisión de 51 casos, *Actas Dermo-Sif.,* 75, 23, 1984.
16. Gooptu, C. and Powell, S.M., The problems of rubber hypersensitivity (types I and IV) in chronic leg ulcer and stasis eczema patients, *Contact Dermatitis,* 41, 89, 1999.
17. Dooms-Goosens, A. et al., Contact dermatitis caused by airborne agents: A review and case reports, *J. Am. Acad. Dermatol.,* 15, 1, 1986.
18. Stankevich, V.V., Vlasiuk, M.G., and Prokofera, L.G., Hygienic evaluation of the organic sulfur vulcanisation accelerators in rubbers for the food industry, *Gig. Sanit.,* 10, 88, 1980.
19. Fisher, A.A., Purpuric contact dermatitis, *Cutis,* 33, 346, 1984.
20. Batschvarov, B. and Minkov, D.M., Dermatitis and purpura from rubber in clothing, *Trans. St. Johns Hosp. Dermatol. Soc.,* 54, 178, 1968.
21. Calnan, C.D. and Peachy, R.D.G., Allergic contact purpura, *Clin. Allergy,* 1, 287, 1971.
22. Burrows, D., Thiuram dermatitis and purpura, *Contact Dermatitis Newsletter,* 12, 333, 1972.
23. Ancona, A., Monroy, F., and Fernandez-Diez, J., Occupational dermatitis from IPPD in tyres, *Contact Dermatitis,* 8, 91, 1982.
24. van Ketel, W.G., Sensitization to hydroquinone and the monobenzylether of hydroquinone, *Contact Dermatitis,* 10, 253, 1984.
25. Goette, D.K., Raccoon-like periorbital leukoderma from contact with swim goggles, *Contact Dermatitis,* 10, 129, 1984.
26. Calnan, C.D., Lichenoid dermatitis from isopropylaminodiphenylamine, *Contact Dermatitis Newsletter,* 10, 237, 1971.
27. Pecegueiro, M. and Brandao, M., Contact plantar pustulosis, *Contact Dermatitis,* 11, 126, 1984.
28. Dooms-Goosens, A. et al., Pustular reactions to hexafluorosilicate in foam rubber, *Contact Dermatitis,* 12, 42, 1985.
29. Bourrain, J.L. et al., Natural rubber latex contact dermatitis with features of erythema multiforme, *Contact Dermatitis,* 35, 55, 1996.
30. Foussereau, J. et al., A case of erythema multiforme with allergy to isopropyl-p-phenylenediamine of rubber, *Contact Dermatitis,* 18, 183, 1988.
31. Nutter, A.F., Contact urticaria to rubber, *Br. J. Dermatol.,* 101, 597, 1979.
32. Wyss, M. et al., Allergic contact dermatitis from natural rubber latex without contact urticaria, *Contact Dermatitis,* 28, 154, 1993.
33. Sugiura, M. et al., Delayed type natural rubber latex allergy not accompanied by immediate type, *Contact Dermatitis,* 43, 370, 2000.
34. Statham, B.N., Concurrent Type 1 and Type IV natural rubber latex sensitivity? *Contact Dermatitis,* 42, 178, 2000.
35. Gottlober, P., Gall, H., and Peter, R.U., Allergic contact dermatitis from natural latex, *Am. J. Contact Derm.,* 12, 135, 2001.
36. Sommer, S. et al., Type IV hypersensitivity reactions to natural rubber latex: Results of a multicentre study, *Br. J. Dermatol.,* 146, 114, 2002.

37. Wilkinson, S.M. and Burd, R., Latex: A cause of allergic contact eczema in users of natural rubber gloves, *J. Am. Acad. Dermatol.,* 39, 36, 1998.
38. Wilkinson, S.M., Patch test reactions to natural rubber latex: Irritant or allergic? *Contact Dermatitis,* 42, 179, 2000.
39. Gortz, J. and Goos, M., Immediate and late type allergy to latex: Contact urticaria, asthma and contact dermatitis, in *Current Topics in Contact Dermatitis,* Frosch, P.J., Dooms-Goosens, A., Lachapelle, J.M., Rycroft, R.J.G., Scheper, R.J., Eds., Springer-Verlag, Berlin, 1989, part 5.

11 Allergic Contact Dermatitis: Tests

Natalie M. Stone

CONTENTS

I. Introduction 127
II. Investigation of Allergic Contact Dermatitis to Rubber Additives 127
III. Rubber Mixes 128
IV. Other Rubber Additives 130
V. Patch Testing with Natural Rubber Latex 130
References 131

I. INTRODUCTION

Allergic contact dermatitis (ACD) is a delayed-type hypersensitivity reaction, investigated by patch testing. This is a specialist investigation mainly performed by dermatologists and occasionally by immunologists. Small quantities of likely allergens are applied under occlusion to intact skin. The patches are removed after a specific time, often 2 days, and readings are preferably taken on the day of removal of the patches and again after 4 days, or sometimes longer. Reactions are interpreted as allergic or irritant depending on the morphology of the reaction. Allergic reactions are then interpreted with respect to their current relevance to the patient's problem. Guidelines for the procedure of patch testing have been suggested.[1]

II. INVESTIGATION OF ALLERGIC CONTACT DERMATITIS TO RUBBER ADDITIVES

ACD to rubber generally occurs to the low molecular weight chemicals added during the manufacture of rubber. They are a common cause of ACD both among workers in the rubber industry and consumers of rubber goods. The most common rubber additive allergens are present on the American, European, and International Standard patch test series.[2]

Standard patch test series have been altered over many years to be most applicable to the individual population being tested. Contact dermatitis groups therefore differ with respect to the allergens in their standard series but all include several rubber allergen mixes as well as individual allergens (Table 11.1). Additional series of extra

0-8493-1670-7/05/$0.00+$1.50

TABLE 11.1
Rubber Allergens in Standard Series

- *n*-isopropyl-*n*-paraphenylenediamine (IPPD) 0.1% pet[a,b]
- mercaptobenzothiazole 1% pet[b]
- mercapto mix 2% pet[a,b]
  n-cyclohexylbenzothiazyl sulfenamide 0.5% pet
  dibenzothiazyl disulfide 0.5% pet
  morpholinylmercaptobenzothiazole 0.5% pet
  mercaptobenzothiazole 0.5% pet
- thiuram mix 1% pet[a,b]
  tetramethylthiuram monosulfide (TMTM) 0.25% pet
  tetramethylthiuram disulfide (TMTD) 0.25% pet
  tetraethylthiuram disulfide (TETD) 0.25% pet
  dipentamethylenethiuram disulfide (PTD) 0.25% pet
- carba mix 3% pet[b]
  1,3-diphenylguanidine (DPG) 1% pet
  zinc diethyldithiocarbamate 1% pet
  zinc dibutyldithiocarbamate 1% pet
- black rubber mix 0.6% pet
  n-phenyl-n-cyclohexylparaphenylenediamine 0.25% pet
  n-isopropyl-n-paraphenylenediamine 0.1% pet
  n,n-diphenyl-paraphenylenediamine 0.25% pet

Additional Rubber Chemicals
  hexamethylenetetramine 2% pet
  diphenylthiourea (DPT) 1% pet
  dibutylthiourea (DBT) 1% pet
  diethylthiourea 1% pet
  n,n-diphenyl paraphenylenediamine 1% pet
  cyclohexyl thiophthalimide 1% pet
  n-phenyl-2-naphtylamine 1% pet
  zinc dimethyldithiocarbamate 1% pet

[a] North American Contact Dermatitis Group Standard Series
[b] British Contact Dermatitis Society Standard Series

rubber allergens may also be used to test patients with a suspected rubber allergy. There are a large number of potential rubber allergens and it is important to test with samples of a patient's own rubber product to ensure that cases are not missed.[1]

III. RUBBER MIXES

Several of the chemically similar rubber additives have been mixed together in a vehicle to form a single patch test application. This adds to ease of application, with the ability to test more chemicals in fewer patch test chambers. When patch testing with allergen mixes there is a risk of false negative reactions if the concentration of a particular component is too low and a risk of irritant reactions if several irritant chemicals are applied at one site. The various mixes of allergens used over the years have been modified and improved to reduce these potential problems. Patients with weak reactions to a rubber mix should be further tested to the individual components of the mix to clarify if an irritant reaction to the mix or an allergic reaction to a component of the mix has occurred.[3]

The North American Contact Dermatitis Group lists thiuram mix and carba mix within the 12 most frequent positive patch test allergens.[4] Thiurams and carbamates are used as accelerators for synthetic and natural rubber. There are 4 thiurams within the thiuram mix. They do not always cross-react with each other and testing with fewer single allergens does lead to cases being missed. The most common individual allergens within the mix vary between different countries and probably reflect the use of different types of rubber products.[5] Thiurams are reported to be the most common of the rubber allergens.[6] They have been widely used as accelerators in rubber gloves. Thiuram allergy has been documented to be increasing within health-care workers with hand eczema, which could reflect the increasing use of gloves in this population.[7] Medical glove manufacturers now often use carbamates instead of thiurams.[8] Chemical analysis has however shown that some gloves labeled as solely containing carbamates may also contain thiurams. This may be a consequence of thiurams added to latex in the country of origin, unknown to the manufacturer, or thiurams being present as impurities within the carbamates.[9] Carba mix has been formulated to contain two related carbamates and diphenylguanidine (DPG). Carba mix is irritant and often causes weak irritant patch test reactions. Carbamates cross-react with thiurams and therefore the two mixes often react together. Due to its irritancy and cross-reactivity with thiuram mix, it has been suggested that carba mix should be dropped from the standard series.[10] Cases where carba mix reacts in isolation from thiuram mix do however occur. This is usually due to allergy to DPG, which is an unrelated compound.[3]

Mercaptobenzothiazole (MBT), and the chemicals in the mercapto mix, are used as accelerators for both natural and synthetic rubber, before vulcanization takes place. Mercapto mix was originally formulated to contain MBT and three of its derivatives, each at 0.25%. Studies showed that the concentration of MBT in the mix was too low and resulted in false negative reactions. In North America, MBT is now tested on the standard series as a single allergen at 1% and the mix is tested containing the three derivatives of MBT, at the higher concentration of 0.33%. In Europe, the mix contains all four chemicals, each at 0.5%, and MBT is tested separately on the standard series at 2%.[11] The mix is included on most standard series as it detects a small number of thiazole sensitive patients who do not react to MBT.[12] Cronin's results suggest that MBT is the most common allergen among the thiazoles.[13]

Vulcanized rubber is known to "perish" over time, by reacting with oxygen and developing cracks and fissures. This process is limited by the addition of antioxidants. N-isopropylphenylenediamine (IPPD) is the main antioxidant found in black or grey coloured rubber. Paraphenylenediamine (PPD) is found on all standard series as a marker of allergy to dyes. PPD does not usually cross-react with IPPD and therefore is not used as a marker for these allergies.[3] Black rubber mix consists of IPPD and two related chemicals. IPPD is the most commonly reacting allergen within the mix. The other two chemicals in the mix, phenyl-cyclohexyl-PPD and diphenyl-PPD, have been difficult to obtain, such that IPPD as a single allergen has replaced the mix on most standard series. It is estimated that by testing with IPPD alone, approximately 10% of allergy to these antioxidants is missed.[14]

IV. OTHER RUBBER ADDITIVES

There are many other rubber additives that are less frequent allergens and are therefore only tested as part of an extended rubber series in patients suspected of having a rubber allergy. Holness and Nethercott found that 11% of patients tested to their extra series of rubber allergens had positive reactions, which would have been missed with their standard series alone.[15]

The thioureas are additives most commonly used as accelerators in high grade, synthetic, neoprene rubber. There are increasing numbers of reports of allergy to thioureas, such as hand eczema due to diethylthiourea in a keyboard wrist support,[16] and generalized eczema due to ethylbutylthiourea in a neoprene wet suit.[17] The thioureas do not always cross-react. Allergy to thioureas is not common but should be considered in patients with a history of rubber allergy who do not have positive reactions to the standard series. Other accelerators include the slow accelerator, hexamethylenetetramine, and the benzothiazolesulfenamides, which are delayed-action accelerators. Most rubber items contain a mixture of different accelerators. Alternative rubber antioxidants include the phenols and quinolones. The most commonly used phenol is butyl hydroxytoluene (BHT). The quinolones may clinically cause hypopigmentation. A further amine antioxidant in frequent use is phenyl-naphthylamine.[3]

Retarders are added to rubber to prevent premature vulcanisation, of which cyclohexylthio-phthalimide is the most common allergen. Organic pigments may be added to rubber as colourants and can cause contact allergy. Glove powder, either within a glove or on the surface of a glove, can contain potential sensitizers. Examples are sorbic acid in glove donning powder[3] and the ammonium salt, cetyl pyridinium chloride, on the surface of a latex glove.[18] Other additives include flame retarders, fungicides, chemical stabilizers, and odorants.

A vast number of rubber additives are potential type IV allergens. It is therefore important to patch test with a patient's own rubber item if allergy is suspected but standard rubber allergens are negative on testing. Patch test reactions from a patient's own products may be improved by soaking the sample for 15 mins before application and by leaving the patch under occlusion for longer than 48 hours.[1]

V. PATCH TESTING WITH NATURAL RUBBER LATEX

There are several difficulties in diagnosing a delayed-type hypersensitivity to natural latex. It can be difficult to obtain a sample of pure latex that is free from additives. Chemicals are often added to natural latex at source[19] and additive-free latex is not commercially available for patch testing. Samples of pure latex preserved in ammonia may be obtained on an individual basis from the large rubber companies. Chemical analyses of some samples have confirmed a lack of additives.[20]

Pure latex is known to cause irritant patch test reactions. Interpreting weak allergic from irritant reactions can be difficult. The use of dry natural latex preserved solely with a high-ammonia preparation is thought to cause fewer irritant reactions.[19]

Positive patch test and prick test reactions to latex are known to be associated. A positive, eczematous patch test reaction to latex in a patient with type I hypersensitivity to latex may be interpreted as a protein contact dermatitis,[21] which is controversial. Cases of positive patch tests to pure latex in the absence of a type I allergy to latex have been reported, suggesting that true delayed type IV reactions to latex do occur.[22] Latex is a natural product that contains many different substances. The exact allergen involved in these cases is therefore unclear, however lymphocyte proliferation tests have suggested that a delayed response to latex protein can occur.[23]

A case of anaphylaxis due to patch testing with latex, in a patient with previously undiagnosed type I latex allergy, has been reported.[24] Care should therefore be taken when patch testing with latex and a type I allergy excluded before patch testing takes place.

REFERENCES

1. Reitschel, R.L. and Fowler, J.F., Jr., Practical aspects of patch testing, in *Fisher's Contact Dermatitis,* Reitschel, R.L. and Fowler, J.F., Jr., Eds., Lippincott Williams and Wilkins, Philadelphia, 2000, chap. 2.

2. Belsito, D.V., Rubber, in *Handbook of Occupational Dermatology,* Kanerva L., Elsner P., Wahlberg J.E., and Maibach H.I., Eds., Springer-Verlag, Berlin, Heidelberg, 2000, chap. 87.

3. Reitschel, R.L. and Fowler, J.F., Jr., Allergy to Rubber, in *Fisher's Contact Dermatitis,* Reitschel, R.L. and Fowler, J.F., Jr., Eds., Lippincott Williams and Wilkins, Philadelphia, 2000, chap. 31.

4. Marks, J.G. et al., North American Contact Dermatitis Group patch test results for the detection of delayed-type hypersensitivity to topical allergens, *J. Am. Acad. Dermatol.,* 38, 911, 1998.

5. Themido, R. and Brandao, F.M., Contact allergy to thiurams, *Contact Dermatitis,* 251, 10, 1984.

6. Conde-Salazar, L. et al., Type IV allergy to rubber additives: A 10 year study of 686 cases, *J. Am. Acad. Dermatol.,* 29, 176, 1993.

7. Gibbon, K.L. et al., Changing frequency of thiuram allergy in healthcare workers with hand dermatitis, *Br. J. Dermatol.,* 144, 347, 2001.

8. Heese, A. et al., Allergic and irritant reactions to rubber gloves in medical health services, *J. Am. Acad. Dermatol.,* 25, 831, 1991.

9. Knudsen, B.B. et al., Release of thiurams and carbamates from rubber gloves, *Contact Dermatitis,* 28, 63, 1993.

10. Logan, R.A. and White, I.R., Carba mix is redundant in patch test series, *Contact Dermatitis,* 18, 303, 1988.

11. Andersen K.E. et al., Recommended changes to the standard series, *Contact Dermatitis,* 5, 389, 1988.

12. Lynde, C.W. et al., Patch testing with mercaptobenzothiazole and mercapto mixes, *Contact Dermatitis,* 8, 273, 1982.

13. Cronin E., Rubber, in *Contact Dermatitis,* Cronin E., Ed., Churchill Livingstone, Edinburgh, 1980, p. 714.

14. Menne, T. et al., Patch test reactivity to the PPD-black-rubber-mix (industrial rubber chemicals) and individual ingredients, *Contact Dermatitis,* 26, 354, 1992.

15. Holness, D.L. and Nethercott, J.R., Results of patch testing with a special series of rubber allergens, *Contact Dermatitis,* 36, 207, 1997.

16. McClewsky, P.E. and Swerlic, R.A., Clinical review: Thioureas and allergic contact dermatitis, *Cutis,* 68, 387, 2001.

17. Reid, C.M., van Grutten, M., and Rycroft, R.J.G., Allergic contact dermatitis from ethylbutylthiourea in neoprene, *Contact Dermatitis,* 28, 193, 1993.

18. Castelain, M. and Castelain, P.-Y., Allergic contact dermatitis from cetyl pyridinium chloride in latex gloves, *Contact Dermatitis,* 28, 118, 1993.

19. Wakelin, S.H. et al., Patch testing with natural rubber latex, *Contact Dermatitis,* 40, 89, 1999.

20. Wilkinson, S.M. and Beck, M.H., Allergic contact dermatitis from latex rubber, *Br. J. Dermatol.,* 134, 910, 1996.

21. Gortz, J. and Goos, M., Immediate and late type allergy to latex: Contact urticaria, asthma and contact dermatitis, in *Current Topics in Contact Dermatitis,* Frosch, P.J., Dooms-Goosens, A., Lachapelle, J.M., Rycroft, R.J.G., and Scheper, R.J., Eds, Springer-Verlag, Berlin, 1989, part 5.

22. Wilkinson, S.M. and Burd, R., Latex: A cause of allergic contact eczema in users of natural rubber gloves, *J. Am. Acad. Dermatol.,* 38, 36, 1998.

23. Raulf-Heimsoth, M. et al., Lymphocyte proliferation response to extracts from different latex materials and to the purified latex allergen Hev b 1 (rubber elongation factor), *J. Allergy Clin. Immunol.,* 98, 640, 1996.

24. Parry, E.J. and Beck, M.H., Acute anaphylaxis resulting from routine patch testing with latex, *Contact Dermatitis,* 41, 236, 1999.

12 Allergic Contact Dermatitis: Prognosis

Natalie M. Stone

CONTENTS

I. Prognosis for Allergic Contact Dermatitis 133
References 134

I. PROGNOSIS FOR ALLERGIC CONTACT DERMATITIS

There is little literature concerning the prognosis of allergic contact dermatitis (ACD) as a whole, and even less concerning the prognosis of ACD to natural rubber latex in particular. The prognosis for complete clearance of ACD is generally considered to be poor, for both occupational and nonoccupational allergic contact dermatitis.[1]

Hogan et al. in 1990 reviewed previous studies concerning the prognosis of irritant and allergic occupational dermatitis. They suggested that less than 50% of patients were completely clear of eczema after several years of follow-up.[2]

The prognosis for improvement of occupational ACD is reported to be worse than for irritant contact dermatitis.[3] Some individual allergens are known to cause more chronic disease than others, of which chromate is the classic example.[4] The black rubber antioxidant, *n*-isopropyl-*n*-paraphenylenediamine (IPPD), has also been reported to cause persistent dermatitis in some patients, despite strict avoidance of the allergen.[5]

Rubber ACD is one of the most common causes of occupational ACD.[6] The majority of patients with occupational ACD are thought to clinically improve after avoidance of the allergen.[7] Recent studies have reported a better prognosis for occupational dermatitis than previously suggested. Nethercott and Holness in 1994 reported a retrospective study where 76% of cases of occupational contact dermatitis improved.[8]

Several recent studies of occupational ACD have suggested that length of time exposed to an allergen, before avoidance, is the most important predictor for prognosis.[9] Early detection of ACD, such as to rubber, may be of vital importance in improving the prognosis for occupational ACD.

Reports of ACD to natural latex in the absence of allergy to a rubber additive are at present few and no long-term follow-up has been discussed. Eczema in some cases has however been reported to clear completely after avoidance of latex, suggesting a good prognosis.[10]

REFERENCES

1. Wall, L.M. and Gebauer, K.A., A follow up study of occupational skin disease in Western Australia, *Contact Dermatitis*, 24, 241, 1991.
2. Hogan, H., Dannaker, C.J., and Maibach, H.I., The prognosis of contact dermatitis, *J. Am. Acad. Dermatol.*, 23, 300, 1990.
3. Meding, B. and Swanbeck, G., Consequences of having hand eczema, *Contact Dermatitis*, 23, 6, 1990.
4. Burry, J.N. and Kirk, J., Environmental dermatitis: Chrome cripples, *Med. J. Aust.*, 2, 720, 1975.
5. Alfonzo, C., Allergic contact dermatitis to isopropylaminodiphenylamine (IPPD), *Contact Dermatitis*, 5, 145, 1979.
6. Meyer, J.D. et al., Occupational contact dermatitis in the UK: A surveillance report from EPIDERM and OPRA, *Occup. Med.*, 50, 265, 2000.
7. Goh, C.L., Prognosis of contact and occupational dermatitis, *Clin. Dermatol.*, 15, 655, 1997.
8. Nethercott, J.R. and Holness, D.L., Disease outcome in workers with occupational skin disease, *J. Am. Acad. Dermatol.*, 30, 569, 1994.
9. Adisesh, A., Meyer, J.D., and Cherry, N.M., Prognosis and work absence due to occupational contact dermatitis, *Contact Dermatitis*, 46, 273, 2002.
10. Gottolober, P., Gall, H., and Peter, R.U., Allergic contact dermatitis from natural latex, *Am. J. Contact Dermatol.*, 12, 135, 2001.

13 Latex-Fruit Syndrome

Tanya D. Wright

CONTENTS

I. Introduction 135
II. Latex-Fruit Syndrome 136
    A. Symptoms 136
    B. Latex Proteins and Latex-Fruit Syndrome 136
        1. Hev b 8 (profilin) 136
        2. Hev b 6.02 (hevein) 137
        3. Hev b 7 (patatin-like protein) 137
        4. Hev b 2 (1,3-β-glucanase) 137
        5. Class 1 chitinases 137
    B. Foods Cross-Reacting with Latex 137
III. Conclusions 138
References 138

I. INTRODUCTION

Allergen cross-reactivity appears to be due to IgE antibodies that recognize homologous or structurally similar epitopes on different proteins that are either phylogenically closely related or represent evolutionary conserved structures. Cross-reactivity is referred to when the IgE to one substance recognizes and binds to the same 3 dimensional 5 amino acid sequence of a different substance. It is this that is responsible for the observed clinical and immunological cross-reactivities between different substances such as the large and growing number of plant-derived foods implicated in latex allergy including banana, avocado, chestnut, and kiwi. The cross-reactions observed between latex and pollen (birch, mugwort, and ragweed) allergens provide further evidence of this. Similarly, pollens[1] that share homology with labile proteins in fresh fruits and vegetables cause isolated oral symptoms, which are classically described as oral allergy syndrome.[2]

Other examples of cross-reactivity that are reported from the same phylogenic group include legumes,[1] tree nuts,[2] milk from different species of mammals and eggs from different species of birds,[3] fish, shellfish, and cereal grains.

It should be noted that the clinical relevance of cross-reactive food proteins can be dependent upon various factors including allergen concentration, cooking,[4] route of ingestion (oral or respiratory), exercise, and alcohol consumption.

0-8493-1670-7/05/$0.00+$1.50
© 2005 by CRC Press LLC

135

The prevalence and magnitude of clinical allergy caused by cross-reacting proteins and panallergens (universal allergens) appears to be increasing.[5] This reflects the general increase in atopy and rise in the incidence of allergic disease.[6]

II. LATEX-FRUIT SYNDROME

It is well reported that a significant number of patients who are allergic to latex are also allergic to various plant derived allergens. Approximately 30 to 50% of individuals who are allergic to latex show an associated hypersensitivity to some plant-derived foods, particularly uncooked fresh fruits and vegetables.[7] The foods most frequently involved are banana, avocado, kiwi, and chestnut, although many others of plant origin have been implicated.

In 1991 the first paper was written to describe a patient with latex- and banana-associated allergy.[8] Other authors soon reported several cases of cross-sensitization between latex and different fruits. This association was then formally recognized in 1994[9] as the "latex-fruit syndrome" on the basis of the clinical observation of an unexpectedly high rate of fruit hypersensitivity in patients allergic to latex. It has since been established that the implicated botanical foods are from both fruit and vegetable origin. Where certain pollens are involved because they share homologous proteins, a diagnosis of "latex-fruit-pollen syndrome" is given.

A. SYMPTOMS

Reactions to foods associated with the latex-fruit syndrome and latex-fruit-pollen syndrome have been reported to include local mouth irritation, angiedema, urticaria, asthma, nausea, vomiting, diarrhea, rhinitis, and anaphylaxis.[10]

B. LATEX PROTEINS AND LATEX-FRUIT SYNDROME

In the extensive work undertaken to determine the molecular features of *Hevea brasiliensis*, many protein structures and individual latex allergens have been identified (see Chapter 2). Thirteen of these have received an international nomenclature designation.[11,12]

Four of these proteins have been associated with the latex-fruit syndrome:[13] Hev b 8 (profilin), Hev b 6.02 (hevein), Hev b 7 (patatin-like protein), and Hev b 2 (a β-1,3-glucanase).

1. Hev b 8 (profilin)

The presence of profilin in latex has been established as an important allergen. Profilins are low molecular weight proteins found in all eukaryotic cells where their function is to regulate the actin cytoskeleton with their actin-binding proteins.[14] A link between latex profilin and food profilins is widely accepted, and it has been suggested that primary sensitization to latex profilin in the majority of cases takes place via pollen or food profilins.[15]

The role of profilin in allergy to certain exotic fruits was investigated[16] and it was concluded that profilin is an important mediator of IgE cross-reactivity between pollen and exotic fruits. Because the ubiquitous profilins share immunogenicity, they have been described as the panallergens of various plant species.[17] This is significant in their role as IgE mediators in allergy, and herein the link with latex allergy lies.

2. Hev b 6.02 (hevein)

Hevein and the hevein precursor prohevein (Hev b 6.01) have been identified as major allergens in latex. At the N-terminus, there is the hevein domain, which binds chitin, a polysaccharide found on the cell walls of fungi.

Certain fruits and vegetables produce an enzyme called a class 1 chitinase in response to a fungal attack. These class 1 chitinases have a chitin-binding domain, which is very similar to the latex protein hevein domain.[18] If an individual develops IgE antibodies to the hevein fragment in latex, it is likely that the IgE will also recognize the homologous protein structure in fruits and vegetables containing these class 1 chitinases and a clinical reaction to these may be evoked.

Identifying these proteins that are homologous to known allergens allows potentially cross-reactive allergens to be predicted. The value of this information in the prevention and management of these clinical reactions should not be underestimated.

3. Hev b 7 (patatin-like protein)

The latex protein Hev b 7 (patatin-like protein) shows cross-reactivity with the analogous protein in potato (patatin). It has been identified as a major cross-reactive protein in latex-associated potato allergy.[19]

4. Hev b 2 (1,3-β-glucanase)

This latex protein has been found to cross-react with proteins present in bell pepper. Clinical reactions from this have been noted.[20]

5. Class 1 chitinases

Chitinases are proteins found in a wide variety of seed-producing plants. They have a defensive role within these plants.

Class 1 chitinases have been described as the most important panallergens in fruits associated with the latex-fruit syndrome and are the major allergens that are responsible for the latex-fruit syndrome. These enzymes contain an N-terminal hevein-like domain homologous to the latex hevein, and a larger catalytic domain. Banana, chestnut, and avocado are examples of plant-derived foods that contain class 1 chitinases with an N-terminal hevein-like domain.

B. FOODS CROSS-REACTING WITH LATEX

It should be noted that the more proteins a food contains that are homologous to latex, the more likely it is that the food will cross-react with latex.

Table 13.1 indicates foods that have been reported to have a high incidence of cross-reactivity with latex and the main protein that has been implicated.

TABLE 13.1
Foods Cross-Reacting with Latex
and the Main Proteins Implicated

Food	Protein
Avocado[23,25,26]	Class 1 chitinase
Banana[24,27]	Class 1 chitinase
Chestnut[23,27,28]	Class 1 chitinase
Kiwi[9,29]	Class 1 chitinase
Passion fruit[29]	Class 1 chitinase
Papaya[29]	Class 1 chitinase
Mango[27,28,29]	Class 1 chitinase
Tomato[27,28,29]	Class 1 chitinase
Bell pepper[22]	1,3-β-glucanase and profilin
Potato[20,21]	Patatin-like protein
Celery[17,20]	Prolifin

III. CONCLUSIONS

Making a diagnosis and clinical evaluation[30] requires a careful and detailed history, physical examination, laboratory evaluation, and in some cases oral food challenges.[31] An experienced practitioner is essential in the execution and interpretation of tests[32] including skin prick tests, specific IgE (RAST), elimination diets, and any challenges undertaken.

It has been recommended that patients allergic to latex are tested for potential sensitivity to foods commonly associated with latex allergy, and also to foods associated with tree or grass pollen allergy.[33]

Unreliable histories and false positive and false negative skin prick tests and specific IgE (RAST) tests can mask or hinder diagnoses.[34] It has been reported that serological tests appear to be of low significance for the prediction of food allergy in latex-allergic patients.[35] It is these limitations that have hindered the progression of evaluating classical allergens and where cross-reactivity exists, these problems are magnified.

Nutritional advice[36] and psychological support should be made available to these patients, particularly if the diagnosis is a recent one.

REFERENCES

1. Valenta, R. and Kraft, D., Type 1 allergic reactions to plant-derived food: A consequence of primary sensitization to pollen allergens, *J. Allergy Clin. Immunol.*, 97, 893, 1996.
2. Yagami, T., Allergies to cross-reactive plant proteins. Latex fruit syndrome is comparable with pollen food allergy syndrome, *Int. Arch. Allergy Immunol.*, 128, 271, 2002.

3. Bernhisel-Broadbent, J. and Sampson, H.A., Cross allergenicity in the legume botanical family in children with food hypersensitivity, *J. Allergy Clin. Immunol.*, 83, 435, 1989.
4. Sicherer, S.H., Burks, A.W., and Sampson, H.A., Clinical features of acute allergic reactions to peanut and tree nuts in children, *Pediatrics*, 102, e6, 1998.
5. Bousquet, J. et al., Scientific criteria and the selection of allergenic foods for product labeling, *Allergy*, 53, 3, 1998.
6. Bernhisel-Broadbent, J., Strausse, D., and Sampson, H.A., Fish hypersensitivity II: Clinical relevance of altered fish allergenicity caused by various preparation methods, *J. Allergy Clin. Immunol.*, 90, 622, 1992.
7. Sicherer, S., Clinical implications of cross-reactive food allergens, *J. Allergy Clin. Immunol.*, 108, 881, 2001.
8. Sicherer, S., Advances in anaphylaxis and hypersensitivity reactions to foods, drugs, and insect venom, *Adv. Asth. Allergy Immunol.*, 111, S829–S834, 2003.
9. Blanco, C., Latex fruit syndrome, *Curr. Allergy Asth. Rep.*, 31, 47, 2003.
10. M'Raihi, L. et al., Cross reactivity between latex and banana, *J. Allergy Clin. Immunol.*, 87, 129, 1991.
11. Blanco, C. et al., Latex allergy: Clinical features and cross reactivity with fruits, *Ann. Allergy*, 73, 309, 1994.
12. Kim, K.T. and Hussain, H., Prevalence of food allergy in 137 latex-allergic patients, *Allergy Asth. Proc.*, 20, 95, 1999.
13. Poley, G.E., Jr. and Slater, J.E., Latex allergy, *J. Allergy Clin. Immunol.*, 105, 1054, 2000.
14. ftp://ftp.biobase.dk/pub/who-iuis/allergen.list.
15. Wagner, S. and Breiteneder, H., The latex-fruit syndrome, *Biochem. Soc. Trans.*, 30, 935, 2002.
16. Carlson, I. et al., Actin polymerization is influenced by profilin, a low molecular weight protein in non-muscle cells, *J. Molec. Biol.*, 115, 465, 1977.
17. Ganglberger, E. et al., Hev b 8, the *Hevea brasiliensis* latex profilin, is a cross-reactive allergen of latex, plant foods and pollen, *Int. Arch. Allergy Immunol.*, 125, 216, 2001.
18. Reindl, J. et al., IgE reactivity to profilin in pollen-sensitized subjects with adverse reactions to banana and pineapple, *Int. Arch. Allergy Immunol.*, 128, 105, 2002.
19. Valenta, R. et al., Profilins constitute a novel family of functional plant pan-allergens. *J. Exp. Med.*, 175, 377, 1992.
20. Ebner, C. et al., Identification of allergens in apple, pear, celery, carrot and potato: Cross-reactivity with pollen allergens, *Monogr. Allergy*, 32, 73, 1996.
21. Schmidt, M.H., Raulf-Heimsoth, M., and Posch, A., Evaluation of patatin as a major cross-reactive allergen in latex-induced potato allergy, *Ann. Allergy Asth. Immunol*, 89, 613, 2002.
22. Wagner, S. et al., Bell pepper is involved in the latex-fruit syndrome based on cross-reactivities to Hev b 2, Hev B 8, and a kDa protein, *J. Allergy Clin. Immunol.*, 109, 1034, 2002.
23. Blanco, C. et al., Class 1 chitinases as potential panallergens involved in the latex-fruit syndrome, *J. Allergy Clin. Immunol.*, 103, 507, 1999.
24. Sanchez-Monge, R. et al., Isolation and characterization of major banana allergens: Identification as fruit class 1 chitinases, *Clin. Exp. Allergy*, 29, 673, 1999.
25. Posch, A. et al., Class 1 endochitinase containing a hevein domain is the causative allergen in latex-associated avocado allergy, *Clin. Exp. Allergy*, 29, 667, 1999.
26. Chen, Z. et al., Identification of hevein (Hev 6.02) in Hevea latex as a major cross-reacting allergen with avocado fruit in patients with latex allergy, *J. Allergy Clin. Immunol.*, 102, 476, 1998.

27. Salcedo, G., Diaz-Perales, A., and Sanchez-Monge, R., The role of plant panallergens in sensitization of natural rubber latex, *Curr. Opin. Allergy Clin. Immunol.*, 1, 177, 2001.

28. Diaz-Perales, A. et al., What is the role of the hevein-like domain of fruit class 1 chitinases in their allergenic capacity? *Clin. Exp. Allergy*, 32, 448, 2002.

29. Diaz-Perales, A. et al., Cross-reactions in the latex-fruit syndrome: A relevant role of chitinases but not of complex asparagine-linked glycans, *J. Allergy Clin. Immunol.*, 104, 681, 1999.

30. Sampson, M.D., Food Allergy, *J. Allergy Clin. Immunol.*, 111, S540–S5477, 2003.

31. Sicherer, S.H., Food allergy: When and how to perform oral food challenges, *Pediatr. Allergy Immunol.*, 10, 226, 1999.

32. Sampson, H.A., Food allergy. Part 2: Diagnosis and management, *J. Allergy Clin. Immunol.*, 103, 981, 1999.

33. Levy, D.A. et al., Allergic sensitization and clinical reactions to latex, food and pollen in adult patients, *Clin. Exp. Allergy*, 30, 270, 2000.

34. Sicherer, S., Clinical implications of cross reactive food allergens, *J. Allergy Clin. Immunol.*, 108, 881, 2001.

35. Brehler, R. et al., "Latex-fruit syndrome": frequency of cross-reacting IgE antibodies, *Allergy*, 52, 404, 1997.

36. Perkin, J.E., The latex and food allergy connection, *J. Am. Diet Assoc.*, 100, 1381, 2000.

14 Irritant Dermatitis Due to Occlusive Gloves: Clinical Manifestations

Priyanka Singh, Mayanka Singh,
Mahbub M. U. Chowdhury,
and Howard I. Maibach

CONTENTS

I.   Introduction 141
II. Symptoms 142
III. Occlusion 142
     A.   Long-Term Study 143
          Group A 143
          Group B 143
     B.   Short-Term Study 143
          Group A 143
          Group B 143
IV. Conclusions 145
References 145

I. INTRODUCTION

Allergic contact dermatitis and contact urticaria have been associated with latex intolerance, however, irritation has been less well studied. Unlike allergic contact dermatitis, irritation is due to nonimmunological factors.

Dermatitis from gloves may be due to allergic contact dermatitis or recurrent immunologic contact urticaria (ICU). The reactions could be due to disinfectants used prior to the use of gloves. Also, repeated handwashing and incomplete drying can lead to irritation. In addition, detergents used can account for further deterioration of skin barrier function. Cumulative irritant dermatitis is the most common type of contact dermatitis.

II. SYMPTOMS

Irritant contact dermatitis (ICD) is inflammation of the skin due to chemicals that directly damage skin, and may be acute and/or chronic. Acute ICD produces a burnlike blistering reaction at the site of contact due to a single strong irritant. Contact with weaker irritant may cause cumulative ICD. Initially, it appears as red, scaly, fissured skin as well as dry scaly eczema on the hands and the finger webs.[1] A study conducted by Field and King correlated irritant contact dermatitis (ICD) with wearing gloves.[1] This questionnaire-based study completed by Swedish periodontists associated latex glove use and/or handwashing to skin problems. Skin irritation ranged from mild dryness and itching of the hands to blistering and, in a few cases, to bleeding and desquamation of the skin.

Shmunes and Darby examined bacterial endotoxin in latex gloves.[2] The reaction due to endotoxin included fever, chills, and hypotension also known as Shwartzman reaction and local Shwartzman reaction. An increase in the production of histamine was also noted. Furthermore, this increase in histamine suggested that endotoxin is one of the factors responsible for the deterioration of the cardiovasculature. However, this paper was published in 1984 when the biochemistry of endotoxins was not clearly known.

In addition to endotoxins, gender plays a role in skin irritation due to rubber gloves. In a questionnaire completed by 1200 practicing dentists, female respondents were more likely to have experienced skin irritation compared to male respondents.[3] As many as 94 (37.6%) female respondents experienced skin irritation in contrast to 27.1% of male respondents. The duration gloves were worn was another factor that affected skin irritation. Routine glove wearers were more likely to experience skin irritation than occasional glove wearers. Of the routine glove wearers, 31.6% complained about skin irritation, whereas only 20% of occasional glove wearers reported similar symptoms including nail splitting, nail dryness, and infection of the fingernail bed. Occlusion was considered an important factor in the production of skin irritation.

The growth of bacteria, which can cause irritation, is supported by occlusion. Occlusion alters hydration, skin pH, CO_2 emission rate, and surface lipids.[4]

III. OCCLUSION

Ramsing and Agner performed two studies based on long-term and short-term experimental exposure.[5,6] In both experiments two groups were formed (Group A and Group B). In Group A, one hand wore an occlusive glove and the other served as a control. In Group B (long-term study) both hands wore occlusive gloves. Also, a cotton glove was worn underneath the occlusive glove on either of the hands. In Group B (short term study) both hands were immersed in sodium lauryl sulfate (SLS) solution to simulate a wet working environment and an occlusive glove was worn on one hand. In the long-term exposure experiment, an occlusive glove was worn for 6 hours a day for 14 days, and in the short-term experiment gloves were worn for 6 hours a day for 3 days. In both experiments, transepidermal water loss

(TEWL), skin hydration by electrical capacitance, and inflammation by erythema index was measured.

A. LONG-TERM STUDY[5]

Group A

At the end of 2 weeks, there was a significant increase in TEWL compared to the control hand, which signified a deteriorating effect on the skin barrier function. In addition, on day 3 and day 8 there was an increase in electrical capacitance, which indicates skin dryness. The erythema index showed no significant difference. Finally, in the clinical observations, volunteers suffered from barely perceptible erythema to well defined erythema, papules, and scaling to slight inflammation.

Group B

There was a significant increase in TEWL on the hand with the occlusive glove compared to the hand with the cotton glove. However, electrical capacitance on the hand with the cotton glove increased significantly on day 11. The erythema index again showed no significant differences between the hands. In contrast, in the clinical observations, three volunteers reported skin irritation. They reported redness at first, then papules, and later scaling and slight inflammation. The hand with the cotton glove remained normal.

B. SHORT-TERM STUDY[6]

Group A

Similar to the other studies there was an increase in TEWL on the occluded hand in comparison to the control. In contrast, electrical capacitance did not change significantly with no significant differences between the two hands. After an hour of glove removal, the erythema index was significantly lower on the occluded hand. In the clinical observations, 70% had a spongy white appearance on the occluded hand.

Group B

The TEWL values were significantly different on day 5, with no significant difference between day 2 and day 7. A significant decrease in electrical capacitance was observed between the hands. No significant difference was found between the hands in the erythema index. The clinical observations included dryness with scaling and slight erythema. In both experiments, deterioration of the skin barrier function was noted, which can lead to irritation.[5,6]

Skin is more permeable to some chemicals secondary to occlusion. 2-mercaptobenzothiazole (MBT) and 2,2-dithio-bis-benzothiazole (MBTS) are suspected irritants, as well as allergens in latex. A study funded by the U.S. Consumer Product Safety Commission quantified the amount of MBT and MBTS leached out of several solutions (see Table 14.1 and Table 14.2).[7]

TABLE 14.1

Total Amount of MBT (μg/ml per cm² of sample) Leached after 7 days from Rubber Products into Various Solutions

Solution	Rubber Heel	Rubber Glove
Normal saline	3.1	96.3
Synthetic sweat (pH 5.6)	0.6	97.7
Synthetic sweat (pH 6.8)	3.2	66.2
Synthetic sweat (pH 7.8)	2.6	67.6
Human plasma	2.6	20.7

TABLE 14.2

Total Amounts of MBT/MBTS Removed from Products in Leachate and by Soxhlet Extraction Given as μg/cm² of Sample and μg/g of Sample

Leaching Solution	MBT	MBTS
Rubber Glove		
Normal saline	0.16	—
Synthetic sweat (pH 5.4)	0.03	—
Synthetic sweat (pH 6.8)	0.13	—
Synthetic sweat (pH 7.80)	0.12	—
Human plasma	0.12	—
Rubber Heel		
Normal saline	29.5	82.2
Synthetic sweat (pH 5.4)	26.8	37.7
Synthetic sweat (pH 6.8)	18.6	65
Synthetic sweat (pH 7.80)	18.7	7.5
Human plasma	8.7	2.9

Source: Modified from Emmett, E. A., 1994.[7]

Stein et al. documented disinfectants increasing the concentration of irritant chemicals that permeate through the skin.[8] Zinc dimethyldithiocarbamate (ZDMC) and mercaptobenzothiazole (MBT) are chemicals found in latex gloves. It was recorded that 0.7 mg of ZDMC and 2 mg of MBT per hand and per day was extracted (see Table 14.3).

Some type of irritation from prolonged rubber occlusion is almost routine. The clinical picture is obfuscated by a biological factor, that is, irritation is not readily observed on the palm or dorsal hand. In a controlled experiment Charbonnier demonstrated that the forearm produced more discernable erythema than the dorsal hand.[9]

TABLE 14.3
Comparison of Concentration and Mass Fraction
Extracted for Both Extraction Methods

	BGA-Method with 100 ml 1hr/40 °C		Extraction with 2.5 ml 45 min/40°C	
Substance	Concentration mg/L	w_{ex} mg/g	Concentration mg/L	w_{ex} mg/g
ZDMC	4.1	0.041	13	0.0053
MBT	6.1	0.061	40	0.017

Source: Modified from Stein, G., Hampel, M., and Wunstel, E., 2002.[8]

IV. CONCLUSIONS

Clearly part of the damage results from occlusion, as evidenced by the controlled experiments that showed that a cotton glove-protected hand had less damage than the noncotton glove-protected hand.[5,6] However, this does not completely indict the occlusion as the cotton glove could absorb the leached irritants.[4,8] Because of the frequency of the symptoms of irritation, we believe that considerable advances in glove technology to decrease irritation could lead to worker satisfaction and financial gain for innovative glove manufacturers.

REFERENCES

1. Field, E.A. and King, C.M., Skin problems associated with routine wearing of protective gloves in dental practice, *Br. Dent. J.,* 168, 281, 1990.
2. Shmunes, E. and Darby, T., Contact dermatitis due to endotoxin in irradiated latex gloves, *Contact Dermatitis,* 10, 240, 1984.
3. Burke, F.J.T., Wilson, N.H.F., and Cheung, S.W., Factors associated with skin irritation of the hands experienced by general dental practitioners, *Contact Dermatitis,* 32, 35, 1995.
4. Aly, R. et al., Effect of prolonged occlusion on the microbial flora, pH, carbon dioxide and transepidermal water loss on human skin. *J. Inv. Dermatol.,* 71, 378, 1978.
5. Ramsing, D.W. and Agner, T., Effect of glove occlusion on human skin (I), *Contact Dermatitis,* 34, 1, 1996.
6. Ramsing, D.W. and Agner, T., Effect of glove occlusion on human skin (II), *Contact Dermatitis,* 34, 258, 1996.
7. Emmett, E.A. et al., Skin elicitation threshold of ethyl butyl thiourea and mercaptobenzothiazole with relative leaching from sensitizing products, *Contact Dermatitis,* 30, 85, 1994.
8. Stein, G., Hampel, M., and Wunstel, E., Latexhandschuche im Hautkontakt-gibt es Risiken? *Allergologie,* 25, 593, 2002.
9. Charbonnier, V. et al., Open application assay in investigation of subclinical irritant dermatitis induced by sodium lauryl sulfate (SLS) in man: Advantage of squamometry, *Skin Res. Technol.,* 4, 244, 1998.

15 Irritation Dermatitis Due to Occlusive Gloves: Predictive Testing

Mayanka Singh, Priyanka Singh,
Mahbub M. U. Chowdhury,
and Howard I. Maibach

CONTENTS

I.   Introduction 147
II. Methods 147
III. Testing Paradigm for Predictive Testing 149
     A.   21-Day Cumulative Irritation Assay 149
     B.   Exaggerated Use Studies 149
IV. Conclusions 149
References 149

I. INTRODUCTION

Clinical intolerance to latex gloves may be due to allergy (allergic contact dermatitis or immunologic contact urticaria) and irritation. Irritant dermatitis is due to nonimmunological factors and it is the most common reaction to latex gloves.[1] Clinical identification of glove-induced irritation is discussed further in Chapter 14.

II. METHODS

Cumulative irritancy tests were developed to identify products causing irritant reaction in users. Patch tests are used to estimate cumulative irritancy. Cumulative irritation may be caused by chemicals that do not produce acute irritation from a single application but induce irritation following repeated application.[2]

Bioengineering devices are used in the following studies to quantify irritant response. These can measure electrical impedance, carbon dioxide emission, electrolyte flux, capacitance, laser Doppler velocimetry, and skin reflectance. A common bioengineering device is the evaporimeter (Tewameter™) used to measure transepidermal water loss (TEWL). The advantage of these devices is a noninvasive quantification of some functional skin parameters that are not visible to the naked eye.

Graves tested the occlusive effects of latex gloves on the barrier properties of the stratum corneum.[3] The method used for the study was patch testing with glove patches. Four patches were situated on volunteers, two on each arm. On day one, the first site had a 4-hour occlusion with glove material, the second had an 8-hour occlusion with glove material, and the third site was an unoccluded control. On day 2, the fourth site was an empty Tegaderm® dressing. Four types of measurements were performed including hyperemic response to topical hexyl nicotinate/percorneal permeability, transepidermal water loss, skin surface roughness and skin surface compliance. The percorneal permeability results showed temporary increase by the use of occlusive gloves. The Tegaderm® had no effect.

The TEWL results for the 4- and 8-hour occlusion showed an increase in barrier permeability. However, the 8-hour glove occlusion did not produce a proportional increase in barrier permeability. The skin roughness was significantly reduced in terms of roughness parameters (Ra) and (Rz) by the 4- and 8-hour occlusion. The parameter Ra (μm) is the arithmetic mean roughness value and the parameter Rz (μm) is the 10-point height, that is the average of the height of the five highest peaks plus the depth of the five deepest valleys over the evaluation length. The conclusion was temporary impairment in barrier function is caused by glove patches.

Metsumura et al. performed a study measuring the effects of simple occlusion.[4] He used polyethylene foam closed chambers for 24 hours. The results showed a decrease in water vapor permeability, which suggests induction of morphological alterations. The study implied simple occlusion could act as a primary irritant.

Another study by Graves required volunteers to wear whole gloves for 6-hour periods for 2 days.[4] The results show significant increase in TEWL readings even after the overnight recovery period. The study also suggested that repeated occlusion by gloves might have a cumulative effect.

The role of endotoxins in irradiated latex gloves causing irritant dermatitis was studied in a worker subjected to minor trauma.[5] The worker performed usage tests with purposeful wearing of the gloves for 20 minutes. Twenty-four hours later the patient showed erythema, which was linked to bacterial endotoxin in latex gloves. The study concluded that irradiated sterilized gloves might contain significant endotoxin levels. The irradiation of the bacteria would increase endotoxin level when the bacterial count is increased. This study was published in 1983 and the data and conclusion of the effects of endotoxins requires updating and further investigation.

Ramsing and Agner performed a study on glove occlusion on normal and compromised human skin.[6] The gloves were hypoallergenic and nonlatex. Two studies were performed. In Study A, volunteers wore a glove on normal skin, 6 hours a day for 3 days. In Study B, volunteers wore a glove on sodium lauryl sulfate (SLS)-compromised skin. The skin barrier function was evaluated by measurement of TEWL, skin hydration by electrical capacitance, and inflammation by erythema index. The results of Study A did not show significant change in water barrier function. Study B showed a significantly negative effect on SLS-compromised skin and, therefore, SLS had an irritant effect in glove-occluded hands.

III. TESTING PARADIGM FOR PREDICTIVE TESTING

Our current paradigm submits test gloves to the following:

- 21 day cumulative irritancy
- Exaggerated use studies (with or without additional irritants such as detergents)

A. 21-DAY CUMULATIVE IRRITATION ASSAY

This assay permits evaluation of multiple samples — in a facile, robust, and comparative manner. Principles are discussed by Phillips et al.[7] and updated by Maibach.[2] New samples are compared to a standard of known clinical performance. Endpoints are visual and via bioinstrumentation.[8,9] Surprisingly, some commercial gloves demonstrate visual changes within 3 weeks.

B. EXAGGERATED USE STUDIES

These studies demonstrate changes on the hands, which are not observed on the back, presumably related to the difference in the functional anatomy of the hands compared to the back. Bioengineering instruments demonstrate functional changes not readily seen by morphology. "Stress" tests such as adding soaps and/or surfactants to the exaggerated use test further magnify alterations.

The goal is to identify glove manufacturing methods leading to a higher clinical tolerance whether the mechanism is leaching of irritants from the gloves and/or occlusion of skin. For additional detail on the clinical complexities of glove-induced irritation and dermatitis see Chapter 14.

IV. CONCLUSIONS

Cumulative irritancy tests are useful in predicting irritant dermatitis caused by chemicals that do not produce acute irritation from a single application but induce irritation following repeated application. Bioengineering methods are useful for predicting irritant dermatitis. Further investigations to identify the mechanisms involved in the induction of irritant dermatitis would provide predictive testing methods for irritant dermatitis.

REFERENCES

1. Hunt, L.W. et al., A medical-center-wide, multidisciplinary approach to the problem of natural rubber latex allergy, *J. O. E. M.,* 38(8), 765, 1996.
2. Patil, M. S., Patrick, P., and Maibach, H.I., Animal, human, and *in vitro* test methods for predicting skin irritation, *Dermatoxicology,* 5, 411, 1995.
3. Graves, C. J., Edwards, C., and Marks, R., The occlusive effects of protective gloves on the barrier properties of the stratum corneum. *Curr. Probl. Dermatol.,* 23, 87, 1995.

4. Matsumara, H. et al., Effect of occlusion on human skin, *Contact Dermatitis,* 33, 231, 1995.

5. Shumnes, E. and Darby, T., Contact dermatitis due to endotoxin in irradiated latex gloves, *Contact Dermatitis,* 10, 240, 1984.

6. Ramsing, D. W. and Agner, T., Effect of glove occlusion on human skin (I): Short-term experimental exposure, *Contact Dermatitis,* 34, 1, 1996.

7. Phillips, L. et al., A comparison of rabbit and human skin responses to certain irritants, *Toxicol. Appl. Pharmacol.,* 21, 369, 1972.

8. Elsner, P., Berardesca, E., and Maibach, H. I., *Bioengineering of the skin: Water and the stratum corneum,* Vol. 1, CRC Press, Boca Raton, FL, 1994.

9. Elsner, P., Berardesca, E., and Maibach, H. I., *Bioengineering of the skin: Cutaneous blood flow and erythema,* Vol. 2, CRC Press, Boca Raton, FL, 1995.

16 Management of Hand Dermatitis

*Graham A. Johnston, Nicolas Nicolaou,
and Mahbub M. U. Chowdhury*

CONTENTS

I. Introduction 151
II. Important Issues in the Management of Hand Dermatitis 152
   A. Hand Protection with Gloves 152
   B. Use of Soap Substitutes and Moisturizers 153
   C. Avoidance of Irritants 155
   D. Prognosis and Ongoing Management 156
III. Treatment of Hand Dermatitis 157
   A. Emollients 157
   B. Corticosteroids 158
      1. Topical Corticosteroids 158
      2. Intralesional Steroids 159
      3. Systemic Corticosteroids 159
   C. Topical and Systemic Antibiotics 159
   D. Photochemotherapy 159
   E. Systemic Immunosuppressives 160
      1. Cyclosporin 160
      2. Azathioprine 160
   F. Topical Immunosuppressives 160
   G. Other Modalities 160
References 160
Appendix 16.1: Information Sheet for Patients with Hand Dermatitis 163

I. INTRODUCTION

This chapter covers the practical management of hand dermatitis. It gives suggestions as to how to best approach a patient who has been diagnosed as having either irritant or allergic contact hand dermatitis. Much of the advice also applies to patients with other dermatitic eruptions of the hand in association with atopy or type I or type IV natural rubber latex allergy.

The chapter offers practical instructions for the patient to follow and, where relevant, gives the background studies and evidence base from which these recommendations are drawn. These suggestions are summarized and simplified in an information sheet that can be given to the patient to reinforce the individual points made during the consultation. The information sheet in use is a modified version of several excellent examples[1,2] already published in the literature and is divided into four subheadings to aid the understanding and focus the actions of the patient with hand dermatitis.

The first part of the chapter is also divided into these four subheadings, and the second part covers the main treatments the physician will want to consider when managing a patient with hand dermatitis. In addition, a suggested treatment algorithm for the clinician is given that is also useful for the patient with more severe disease when discussing a treatment plan.

II. IMPORTANT ISSUES IN THE MANAGEMENT OF HAND DERMATITIS

A. HAND PROTECTION WITH GLOVES

An increased awareness of the risks of developing irritant and allergic contact dermatitis in the home and the workplace has led to an increased interest in both the usage of gloves and adverse events attributable to the usage of these gloves.

Protective gloves are one of the key elements in the management of primary and secondary contact dermatitis. Gloves intended for the protection of the skin of the user are referred to as personal protective equipment (PPE) unless they are used for medical applications to prevent contamination and infection where they are referred to as medical devices.[3] Both uses are covered by extensive legislation concerning the design, construction, and suitability for the various tasks required of them (see Chapter 19).

The materials used for the manufacture of protective gloves are natural rubber latex, synthetic rubber, textile fibers, leather, and several polymeric materials. The protective effect of these different glove materials is dependent on both the thickness of the glove and composition of these materials. The breakthrough time increases as the thickness of the glove increases but this does not occur in a linear fashion.[4] The same generic material obtained from different manufacturers can have different chemical resistance due to variation in polymer formulation. In addition, the barrier effect of different generic materials can be very variable. Finally, the quality and therefore protective effect of gloves of the same material can differ due to variations in the manufacturing process and the composition of additives.[5]

If the patient is to use gloves for domestic tasks such as washing dishes and clothes they should be asked to purchase plastic or polyvinyl chloride (PVC) gloves rather than rubber since the latter can cause an allergic contact dermatitis.[6] Indeed gloves are the commonest cause of rubber dermatitis and the allergen is usually a thiuram.[7]

The patients should be informed that gloves should not be worn for more than 15 to 20 minutes at a time and that if water enters the glove it should be taken off immediately. The patient can help to minimize the effects of contaminants by turning the gloves inside out and rinsing them in hot running water several times a week before allowing them to dry completely.

The penetration (leakage) of chemicals refers to the flow through seams, pinholes, and other imperfections. Gloves for industrial and medical use are subject to tests to assess penetration and leakage respectively. However the inside surface of gloves commonly becomes contaminated with the chemicals covering the outside when users take the glove on and off during the course of a working day for changes in tasks, mealtimes, and so forth. This negates any benefits of glove usage and hastens the development of irritant or allergic contact dermatitis due to the occlusive effect of the glove. The patient needs to be made aware of this problem and instructed that if the inside of the glove becomes contaminated with chemicals or soaps both gloves are to be rinsed out immediately and left to dry inside out. The patient should be reminded that if the gloves develop a hole or tear they should be discarded immediately.

Cotton gloves can be used under plastic gloves to soak up sweat that would otherwise irritate the skin although some authorities believe that this simply potentiates the occlusive effect of gloves on sweat.[8] These cotton liners should only be worn a few times before they are washed. Cotton gloves can also be very useful for "dry" household chores. The patient should be told to purchase several pairs of plastic and cotton gloves at a time for use in the kitchen, bathroom, and at work. They should also be reminded to use heavy duty fabric gloves when doing any gardening, "do-it-yourself," and outdoor work and to wear gloves when outdoors in cold weather to prevent the hands drying, cracking, and chapping.

Recommendations have been made on the suitability of different glove materials for handling different groups of chemicals. For example, gloves made of polyvinyl alcohol materials are suitable for the handling of hydrocarbons whereas gloves made of neoprene rubber are more suitable for contact with alkalis, organic, and inorganic acids.[9] Many acrylates rapidly penetrate through the majority of surgical rubber and vinyl gloves.[10]

As has been stated previously, while extensive data is available on the penetration of clothing and gloves by contactants, prevention of contamination of the inside of the glove when putting them on and taking them off is often of far more importance. The actual protection afforded by gloves depends also on manufacturing quality, glove thickness, concentration of contactant, the duration of contact, and environmental temperature and humidity.[11] It should also be remembered that talcum powder (talc) used in many gloves is also a skin irritant.[12] Up-to-date information on protective gloves and their uses can be obtained from several databases.[13]

B. USE OF SOAP SUBSTITUTES AND MOISTURIZERS

Moisturizers, which may contain lipids and humectants, are applied to the skin to improve the signs and symptoms of dry skin conditions (see Chapter 17).[14] Lipids such as petrolatum act by forming an inert occlusive membrane on the epidermal surface. Low molecular weight humectants such as glycerine, lactic acid, and urea are absorbed into the stratum corneum and increase hydration by attracting water.[15]

As well as binding water, urea is also thought to increase penetration of other topically applied substances, reduce the effect of irritant stimuli, and be antipruritic.[16]

Normal soap and water can be very irritating to the hands of a patient with dermatitis. Patients should be told that when washing their hands, either at work or at home, to always use lukewarm (preferably running) water and a moisturizer as a soap substitute. They should be advised to dry the skin carefully with a clean towel and pay particular attention to the interdigital spaces where irritants can accumulate.

Moisturizers used as soap substitutes can either be a water-based paraffin containing cream such as Aqueous Cream BP or, for more heavy duty uses, the paraffin-based Emulsifying Ointment BP. Conversely, and for the ease of application and increased patient compliance, soap substitutes should be chosen so that they can also be used as moisturizers applied directly to the skin to form a protective layer. Moisturizers have not only been shown to be important in the treatment of established soap or detergent induced irritant contact dermatitis,[17] but have also been shown to have a preventative role in the development of irritant dermatitis both in experimental domestic situations and in real-life work situations.[18]

Ideally, the patient should be prescribed several large tubs of moisturizer/soap substitute, which can then be placed next to every sink both at home and at work. Smaller tubes to carry around in a bag or in the car should also be given. The patient should also be instructed to use the soap substitute as a general moisturizer and be reminded that these products are safe to apply to all areas of the skin even in children. The patient should be instructed to apply them several times a day or whenever their skin feels dry or itchy.

While experimental single applications of moisturizers do not cause long-lasting effects, the repeated application of a moisturizer for as little as twice daily for one week produces prolonged increases in physiological markers such as skin conductance and, by implication, skin hydration.[19]

Barrier creams are also referred to as protective ointments or "invisible gloves" (see Chapter 17). They are designed to prevent or reduce the penetration and absorption of various hazardous materials into the skin and replace protective clothing in situations where personal protective equipment such as gloves, sleeves, or faceguards cannot be safely or conveniently used.[20] While they are often used in the management of contact dermatitis, actual benefits have not been conclusively proven and indeed some authorities argue that they exacerbate rather then ameliorate the situation.[15] Any benefit is probably due to their beneficial effects on the stratum corneum as moisturizers rather than as barriers in their own right.[9] They are therefore recommended only for use with low-grade irritants such as water, detergents, and cutting oils.

Active barrier creams are proposed to work by the use of active ingredients that trap or transform allergens but they are also now thought to be generally ineffective.[20] Barrier creams do not offer complete skin protection if this is assessed solely as protection of the barrier function of the skin or protection of skin hydration,[21] but they do offer partial protection that may be useful. Water-in-oil creams can be protective against irritants such as alkalis and detergents present in water but only for a limited time period. Oil-in-water creams however are of no use against solvents.[20]

The prescriber must remember that some commercially obtainable creams contain fragrances and preservatives such as bronopol or lanolin and be alert to the possibility of contact sensitization to the barrier cream itself. Recent experimental data on the efficacy of barrier creams is available[15,21]

C. AVOIDANCE OF IRRITANTS

Irritant contact dermatitis is the commonest cause of exogenous hand dermatitis. In a study of hand eczema in over 1900 patients in the Netherlands,[22] 50% of cases were diagnosed as irritant contact dermatitis. Medical workers, caterers, cleaners, and housekeepers are particularly at risk. Indeed anyone who, in the course of their occupational or domestic tasks, washes his or her hands frequently may develop hand dermatitis leading to the use in the past of such terms as "housewife's eczema" or "dishpan hands."

Individuals vary in their ability to react to irritants. One prospective study of trainee hairdressers observed the development of clinical hand dermatitis and sensitization and compared this with the subjects' irritant threshold to sodium lauryl sulphate (SLS). The development of hand dermatitis was associated with a lower irritant threshold.[23] A similar association was not found for sensitization.

Eliminating the cause (or more often causes) of irritant contact dermatitis is not a simple task. However, since endogenous factors such as constitutional hand dermatitis cannot be changed, it becomes clear that avoidance of irritants is of paramount importance. The success of irritant avoidance depends greatly on the compliance of the patient. It is important to counsel the patient that systematic protection of the hand is important, and that avoidance of irritants plays a large part in this. It also has to be realistically assumed that some patients will find it impossible to follow these instructions categorically. For these patients, partial irritant avoidance is still important.

All patients should be given a hand care information sheet (Appendix 16.1). The patient should be asked to read this carefully several times and then try to use these guidelines as fastidiously as possible. The patient should be encouraged to use only the emollients and soap substitutes that have been prescribed, as over-the-counter products may contain many different irritants.

Patients should be instructed to avoid direct contact with detergents and other cleansing agents, which all contain strong irritants. They can measure out washing powder and detergents carefully using only the amount recommended on the packaging and keep the outside of the packaging free of spillage to avoid direct contact with the detergents and cleansing agents. Skin cleansers used at work are also harsh on the hands and direct contact with these is best avoided altogether.[20]

Soap and detergents may damage the skin by several mechanisms: alkali-induced damage of the stratum corneum increases permeability of the horny layer. Removal of lipids and the protective lipid layer of the skin by soaps and detergents is exacerbated by the prevention of reestablishment of the lipid layer and its normal acidity. Removal of amino acids damages the water-holding capacity of the horny layer.[24] In addition, certain components of soaps such as fatty acids may be directly irritant. For these reasons, patients should be instructed to always use a soap substitute.

TABLE 16.1
List of Example Irritants to Avoid

Shampoos and conditioners
Hair products such as hair lotions and hair dyes
Polishes including metal, wax, shoe, floor, car, furniture, and window polishes
Solvents and stain-removers such as white spirit, petrol, trichloroethylene, turpentine, and thinners
Foods such as oranges, lemons, grapefruit, potatoes, or tomatoes

To avoid any prolonged contact with irritants, patients should also be instructed to use running water if possible when washing up and reminded that rings should not be worn at all during housework or other wet work even after their dermatitis has clinically disappeared and healed. Rings should be cleaned on the inside frequently with a brush then rinsed thoroughly and patients should not wash their hands with soap when wearing a ring. Washing machines and dishwashers are the ideal way of protecting hands from irritants.

The patient can be supplied with a list of irritants that should be avoided in the domestic situation (Table 16.1). This is important not only for those who perform traditional household tasks but also in more heavy-duty domestic chores such as car washing, painting, and decorating.

It is also appropriate to ask the patient with hand dermatitis if another member of the household could do these types of chores for them. This particular suggestion is usually very well received by the patient! It is important for the patient to be made familiar with these irritants and recognize where they are likely to come into contact with them, as this understanding will improve compliance. A full explanation by the physician is also more likely to improve compliance and therefore outcome.

D. PROGNOSIS AND ONGOING MANAGEMENT

It is good practice to give the patient realistic advice with respect to the prognosis of their hand dermatitis and the importance of continuing the above measures indefinitely. Many patients expect only to carry out these measures for the duration of the clinical disease and do not realize that their tendency to develop irritant hand dermatitis will be lifelong, especially if they have an atopic background, and ongoing management is essential.

It is important for the patient to consider any triggering events that may have been responsible for the initial appearance of an episode of hand dermatitis. Irritant dermatitis can appear for the first time after the birth of a child or when an elderly relative is requiring care. Retirement with an increase in housework, maintenance, or gardening duties can also precipitate hand dermatitis.[25] The patient may associate these events with increased "stress" and blame their skin condition on this.

The patient should be told that it will take some months for their skin to return to below the irritant threshold and for clinical dermatitis to disappear. Patients should be informed that the skin will remain vulnerable for at least 4 to 6 months after the dermatitis appears to be completely healed and, therefore they must continue to

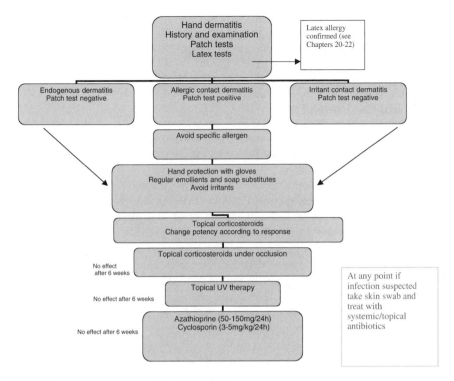

FIGURE 16.1 Management of hand dermatitis.

follow the above instructions. A minority of patients may continue to develop problems despite following this advice and will require more aggressive second-line therapy. For those with an underlying atopic diathesis, especially if in occupations associated with a high risk of hand dermatitis such as nursing, it is recommended hand care guidelines described above be followed indefinitely.

III. TREATMENT OF HAND DERMATITIS

Topical emollients and corticosteroids are the mainstays in the treatment of hand dermatitis (Figure 16.1).

A. EMOLLIENTS

Most hand dermatitis is characterized by dryness and scaling that requires regular reapplication of moisturizers. The patient should be offered a selection of emollients with different characteristics. In general terms, the greasier the emollient the better its effect on dry skin, but the messier an emollient is, the less likely the patient is to apply it regularly. A useful compromise is to prescribe both a less greasy product such as Aqueous Cream BP for use in the morning and throughout the day and to prescribe an oilier emollient such as Emulsifying Ointment BP for use once the patient has finished the day's work. Patients can be offered a number of different emollient samples to try in order to strike a balance between the emollient needs of the skin and what is acceptable to the individual patient to optimize compliance. Emollients and soap substitutes have been discussed in detail previously in this chapter.

B. Corticosteroids

1. Topical Corticosteroids

These are often one of the key elements in treating patients with hand dermatitis. Issues to consider when assessing the patient include whether to treat with cream or ointment and what strength of topical steroid to use.

Most corticosteroid creams are insufficiently lubricating, but corticosteroid ointments, the clinicians preferred option, may be unacceptably greasy to some patients and again a balance must be struck. Different hand sites respond differently to the same strength of topical steroids. The choice of topical corticosteroid therapy depends on the location and severity of the dermatitis. Dermatitis on the dorsum of the hands responds more readily than palmar dermatitis due to the differences in skin thickness. Furthermore, frequent use of a potent topical steroid may cause cutaneous atrophy. In addition, the question of whether topical steroids should be used once or more frequently every day, and whether short bursts of topical steroids are preferable to constant treatment has not been addressed in patients with hand dermatitis.

In a randomized, double blind, parallel group study to determine whether a 3-day burst of a potent corticosteroid is more effective than a mild preparation used for 7 days in children with mild or moderate atopic eczema, no differences were found between the two groups.[26] Therefore a short burst of a potent topical corticosteroid is just as effective as prolonged use of a milder preparation for controlling mild or moderate atopic eczema in children.

In another controlled, double blind study of 76 patients with allergic or irritant contact dermatitis or atopic dermatitis, two corticosteroid creams, Betnovate ® (group III) and Corticoderm® (group II), were compared. Statistical evaluation of the commencement of relief of symptoms and the proportion of healed dermatitis after 1 week and 3 weeks' treatment showed no difference between the groups. The authors concluded that Betnovate® cream and Corticoderm® cream once a day (combined with the emollient Unguentum Merck® when required), have an equivalent clinical effect in the short-term treatment of subacute and chronic dermatitis.[27]

Recommendations for treatment can include potent topical steroid clobetasol propionate 0.05% in an ointment formulation once daily for 2 to 6 weeks, before decreasing the potency to betamethasone valerate 0.1% ointment once daily, and then clobetasone butyrate 0.05% ointment once daily as the patient responds. Subsequent flares are treated with an ascent up the steroid ladder to greater potency steroids in short bursts of no longer than 6 weeks. In patients unresponsive to this regime the effectiveness of topical therapy can be increased by occlusion.[8]

Plastic occlusion increases corticosteroid penetration approximately 10-fold.[2] In hand dermatitis, occlusion can lead to rapid healing of fissures and dramatically improves psoriasiform and atopic hand dermatitis. Unfortunately it also increases the risk of unwanted side effects such as skin atrophy, especially if combined with very potent steroids. Occlusion of the hands is best accomplished by wearing thin plastic (not rubber) gloves overnight. This technique is initially uncomfortable to the patient, but is very beneficial after a few days. The brand is unimportant but they need to be as comfortable as possible to improve compliance. In patients with low grade but very dry hand dermatitis, emollients alone can be used under occlusion to improve their efficacy.

2. Intralesional Steroids

These can be useful in treating hand dermatitis when there is a small but active area of dermatitis and if the dermatitis does not respond to occlusion.[8] Intralesional therapy should be used reluctantly as it can predispose to infection.

3. Systemic Corticosteroids

In acute, severe, blistering hand dermatitis, a brief course of systemic corticosteroids often has a dramatic effect.[8] The aim is to improve the dermatitis sufficiently for topical treatment to be effective. One recommended regime is to use a 10-day tapering course of prednisolone, starting at 40 mg and reducing by 5 mg each day. Topical corticosteroids should be added as soon as the blistering and edema starts to decrease. Long-acting triamcinolone injections should be avoided, because of the risk that the patient relies on these rather than proper hand care and topical therapy, and because of the higher risk of adrenal suppression and other unwanted steroid effects.

C. Topical and Systemic Antibiotics

Hand dermatitis can become secondarily infected and require recurrent courses of oral antibiotics. Some authors prefer a systemic antibiotic and a topical corticosteroid, although there is some evidence for the efficacy of topical antibiotic and corticosteroid treatment in atopic and contact dermatitis.[28,29]

Topical antiseptic soaks such as potassium permanganate are useful in acutely inflamed or infected hand dermatitis where they help to combat infection and dry up the hands in acute blistering hand dermatitis.[1] Practical issues include taking skin swabs for culture and sensitivity.

D. Photochemotherapy

Psoralen ultraviolet A (PUVA) treatment is a useful option for unresponsive hand dermatitis.[30] In a left-right comparison of Ultra Violet B (UVB) phototherapy and topical photochemotherapy (PUVA) in bilateral chronic hand dermatitis for 6 weeks, there was no significant differences in improvement, but side effects occurred more often on the PUVA-treated side such as burning sensation, discomfort, and increased erythema.[31] Taking into account the similar responses and relative incidence of side effects, it is advisable to start treatment with UVB phototherapy and progress to topical photochemotherapy if this fails.

E. Systemic Immunosuppressives

1. Cyclosporin

Cyclosporin has been shown to be effective in the management of hand dermatitis. In a comparison of cyclosporin and topical betamethasone-17,21-dipropionate in the treatment of severe chronic hand dermatitis, cyclosporin at 3 mg/kg/day was as effective as topical betamethasone-17,21-dipropionate.[32] Low-dose cyclosporin is a useful addition for the short-term treatment of severe chronic hand dermatitis in patients unresponsive to conventional therapy, but is contraindicated in patients with hypertension or renal disease, and requires regular, careful monitoring of serum electrolytes and blood pressure.

2. Azathioprine

Azathioprine can be used to establish control of atopic dermatitis, although no controlled studies have been performed in hand dermatitis, and it can take more than four weeks to be effective. In a double blind, randomized, placebo-controlled, cross-over trial of azathioprine in adult patients with severe atopic dermatitis, there was significant improvement in the active treatment group compared to placebo.[33] This improvement must be balanced against the drug's hepatotoxicity, potential for bone marrow suppression, and gastrointestinal side effects, and therapy requires regular monitoring of the full blood count and liver enzymes.

F. Topical Immunosuppressives

Tacrolimus ointment has been shown to have some beneficial effect in long-standing cases of chronic dyshidrotic palmar eczema,[34] and the emerging group of topical immunosuppressive drugs may prove to be very helpful in the future management of hand dermatitis.

G. Other Modalities

Evening primrose oil has not been shown to be beneficial in the treatment of chronic hand dermatitis as orally administered evening primrose oil is not superior to placebo.[35]

Botulinum toxin injections have been shown, in a small study, to be beneficial in 10 patients with dyshidrotic eczema, but are potentially uncomfortable for patients.[36]

REFERENCES

1. Rietschel, R.L. and Fowler, J.F., Jr., Treatment of contact dermatitis, in *Contact Dermatitis,* 5th Ed., Rietschel R.L., Fowler J.F., Jr., Eds., Lippincott Williams and Wilkins, Philadelphia, 2001, chap. 38.
2. Epstein, E., Hand dermatitis, in *Common Skin Disorders,* 5th Ed., W.B. Saunders, New York, 2000, chap. 15.

3. Mellström, G.A. and Boman, A., Protective gloves, in *Handbook of Occupational Dermatology*, Kanerva, L., Elsner, P., Wahlberg, J.E., Maibach, H.I., Eds., Springer-Verlag, Berlin, 2000, chap. 53.

4. Jencen, D.A. and Hardy. J.K., Effect of glove material thickness on permeation characteristics, *Am. Ind. Hyg. Assoc. J.*, 50, 623, 1989.

5. Mellström, G.A. and Boman, A.S., Gloves: Types, materials and manufacturing, in *Protective Gloves for Occupational Use*, Mellström, G.A., Wahlberg, J, E., Maibach, H.I., Eds., CRC Press, Boca-Raton, FL, 1994, p. 21.

6. Estlander, T., Jolanki, R., and Kanerva, L., Allergic contact dermatitis from rubber and plastic gloves, in *Protective Gloves for Occupational Use*, Mellström, G.A., Wahlberg, J.E., Maibach, H.I., Eds., CRC Press, Boca Raton, FL, 1994, p. 221.

7. Estlander, T., Jolanki, R., and Kanerva, L., Dermatitis and urticaria from rubber and plastic gloves. *Contact Dermatitis*, 14, 20, 1986.

8. Epstein, E., Hand dermatitis: Practical management and current concepts, *J. Am. Acad. Dermatol.*, 10, 395, 1984.

9. Rycroft, R.J.G., Occupational contact dermatitis, in *Textbook of Contact Dermatitis*, Rycroft, R.J.G., Menné, T., Frosch, P.J., Lepoittevin J-P., Eds., Springer-Verlag, Berlin, 2001, chap. 29.

10. Munksgaard, E.C., Permeability of protective gloves to (di)methacrylates in resinous dental materials, *Scand. J. Dent. Res.*, 100, 189, 1992.

11. Estlander, T. and Jolanki, R., How to protect the hands, *Dermatol. Clin.*, 6, 105, 1988.

12. Kanerva, L., Skin disease from dental materials, in *Textbook of Contact Dermatitis*, Rycroft, R.J.G., Menné, T., Frosch, P.J., Lepoittevin J.-P., Eds., Springer-Verlag, Berlin, 2001, chap. 39.

13. Mellström, G.A., Lindahl, G., and Wahlberg, J.E., DAISY: Reference database on protective gloves, *Semin. Dermatol.*, 8, 75, 1989.

14. Zhai, H. and Maibach, H.I., Moisturisers in preventing irritant contact dermatitis: An overview, *Contact Dermatitis*, 38, 241, 1998.

15. Zhai, H., Anigbogu. A., and Maibach, H.I., Treatment of irritant and allergic contact dermatitis, in *Handbook of Occupational Dermatology*, Kanerva, L., Elsner, P., Wahlberg, J.E., Maibach, H.I., Eds., Springer-Verlag, Berlin, 2000, chap. 51.

16. Serup, J. A., Double-blind comparison of two creams containing urea as the active ingredient: Assessment of efficacy and side effects by non invasive techniques and a clinical scoring scheme, *Acta Derm. Venereol. Suppl. (Stockholm)*, 177, 33, 1992.

17. Halkier-Sørensen, L. and Thestrup-Pedersen, K., The efficacy of a moisturizer (Locobase) among cleaners and kitchen assistants during everyday exposure to water and detergents, *Contact Dermatitis*, 29, 266, 1993.

18. Hannuksela, A. and Kinnunen, T., Moisturisers prevent irritant dermatitis, *Acta Derm. Venereol.*, 72, 42, 1992.

19. Serup, J., Winther, A., and Blichmann, C.W., Effects of repeated application of a moisturiser, *Acta Derm. Venereol.*, 69, 457, 1989.

20. Lachapelle, J-M., Principles of prevention and protection in contact dermatitis, in *Textbook of Contact Dermatitis*, Rycroft, R.J.G., Menné, T., Frosch, P.J., Lepoittevin, J-P., Eds., Springer-Verlag, Berlin, 2001, chap. 42.

21. Grunewald, A.M. et al., Efficacy of barrier creams, in *Irritant Dermatitis: New Clinical and Experimental Aspects*, Elsner, P., and Maibach, H.I., Eds., Karger, Basel, 1995, 187.

22. Lantinga, H., Nater, J.P., and Coenraads, P.J., Prevalence, incidence and course of eczema on the hands and forearms in a sample of the general population, *Contact Dermatitis*, 10, 135, 1984.

23. Smith, H.R. et al., Skin irritation thresholds in hairdressers: Implications for the development of hand dermatitis, *Br. J. Dermatol.,* 146, 849, 2002.

24. Rietschel, R.L. and Fowler, J.F., Jr., Hand dermatitis due to contactants: Special considerations, in *Contact Dermatitis,* 5th ed., Rietschel, R. L., Fowler, J.F. Jr., Eds., Lippincott Williams and Wilkins, Philadelphia, 2001, chap. 18.

25. McFadden, J.P., Hand eczema, in *Textbook of Contact Dermatitis,* Rycroft, R.J.G., Menné, T., Frosch, P.J., Lepoittevin J-P., Eds., Springer-Verlag, Berlin, 2001, chap. 19.

26. Thomas, K.S. et al., Randomised controlled trial of short bursts of a potent topical corticosteroid versus prolonged use of a mild preparation for children with mild or moderate atopic eczema. *Br. Med. J.,* 324, 768, 2002.

27. Bleeker, J. et al., Double blind comparative study of Corticoderm™ cream + Unguentum Merck™ and Betnovate™ cream + Unguentum Merck™ in hand dermatitis, *J. Dermatol. Treat.,* 1, 87, 1989.

28. Strategos, J., Fusidic acid-betamethasone combination in infected eczema: An open, randomised comparison with gentamicin-betamethasone combination, *Pharmatherapeutica,* 4, 601. 1986.

29. Hjorth, N., Schmidt, H., and Thomsen, K., Fusidic acid plus betamethasone in infected or potentially infected eczema, *Pharmatherapeutica,* 4, 126, 1985.

30. Tegner, E. and Thelin, I., PUVA treatment of chronic eczematous dermatitis of the palms and soles, *Acta Derm. Venereol.,* 61, 570, 1981.

31. Simons, J.R., Bohnen, I.J., and van der Valk, P.G., A left-right comparison of UVB phototherapy and topical photo chemotherapy in bilateral chronic hand dermatitis after 6 weeks' treatment, *Clin. Exp. Dermatol.,* 22, 7, 1997.

32. Granlund, H. et al., Comparison of cyclosporine and topical betamethasone-17, 21-dipropionate in the treatment of severe chronic hand eczema, *Acta Derm. Venereol.,* 76, 371, 1996.

33. Berth-Jones, J. et al., Azathioprine in severe adult atopic dermatitis: A double blind, placebo-controlled, crossover trial, *Br. J. Dermatol.,* 147, 324, 2002.

34. Schnopp, C. et al., Topical tacrolimus (FK506) and mometasone furoate in treatment of dyshidrotic palmar eczema: A randomised, observer-blinded trial, *J. Am. Acad. Dermatol.,* 46, 73, 2002.

35. Whitaker, D.K., Cilliers, J., and de Beer. C., Evening primrose oil (Epogam) in the treatment of chronic hand dermatitis: Disappointing therapeutic results, *Dermatology,* 193, 115, 1996.

36. Swartling, C. et al., Treatment of dyshidrotic hand dermatitis with intradermal botulinum toxin, *J. Am. Acad. Dermatol.,* 47, 667, 2002.

APPENDIX 16.1
Information Sheet for Patients with Hand Dermatitis

DEPARTMENT OF DERMATOLOGY

HAND DERMATITIS INFORMATION SHEET

Here are four important tips to speed healing and prevent relapse of your hand dermatitis.

1. Protect your hands with gloves
   - If gloves are used for washing dishes and clothes they should be *plastic or PVC* and not rubber since rubber can cause dermatitis. Gloves should not be worn for more than 15 to 20 minutes at a time. If water enters a glove, take the glove off immediately. Turn the gloves inside out and rinse them under the hot water tap several times a week and then allow them to dry completely.
   - *Cotton gloves* can be used under plastic ones to soak up sweat that would otherwise irritate your skin. They should only be worn a few times before they are washed.
   - Buy several pairs of plastic and cotton gloves at a time for use in the kitchen, bathroom, and at work.
   - Beware of contaminating the *insides* of gloves with chemicals and soaps. If gloves become contaminated, rinse out immediately and leave to dry inside out. If gloves develop a hole discard immediately. Wearing a glove with a hole is worse than no gloves at all.
   - Wear cotton gloves for housework. Wash them in the washing machine regularly.
   - Use heavy duty fabric gloves when doing any gardening, do-it-yourself projects, and outdoor work.
   - Wear gloves when outdoors in cold weather to prevent your hands drying, cracking, and chapping.
2. Use soap substitutes
   - Normal soap and water can be very irritating to your hands.
   - When washing your hands use lukewarm water and a soap substitute such as Aqueous Cream or Emulsifying Ointment. Soap substitutes are also excellent moisturizers and form a protective layer over the skin. Dry carefully with a clean towel, not forgetting to dry between the fingers.
   - Have several tubs of these soap substitutes both at home and at work, one next to each sink. Smaller tubes to carry around with you are also a good idea.
   - Use your soap substitute as a general moisturizer as well. They are safe to apply to all areas of the skin even in children. They should be used whenever your skin feels dry or itchy.

3. Avoid irritants
   - Avoid direct contact with *detergents and other cleansing agents.* These are all irritants. Measure out washing powder and detergents carefully using only the amount recommended on the packaging. Keep the outside of the packaging free of spillage to avoid direct contact with the detergents and cleansing agents.
   - Skin cleansers used at work are also harsh on the hands and best avoided. Use a soap substitute instead.
   - For washing up, use running water if possible.
   - Rings should not be worn during housework or other work, even when the dermatitis has healed. Rings should be cleaned on the inside frequently with a brush then rinsed thoroughly.
   - Never wash your hands with soap when wearing a ring.
   - Washing machines and dishwashers are the ideal way of protecting your hands from irritants.
   - Avoid direct contact with *shampoo.* Let somebody else shampoo your hair or use plastic or PVC gloves.
   - Avoid direct contact with polishes including *metal, wax, shoe, floor, car, furniture, and window polishes.*
   - Avoid direct contact with *solvents and stain-removers* such as white spirit, petrol, trichloroethylene, turpentine, and thinners.
   - Do not peel or squeeze *oranges, lemons, grapefruit, potatoes, or tomatoes* with bare hands.
   - Do not apply *hair lotion, hair cream, or hair dye* with bare hands.
   - Could another family member do these chores for you?
4. Keep going
   - It takes time for your skin to recover from dermatitis. Do not forget that the skin will remain vulnerable for at least 6 months after the dermatitis appears to be completely healed, so continue to follow the above instructions.

17 Barrier Creams/Moisturizers

Hongbo Zhai, Mahbub M. U. Chowdhury, and Howard I. Maibach

CONTENTS

I. Introduction...165
II. Barrier Creams (BC) 166
    A. Definition and Terms...166
    B. Reasons to Use Barrier Creams...166
    C. Mechanism of Action and Duration 166
    D. Application Methods and Efficacy..167
    E. U.S. Food and Drug Administration Monograph Skin
        Protectants 167
III. Moisturizers 167
    A. Definition and Terms...167
    B. Effect of Moisturizers on Skin...168
    C. Moisturizers in Preventing Irritant Contact Dermatitis...................168
IV. Conclusions..171
References..173

I. INTRODUCTION

From etiological grounds, contact dermatitis (CD) is divided into irritant contact dermatitis (ICD) and allergic contact dermatitis (ACD). ICD results from contact with irritants, while ACD is an immunological reaction in response to contact with an allergen in sensitized individuals.[1] CD comprises 90 to 95% of work-related dermatoses,[1] therefore, various prophylactic measures have been used to reduce the risk of developing such CD.[1-6] Barrier creams (BC) as well as moisturizers may play an important role in this strategy. Due to ambiguous definitions, the terms of BC and moisturizers are often confused in the literature and workplace. Moisturizers and BC may share characteristics, and thus to strictly distinguish between them may be difficult. Barrier creams target the prevention of external noxious substances penetrating skin, used usually in occupational settings to prevent contact dermatitis.[2-8] Moisturizers are frequently used for the treatment or prevention of "dry" skin conditions as well as to maintain healthy skin, which may be an attribute of cosmetic products.[9–11]

II. BARRIER CREAMS (BC)

A. DEFINITION AND TERMS

BC, in theory, are designed to prevent or reduce the penetration of harmful agents.[2–8,12,13] BC are also called "skin protective creams (SPCs)" or "protective creams (PCs)," as well as "protective ointments," "invisible glove," "barrier," "protective" or "pre-work" creams and/or gels (lotions), and "antisolvent" gels.[12,14–17] Frosch et al.[12] consider "skin protective creams" a more appropriate terminology since most creams do not provide a real barrier, at least not comparable to stratum corneum.

B. REASONS TO USE BARRIER CREAMS

Avoiding some irritants or allergens may not be practical for persons whose occupation or activities involve working in certain environments. Protective clothing as well as other personal devices may provide protective effects in industry.[18,19] However, protective clothing may trap moisture and occlude potentially damaging substances next to the skin for prolonged periods and increase the likelihood that dermatitis will develop.[18,19] In practice, BC are recommended only for low-grade irritants (water, detergents, organic solvents, cutting oils).[2,20–23] The first line of defense against hand dermatitis is to wear gloves, but in many professions it is impossible to wear gloves because of the loss of dexterity. In some instances, an alternative could be to apply BC. BC are also used to protect the face and neck against chemical and resinous dust and vapors.[24] Many workers prefer a barrier cream instead of gloves because they do not want the hand continuously sealed inside a glove. Furthermore, gloves can inhibit skin barrier function.[2] Additionally, gloves often do not resist the penetration of low molecular weight chemicals. Some allergens are soluble in rubber gloves, and may penetrate the glove and produce severe dermatitis.[2,24,25] Another reason to avoid wearing gloves is the fact that an allergic reaction to rubber latex has become a growing problem.[24,25] Furthermore, due to continuous glove wearing, workers can develop serious symptoms including generalized urticaria, conjunctivitis, rhinitis, and asthma (contact urticaria syndrome).[2,26]

C. MECHANISM OF ACTION AND DURATION

There is little information on the mechanisms of action of barrier creams. The frequently quoted general rule is that water-in-oil (W/O) emulsions are effective against aqueous solutions of irritants and oil-in-water (O/W) emulsions are effective against lipophilic materials.[8,12,19] Some studies have demonstrated exceptions to this rule.[27,28] BC may contain active ingredients that are presumed to work by trapping or transforming allergens or irritants.[7,28] Most believe they interfere with absorption and penetration of the allergen or irritants with physical blocking by forming a thin film that protects the skin.[7,28–30]

In order to avoid frequent interruptions for reapplication, BC are expected to remain effective for 3 or 4 hours. Most manufacturers claim that their products last around 4 hours. Others suggest use "as often as necessary."[19] Several studies document duration of action with varying results.[20,23,31,32]

D. APPLICATION METHODS AND EFFICACY

BC effectiveness may be influenced by application methods.[33–,35] Wigger-Alberti et al.[34] determined which areas of the hands were likely to be missed on self-application of BC by a fluorescence technique at the workplace. BC application was incomplete, especially on the dorsal aspects of the hands. Most manufacturers suggest rubbing thoroughly onto skin and to pay special attention to cuticles and skin under nails with drying for approximately 5 minutes. A thin layer of BC should be applied to all appropriate skin surfaces 3 to 4 times daily. Further controlled experiments are indicated to support these recommendations.

BC efficacy in preventing or reducing ICD and ACD has been documented in many experimental environments.[2–8,12,13] However, some reports document that inappropriate BC application may exacerbate rather than ameliorate.[7,12,23,27,36–38]

E. U.S. FOOD AND DRUG ADMINISTRATION MONOGRAPH SKIN PROTECTANTS

U.S. Food and Drug Administration (FDA) defines 13 skin protectants for over-the-counter (OTC) products.[39] These ingredients are allantoin (0.5 to 2%), aluminum hydroxide gel (0.15 to 5%), calamine (1 to 25%), cocoa butter (50 to 100%), dimethicone (1 to 30%), glycerin (20 to 45%), kaolin (4 to 20%), petrolatum (30 to 100%), shark liver oil (3%), white petrolatum (30 to 100%), zinc acetate (0.1 to 2%), zinc carbonate (0.2 to 2%), and zinc oxide (1 to 25%).

In addition, an OTC lotion (containing quaternium-18 bentonite) against poison ivy, oak, or sumac has been approved by the U.S. FDA and has been commercialized.

III. MOISTURIZERS

A. DEFINITION AND TERMS

The term moisturizer was generated by Madison Avenue marketers.[10] The definition of "moisturizers are substances used to reduce the signs and symptoms of dry, scaly skin, making the rough surface soft and smooth" may lack specificity. In addition, the term "dry skin" is not generally accepted.[10,11] No consensus exists regarding the definition of a moisturizer.[10] Moisturizers are used daily to alleviate or improve "dry" skin symptoms such as chapped hands and heels, ichthyosis, asteatosis, atopic dermatitis, and atopic dry skin.[9–11] Application of moisturizers may increase skin hydration and therefore may modify the physical and chemical nature of the skin surface, so as to smooth, soften and make more pliable.[9,11]

B. EFFECT OF MOISTURIZERS ON SKIN

Natural moisturizing factors (NMF), stored in the stratum corneum (SC), aid horny layer hydration and flexibility and consist of a mixture of low molecular weight soluble hygroscopic substances.[10,11] They include amino acids, lactic acid, pyrrollidone carboxylic acid (PCA), and urea. A deficiency of NMF is linked to dry skin conditions.[11] Skin function maintenance is important in protecting the skin against many disorders which cause dry, chapped and cracked skin, sensitivity, irritation or inflammation, and also against the repeated use of water, detergents, and other irritants.

Moisturizers often contain humectants of low molecular weight and lipids. Humectants, such as urea, glycerin, lactic acid, PCA, and salts are absorbed into the SC, and at that site, attract water to increase hydration.[11,40] Lipids, for instance petrolatum, beeswax, lanolin, and various oils in moisturizers, have traditionally been considered to exert their effects on the skin solely by forming an inert, epicutaneous, occlusive membrane. They are therefore incorporated into formulations on the basis of their technical and sensory properties rather than on their possible epidermal impact.[40,41] However, topically applied lipids may also penetrate down to the living cells of normal epidermis, enter into metabolism and significantly modify endogenous epidermal lipids.[42] In normal skin, a single application of a moisturizer did not cause long-lasting effects expressed as skin capacitance and conductance,[43,44] whereas repeated applications of a moisturizer twice daily for 1 week produced a significant increase in the skin conductance for at least 1 week posttreatment.[45]

Urea is a unique physiological, nonallergic substance,[46,47] and has been used in dermatologic therapy for decades. Urea can decrease reversibly the turnover of epidermal cells,[48] and may enhance the penetration of other substances into skin.[46,49,50] Other effects include binding water in the horny layer, antipruritic properties, and reducing contact dermatitis from irritant stimuli.[46,47,51,52] High concentrations of urea can be irritant and thereby cause irritant dermatitis and sensory irritation.[10]

C. MOISTURIZERS IN PREVENTING IRRITANT CONTACT DERMATITIS

Hannuksela and Kinnunen[53] developed a wash test method to determine the effect of moisturizers in preventing ICD on 12 healthy female students. The participants washed the outer aspects of their upper arms with a liquid dishwashing detergent for one minute twice daily for 1 week. Eight commercial moisturizers were applied to the left upper arm just after each washing, while the other arm was left untreated. During the second week, the left upper arm only was treated with the moisturizers twice daily. Transepidermal water loss (TEWL) increased during the washing period by 13 $g/m^2/h$ in the untreated arm, while the increase in the treated areas was only 3 $g/m^2/h$. Visible dermatitis appeared on the untreated arm, while the treated areas remained objectively and subjectively free of symptoms and signs. Blood flow also increased significantly in the washed, untreated arm, but did not change in the arm treated with moisturizer.

During the second week, the dermatitis on the washed, untreated arm disappeared and the laser Doppler values normalized. The TEWL values also decreased to near normal. The mean decrease was more pronounced when moisturizers with a high fat content were used but, due to interindividual variation, the differences between the results for the eight moisturizers were not statistically significant. When the effect of a moisturizer was compared to no treatment after the 1 week wash out period, the use of the moisturizers enhanced the healing process significantly.

Halkier-Sørensen and Thestrup-Pedersen[54] utilized a crossover design to evaluate the efficacy of a moisturizer (Locobase®) among 111 cleaners and kitchen assistants during everyday work. The population was divided into two groups: 56 workers used the test moisturizer only on their hands for the first 2 weeks and stopped this during the subsequent 2 weeks, and vice versa (n = 55). The moisturizer prevented the development of skin dryness. Electrical capacitance (epidermal hydration) decreased significantly when the study subjects were not using the moisturizer.

Lane and Drost[55] examined the effect of a water-in-oil moisturizer in comparison with its blank control on 34 premature newborns. One-half of the neonates were treated twice daily with test moisturizer for up to 16 days, and the other half served as controls. They demonstrated statistically less dermatitis of the hand (day 2 through day 11), feet (day 2 through 16), and abdomen (day 7 through day 11) of sites treated with moisturizer.

Lodén[51] showed that repeated applications of urea-containing moisturizers to influence both TEWL and the apparent susceptibility to sodium laurel sulphate (SLS)-induced irritation. Three applications of 5% urea increased TEWL, whereas treatment with 10% urea for 10 and 20 days decreased TEWL. It is possible that a greater amount of urea alters the binding capacities of the SC, retarding SLS penetration.

Lodén and Andersson[56] observed the effect of topically applied lipids on surfactant-irritated skin in 21 healthy subjects, showing that canola oil and its sterol-enriched fraction reduced the degree of SLS-induced irritation. Neither fish oil (rich in eicosapentaenoic acid) nor borage oil (rich in γ–linolenic acid and linoleic acid) influenced inflammation caused by SLS.

Olivarius et al.[57] evaluated the effect of moisturizing creams against water in an *in vivo* human model. This was based on the color intensities when an aqueous solution of crystal violet is applied to the dorsal and volar aspects of hand skin in 12 subjects pretreated with test creams. The test moisturizer showed certain protective effects (dorsal 57%, volar 34%) against water.

Gammal et al.[58] assessed the efficacy of moisturizers by a soap-induced xerosis human model. The lower legs of 22 women were washed daily for 10 days with soap to induce the xerosis. After washing, one side received a moisturizer, the other served as an untreated control. The values of clinical scaling, electrical conductance, and image analysis of adhesive-coated discs (D-Squames®) were compared on each evaluation day. On the moisturizer-treated legs there was a significant decrease in dryness grades and scaling indicators at all time points. Conductance was significantly increased on days 8 and 11.

Ramsing and Agner[59] tested the effect of a moisturizer on experimentally irritated human skin in two studies. In a prevention study, both hands of 12 volunteers were immersed in a 0.375% SLS solution, 10 min twice daily for 2 days. Before each immersion, one hand was treated with the moisturizer; the other hand served as control. In a therapeutic study, the immersion procedure was the same as mentioned above. After the last immersion, one hand was treated with the moisturizer for 5 days; the other served as control. A significant preventive effect was obtained on the treated hand, while TEWL and blood flow were significantly increased and electrical capacitance was significantly decreased on the control hand. A significant therapeutic effect was also observed on the treated hand, while TEWL was significantly increased and electrical capacitance was significantly decreased on the control hand on day 8.

Lodén et al.[60] measured the efficacy of a moisturizer on patients with atopic skin. One forearm was treated with a moisturizing cream twice daily for 20 days. On day 21, the skin was exposed to SLS and on day 22, the irritant reaction was measured noninvasively. Skin capacitance was significantly increased by the treatment, indicating increased skin hydration. As reflected by TEWL and superficial skin blood flow values, the skin susceptibility to SLS was significantly reduced. They concluded that certain moisturizers could improve skin barrier function in atopics and reduce skin susceptibility to irritants.

Held and Agner[61] compared two experimental models of moisturizer efficacy on the recovery of irritated skin on the hands and the volar forearms. Twelve healthy volunteers had their hands immersed in SLS 10 minutes twice daily for 2 days, and at the same time the volunteers had patch tests with SLS (0.125%, 0.25%, and 0.5%) applied on their forearms for 24 hours. After irritation of the skin, the volunteers had a moisturizer applied on one arm/hand three times daily for the following 9 days. The other arm/hand served as untreated control. Both models were found useful, and the moisturizer was found to accelerate regeneration of the skin barrier function in both hands (day 8, $p < 0.05$) and the volar forearms (0.5% SLS, day 5 and day 8, $p < 0.01$).

Held and Jorgensen[62] investigated whether applying a moisturizer to compromised skin before wearing an occlusive glove could reduce skin irritation. Healthy volunteers had both hands immersed in a SLS solution twice daily for 2 days. After each immersion, one hand had a moisturizer applied and both hands were put in occlusive gloves for 2 hours. They found moisturizer had a statistically significant positive effect on both the water barrier function and the hydration level of the skin. Although not statistically significant, less inflammation was observed on the moisturizer-treated hand. They suggested that use of a moisturizer under an occlusive glove may diminish irritation from exposure to a detergent followed by glove wearing.

Held et al.[63] evaluated the effect of six commercial moisturizers on the recovery of irritated human skin. Thirty-six healthy volunteers had patch tests with SLS 0.5% applied on their forearms/upper arms for 24 hours. After irritation of the skin, all volunteers had a moisturizer applied on one forearm/upper arm only, 3 times daily, for the following 5 days. The other forearm/upper arm served as an untreated control. Each moisturizer was tested on 12 volunteers and each volunteer tested two moisturizers at the same time. All six moisturizers were found to accelerate regeneration of the skin barrier function when compared to irritated nontreated skin. The most lipid-rich moisturizers improved barrier restoration more rapidly than the less lipid-rich moisturizers.

Zhai et al.[64] conducted a study of prevention of irritant dermatitis by applying a model lipid emulsion before wearing occlusive gloves. In addition, its therapeutic effect on moderately dry skin was determined. Fifteen volunteers with normal hands were enrolled in a primary prevention assay and another 15 with dry skin for a therapeutic study. In the prevention group, test emulsion was applied to one hand while the opposite remained untreated; 30 minutes later, both were gloved for 3 hours. Skin condition was evaluated by visual scoring, water sorption-desorption test (SDT), TEWL, and skin capacitance, and repeated for 5 days. In the therapeutic group, one hand received the test emulsion, while the other remained untreated daily, up to 5 days. In the prevention group, after glove occlusion, untreated hands showed significantly higher TEWL values ($p < 0.01$ on day 4 and $p < 0.05$ on day 5) compared to emulsion treated hands. Glove occlusion caused dehydration on both hands, but the untreated showed more dehydration. Emulsion treated hands showed a significantly greater water holding capacity compared to untreated hands from 0-second up to 120-second measurements. In the therapeutic group, emulsion treated hands showed significantly decreased dryness ($p < 0.05$) compared to untreated hands from day 3 to day 5. Also, the emulsion treated side showed significantly increased skin hydration compared to untreated hands. They concluded the test emulsion minimized glove induced-ICD and decreased dry skin.

The effects of moisturizers in the prevention of ICD are summarized in Table 17.1.

IV. CONCLUSIONS

BC and moisturizers are frequently dispensed by healthcare personnel to workers to prevent occupational dermatitis. Though BC and moisturizers may share some characteristics, they exist for different applications. BC are focused on prevention, and moisturizers are utilized for "dry" skin as well as to maintain healthy skin.

BC may protect against low-grade irritants, but should be not used as primary protection against high-risk substances including corrosive agents. However, wet workers utilizing water, soaps, and detergents daily may benefit by applying BC frequently. Furthermore, BC may also shield skin from chemicals, oils, and other substances and make them easier to clean at the end of the workday.[19] To achieve optimal protective effects, BC should be used with careful consideration of the types of substances they are designed to protect against based on a specific exposure conditions. Proper and full education in use is essential.[34,35] Inappropriate BC application may exacerbate irritation;[7,12,23,27,36–38] and using BC on diseased skin may lead to increased irritation.[7,18]

The efficacy of moisturizers in the prevention of ICD has been well documented.[9,48] Application of appropriate moisturizers may also accelerate the rate of healing on damaged skin.[53,58,59,61,63,64] Use of a moisturizer under an occlusive glove may diminish irritation from exposure to a detergent[62] and can minimize glove-induced ICD as well as decreasing skin dryness.[64] Individuals regularly exposed to irritants should be encouraged to apply moisturizers frequently to reduce such dermatitis. However, controversial results have indicated that daily use moisturizers on normal skin might increase skin susceptibility to irritants even after 5 consecutive daily application.[65,66] The potential irritant effect of moisturizers needs to be evaluated further.[67]

Optimal BC and moisturizers use not only prevents, but also treats mild ICD. Mixture of water-binding ingredients in the formulations may provide beneficial

TABLE 17.1
Effects of Moisturizers in the Prevention of ICD

Irritants	Moisturizers	Results	Authors and References
Liquid dishwashing detergent	8 commercial moisturizers (3 O/W creams, 1 skin oil, 4 double emulsions)	Significant prevention ICD, enhanced healing process	Hannuksela and Kinnunen[53]
Water and detergents	Locobase®	Prevented the development of skin dryness	Halkier-Sørensen and Thestrup-Pedersen[54]
Dermatitis with premature newborns	Water-in-oil emollient	Significant decrease dermatitis	Lane and Drost[55]
SLS	3 cream emulsions, 3 gels	5% urea increased TEWL, 10% urea for 10 and 20 days decreased TEWL	Lodén[51]
SLS	Hydrocortisone cream, fish oil, borage oil, petrolatum, canola oil, canola USF, shea butter USF, sunflower oil	Canola oil and its sterol-enriched fraction reduced SLS-induced irritation	Lodén and Andersson[56]
Water	Plutect 22®, Kerodex 71®, Locobase®	Protective effect against water	Olivarius et al.[57]
Soap	Vaseline Intensive Care Lotion®	Significant decrease dryness and scaling	Gammal et al.[58]
SLS	Locobase®	Significant preventive and therapeutic effects	Ramsing and Agner[59]
SLS	Canoderm®	Skin hydration significant increase and reduced skin susceptibility to irritants	Lodén et al.[60]
SLS	1 moisturizer	Accelerated regeneration of skin barrier function	Held and Agner[61]
SLS	1 moisturizer	Moisturizer, under occlusive glove, diminished irritation from exposure to detergent followed by glove wearing	Held and Jorgensen[62]
SLS	6 moisturizers	Accelerated regeneration of the skin barrier function when compared to irritated non-treated skin. Most lipid-rich moisturizers improved barrier restoration more rapidly than the less lipid-rich moisturizers	Held et al.[63]
Occlusive glove induced-ICD	1 model lipid emulsion	Minimized glove induced-ICD and decreased dry skin	Zhai et al.[64]

synergy.[68] Cosmetically functional BC or moisturizers, in particular containing cosmetic active components, are more acceptable to the public.[69,70] The optimum time to use moisturizers remains to be determined. In industries and individuals at low risk, dosing will probably be started after dermatitis develops. Conversely, in some industries and individuals at high risk, prophylaxis such as BC may be applied prior to work.

REFERENCES

1. Diepgen, T.L. and Coenraads, P.J., The epidemiology of occupational contact dermatitis, in *Handbook of Occupational Dermatology,* Kanerva, L. et al., Eds., Springer, Berlin, 2000, p. 3.
2. Wigger-Alberti, W. and Elsner, P., Do barrier creams and gloves prevent or provoke contact dermatitis? *Am. J. Contact Dermatitis,* 9, 100, 1998.
3. Zhai, H. and Maibach, H.I., Efficacy of barrier creams (skin protective creams), in *Cosmetics: Controlled Efficacy Studies and Regulation,* Elsner, P., Merk, H.F., and Maibach, H.I., Eds., Springer, Berlin, 1999, p. 156.
4. Wigger-Alberti, W. and Elsner, P., Protective creams, in *Cosmeceuticals: Drugs vs. Cosmetics,* Elsner, P. and Maibach, H.I., Eds., Marcel Dekker, New York, 2000, p. 189.
5. Zhai, H., Anigbogu, A., and Maibach, H.I., Treatment of irritant and allergic contact dermatitis, in *Handbook of Occupational Dermatology,* Kanerva, L. et al., Eds., Springer, Berlin, 2000, p. 402.
6. Wigger-Alberti, W. and Elsner, P., Barrier creams and emollients, in *Handbook of Occupational Dermatology,* Kanerva, L. et al., Eds., Springer, Berlin, 2000, p. 490.
7. Lachapelle, J.M., Efficacy of protective creams and/or gels, in *Prevention of Contact Dermatitis: Current Problems in Dermatology,* Elsner, P. et al., Eds., Karger, Basel, 1996, p. 182.
8. Zhai, H. and Maibach, H.I., Percutaneous penetration (Dermatopharmacokinetics) in evaluating barrier creams, in *Prevention of Contact Dermatitis: Current Problems in Dermatology,* Elsner, P. et al., Eds., Karger, Basel, 1996, 193.
9. Zhai, H. and Maibach, H.I., Moisturizers in preventing irritant contact dermatitis: An overview, *Contact Dermatitis,* 38, 241, 1998.
10. Kligman, A., Introduction, in *Dry skin and moisturizers,* Lodén, M. and Maibach, H.I., Eds., CRC Press, Boca Raton, FL, 2000, p. 3.
11. Lodén, M., Moisturizers, in *Cosmeceuticals: Drugs vs. Cosmetics,* Elsner, P. and Maibach, H.I., Eds., Marcel Dekker, New York, 2000, p. 73.
12. Frosch, P.J., Kurte, A., and Pilz, B., Biophysical techniques for the evaluation of skin protective creams, in *Noninvasive Methods for the Quantification of Skin Functions,* Frosch, P.J. and Kligman, A.M., Eds., Springer, Berlin, 1993, p. 214.
13. Zhai, H. and Maibach, H.I., Models assay for evaluation of barrier formulations, in *Hand Eczema,* Menné, T. and Maibach, H.I., Eds., CRC Press, Boca Raton, FL, 2000, p. 333.
14. Goh, C.L. and Gan, S.L., Efficacies of a barrier cream and an afterwork emollient cream against cutting fluid dermatitis in metalworkers: A prospective study, *Contact Dermatitis,* 31, 176, 1994.
15. Guillemin, M. et al., Simple method to determine the efficiency of a cream used for skin protection against solvents, *Br. J. Ind. Med.,* 31, 310, 1974.
16. Mahmoud, G. and Lachapelle, J.M., Evaluation of the protective value of an antisolvent gel by laser Doppler flowmetry and histology, *Contact Dermatitis,* 13, 14, 1985.

17. Lodén, M., The effect of 4 barrier creams on the absorption of water, benzene, and formaldehyde into excised human skin, *Contact Dermatitis,* 14, 292, 1986.

18. Mathias, C.G.T., Prevention of occupational contact dermatitis, *J. Am. Acad. Dermatol.,* 23, 742, 1990.

19. Davidson, C.L., Occupational contact dermatitis of the upper extremity, *Occup. Med.,* 9, 59, 1994.

20. Boman, A., Wahlberg, J.E., and Johansson, G., A method for the study of the effect of barrier creams and protective gloves on the percutaneous absorption of solvents, *Dermatologica,* 164, 157, 1982.

21. McClain, D.C. and Storrs, F., Protective effect of both a barrier cream and a polyethylene laminate glove against epoxy resin, glyceryl monothioglycolate, frullania, and tansy, *Am. J. Contact Dermatitis,* 13, 201, 1992.

22. Mellström, G.A., Johansson, S., and Nyhammar, E., Barrier effect of gloves against cytostatic drugs, in *Prevention of Contact Dermatitis: Current Problems in Dermatology,* Elsner, P. et al., Eds., Karger, Basel, 1996, p. 163.

23. Zhai, H. and Maibach, H.I., Effect of barrier creams: Human skin *in vivo, Contact Dermatitis,* 35, 92, 1996.

24. Birmingham, D., Prevention of occupational skin disease, *Cutis,* 5, 153, 1969.

25. Estlander, T., Jolanki, R., and Kanerva, L., Rubber glove dermatitis: A significant occupational hazard-prevention, in *Prevention of Contact Dermatitis: Current Problems in Dermatology,* Elsner, P. et al., Eds., Karger, Basel, 1996, p. 170.

26. Amin, S. and Maibach, H.I., Immunologic contact urticaria definition, in *Contact Urticaria Syndrome,* Amin, S., Lahti, A., and Maibach, H.I., Eds., CRC Press, Boca Raton, FL, 1997, p. 11.

27. Frosch, P.J. et al., Efficacy of skin barrier creams (II): Ineffectiveness of a popular "skin protector" against various irritants in the repetitive irritation test in the guinea pig, *Contact Dermatitis,* 29, 74, 1993.

28. Frosch, P.J. and Kurte, A., Efficacy of skin barrier creams (IV): The repetitive irritation test (RIT) with a set of 4 standard irritants, *Contact Dermatitis,* 31, 161, 1994.

29. Orchard, S., Barrier creams, *Dermatol. Clin.,* 2, 619, 1984.

30. Marks, J.G. Jr. et al., Prevention of poison ivy and poison oak allergic contact dermatitis by quaternium-18 bentonite, *J. Am. Acad. Dermatol.,* 33, 212, 1995.

31. Reiner, R. et al., Ointments for the protection against organophosphate poisoning, *Arzneim-Forsch/Drug Res.,* 32, 630, 1982.

32. Zhai, H. et al., In vitro percutaneous absorption of sodium lauryl sulfate (SLS) in human skin decreased by quaternium-18 bentonite gels, *In Vitro Molecul. Toxicol.,* 12, 11, 1999.

33. Packham, C.L., Evaluation of barrier creams: An *in vitro* technique on human skin (letter), *Acta Derm. Venereol.,* 74, 405, 1994.

34. Wigger-Alberti, W. et al., Self-application of a protective cream: Pitfalls of occupational skin protection, *Arch. Dermatol.,* 133, 861, 1997.

35. Wigger-Alberti, W. et al., Training workers at risk for occupational contact dermatitis in the application of protective creams: Efficacy of a fluorescence technique, *Dermatology,* 195, 129, 1997.

36. Goh, C.L., Cutting oil dermatitis on guinea pig skin (I): Cutting oil dermatitis and barrier cream, *Contact Dermatitis,* 24, 16, 1991.

37. Frosch, P.J. et al., Efficacy of skin barrier creams (I): The repetitive irritation test (RIT) in the guinea pig, *Contact Dermatitis,* 28, 94, 1993.

38. Treffel, P., Gabard, B., and Juch, R., Evaluation of barrier creams: An *in vitro* technique on human skin, *Acta Derm. Venereol.,* 74, 7, 1994.

39. Federal Register, Skin protectant drug products for over-the-counter human use, 48, 6832, 1983.

40. Lodén, M., Barrier recovery and influence of irritant stimuli in skin treated with a moisturizing cream, *Contact Dermatitis,* 36, 256, 1997.

41. Lodén, M., Biophysical properties of dry atopic and normal skin with special reference to effects of skin care products, *Acta Derm. Venereol. (Suppl.),* 192,1, 1995.

42. Wertz, P.W. and Downing, D.T., Metabolism of topically applied fatty acid methyl esters in BALB/C mouse epidermis, *J. Dermatol. Sci.,* 1, 33, 1990.

43. Blichmann, C.W., Serup, J., and Winther, A., Effects of single application of a moisturizer: Evaporation of emulsion water, skin surface temperature, electrical conductance, electrical capacitance, and skin surface (emulsion) lipids, *Acta Derm. Venereol.,* 69, 327, 1989.

44. Lodén, M. and Lindberg, M., The influence of a single application of different moisturizers on the skin capacitance, *Acta Derm. Venereol.,* 71, 79, 1991.

45. Serup, J., Winther, A., and Blichmann, C.W., Effects of repeated application of a moisturizer, *Acta Derm. Venereol.,* 69, 457, 1989.

46. Serup, J., A double-blind comparison of two creams containing urea as the active ingredient, assessment of efficacy and side-effects by non-invasive techniques and a clinical scoring scheme, *Acta Derm. Venereol. (Suppl.),* 177, 34, 1992.

47. Swanbeck, G., Urea in the treatment of dry skin, *Acta Derm. Venereol. (Suppl.),* 177, 7, 1992.

48. Hannuksela, A., Moisturizers in the prevention of contact dermatitis, in *Prevention of Contact Dermatitis: Current Problems in Dermatology,* Elsner, P. et al., Eds., Karger, Basel, 1996, p. 214.

49. Feldmann, R.J. and Maibach, H.I., Percutaneous penetration of hydrocortisone with urea, *Arch. Dermatol.,* 109, 58, 1974.

50. Wohlrab, W., Effect of urea on penetration kinetics of vitamin A acid in human skin, *Z. Hautkr.,* 65, 803, 1990.

51. Lodén, M., Urea-containing moisturizers influence barrier properties of normal skin, *Arch. Dermatol. Res.,* 288, 103, 1996.

52. Serup, J., A three-hour test for rapid comparison of effects of moisturizers and active constituents (urea), Measurement of hydration, scaling and skin surface lipidization by noninvasive techniques, *Acta Derm. Venereol. (Suppl.),* 177, 29, 1992.

53. Hannuksela, A. and Kinnunen, T., Moisturizers prevent irritant dermatitis, *Acta Derm. Venereol.,* 72, 42, 1992.

54. Halkier-Sørensen, L. and Thestrup-Pedersen, K., The efficacy of a moisturizer (Locobase) among cleaners and kitchen assistants during everyday exposure to water and detergents, *Contact Dermatitis,* 29, 266, 1993.

55. Lane, A.T. and Drost, S.S., Effects of repeated application of emollient cream to premature neonates' skin, *Pediatrics,* 92, 415, 1993.

56. Lodén, M. and Andersson, A.C., Effect of topically applied lipids on surfactant-irritated skin, *Br. J. Dermatol.,* 134, 215, 1996.

57. Olivarius, F.D.F. et al., Water protective effect of barrier creams and moisturizing creams: A new *in vivo* test method, *Contact Dermatitis,* 35, 219, 1996.

58. Gammal, C.E. et al., A model to assess the efficacy of moisturizers — The quantification of soap-induced xerosis by image analysis of adhesive-coated discs (D-Squames®), *Clin. Exp. Dermatol.,* 21, 338, 1996.

59. Ramsing, D.W. and Agner, T., Preventive and therapeutic effects of a moisturizer: An experimental study of human skin, *Acta Derm. Venereol.,* 77, 335, 1997.

60. Lodén, M., Andersson, A.C., and Lindberg, M., Improvement in skin barrier function in patients with atopic dermatitis after treatment with a moisturizing cream (Cano-derm®), *Br. J. Dermatol.*, 140, 264, 1999.

61. Held, E. and Agner, T., Comparison between 2 test models in evaluating the effect of a moisturizer on irritated human skin, *Contact Dermatitis*, 40, 261, 1999.

62. Held, E. and Jorgensen, L.L., The combined use of moisturizers and occlusive gloves: An experimental study, *Am. J. Contact Dermatitis*, 10, 146, 1999.

63. Held, E., Lund, H., and Agner, T., Effect of different moisturizers on SLS-irritated human skin, *Contact Dermatitis*, 44, 229, 2001.

64. Zhai, H. et al., Prevention and therapeutic effects of a model emulsion on glove-induced irritation and dry skin in man, *Dermatol. Beruf Umwelt/Occup. Environ. Deramtol.*, 4, 134, 2002.

65. Held, E., Sveinsdóttir, S., and Agner, T., Effect of long-term use of moisturizer on skin hydration, barrier function and susceptibility to irritants, *Acta Derm. Venereol.*, 79, 49, 1999.

66. Held, E. and Agner, T., Effect of moisturizers on skin susceptibility to irritants, *Acta Derm. Venereol.*, 81, 104, 2001.

67. Agner, T. et al., Evaluation of an experimental patch test model for the detection of irritant skin reactions to moisturisers, *Skin Res. Technol.*, 6, 250, 2000.

68. Miettinen, H. et al., Studies on constituents of moisturizers: water-binding properties of urea and NaCl in aqueous solutions, *Skin Pharmacol. Appl. Skin Physiol.*, 12, 344, 1999.

69. Kobayashi, R. et al., Neoagarobiose as a novel moisturizer with whitening effect, *Biosci. Biotechnol. Biochem.*, 61, 162, 1997.

70. Jemec, G.B. and Wulf, H.C., Correlation between the greasiness and the plasticizing effect of moisturizers, *Acta Derm. Venereol.*, 79, 115, 1999.

18 Occlusive Effects: Man vs. Animal

Hongbo Zhai, Mahbub M. U. Chowdhury, and Howard I. Maibach

CONTENTS

I. Introduction..177
II. Skin Barrier Function..178
III. Effects of Occlusion on Barrier Function...178
IV. Evaluating Methods...179
    A. Animal Models...179
    B. Human Models...181
V. Conclusions..183
References..185

I. INTRODUCTION

Occlusion means the skin covered directly or indirectly by impermeable films or substances including diapers, tape, chambers, gloves, textiles, garments, wound dressings, and transdermal devices.[1] In addition, certain topical vehicles that contain fats and/or polymer oils (petrolatum, paraffin) may also generate occlusive effects.[2]

Occlusion, because of its simplicity, is widely utilized to enhance the penetration of applied drugs in clinical practice. However, occlusion does not increase percutaneous absorption to all chemicals.[3–5] It may increase penetration of lipid-soluble, nonpolar molecules but has less effect on polar molecules, with a trend of enhanced occlusion-induced absorption with increasing penetrant lipophilicity.[5–7] In practice, increasing skin penetration rates of applied drug is far from simple. Skin barrier function can be ascribed to the macroscopic structure of the stratum corneum, consisting of alternating lipoidal and hydrophilic regions. For this reason, physico-chemical characteristics of the chemical, such as partition coefficient, structure, and molecular weight, play an important role in determining the facility of absorption.[8,9] Another factor to consider in drug percutaneous absorption is the vehicle in which the drug is formulated, as it acts on drug release from the formulation.[7,10] In addition, the anatomical site may also influence the effects of occlusion on percutaneous absorption.[11]

In many industrial and food fields, protective gloves or clothing are required to protect the workers from hazardous materials or for hygiene. In turn, these protective measures may also produce negative effects due to the nature of occlusion, which often causes stratum corneum hyperhydration and reduces the protective barrier properties of the skin.[12] Many gloves do not resist the penetration of low molecular weight chemicals and, therefore, these chemicals may enter the glove and become trapped on the skin under occlusion for many hours leading to irritation, dermatitis, or eczematous changes.[13–15]

Wound dressings have been employed to speed the healing processes in acute and chronic wounds. They keep healing tissues moist and increase superficial wound epithelialization.[2,16,17] However, occlusive or semiocclusive dressings can increase microorganisms and hence induce wound infections.[2,18–21] A significant increase in the density of *Staphylococcus aureus* and lipophilic diphtheroids were observed after 24 hours (h) occlusion in eczematous and psoriatic skin.[19]

Thus, the effects of occlusion on skin are complex and may produce profound changes that include altering epidermal lipids, DNA synthesis, epidermal turnover, pH, epidermal morphology, sweat glands, and Langerhans cells stresses.[1–4,20,22–29] Evaluation and investigation of the impact of occlusion on barrier function are important in many fields including skin physiology, pathology, pharmacology, and dermatology. This chapter focuses on the effect of occlusion on percutaneous absorption only and also summarizes relevant animal and human models.

II. SKIN BARRIER FUNCTION

Stratum corneum (horny layer) has been well recognized as a principle barrier of the skin. It is a cellular tissue with a fabric of cornified cells creating a tough, flexible, coherent membrane.[29] This acts as a two-way barrier minimizing loss of water, electrolytes, and other body constituents, and decreasing the entry of noxious substances from the external environment.[30] Topical application of pharmaceutical agents to this semipermeable membrane has been shown to be a route of entry into the systemic circulation as well as an obvious choice in the treatment of dermatological disease.[3,4,29] Physical, chemical and pathological factors can disturb barrier function with even changes in environmental humidity inducing pathophysiologic alterations.[25] Maintenance of the stratum corneum structural integrity is critical to barrier function. Increasing stratum corneum hydration can progressively reduce its barrier efficiency.[1,3–5,22–24,27–29,31,32] Stratum corneum is extremely hygroscopic: it can pick up 500% of its dry weight in less than 1 h following immersion in water, swelling vertically up to five times its original width.[29]

III. EFFECTS OF OCCLUSION ON BARRIER FUNCTION

Healthy stratum corneum typically has a water content of 10 to 20%.[30] Occlusion can block diffusional water loss from skin surface, increasing stratum corneum hydration, thereby swelling the corneocytes, and promoting water uptake into intercellular lipid domains.[3,4] Water content can be increased up to 50% with occlusion[3,4] with even short time (30 minutes) exposure resulting in significantly increased stratum corneum hydration.[33] With 24 hour occlusion, the relative water content in stratum corneum can be increased significantly from 53% before occlusion to 59%.[20] Twenty-four hour occlusion can induce morphological changes on the surface deepening skin furrows.[22] Water under occlusion may disrupt barrier lipids and damage stratum corneum similar to surfactants.[28] Kligman[1] studied hydration dermatitis in man: 1 week of an impermeable plastic film did not injure skin, 2 weeks was moderately harmful to some but not all subjects, 3 weeks regularly induced dermatitis. Hydration dermatitis was independent of race, sex, and age. They examined the potential role of microorganisms in developing hydration dermatitis by using antibiotic solutions immediately following occlusion with plastic wrapping and showed microorganisms had no impact. In addition, hydrogels did not appreciably hydrate or macerate the surface by visual inspection when left in place for 1 week. However, some transdermal drug delivery systems (TDDS) may indeed provoke a dermatitis when applied twice weekly to the same site. These occlusive devices demonstrated marked cytotoxicity to Langerhans cells, melanocytes and keratinocytes.

Nieboer et al.[34] evaluated the effects of occlusion with transdermal therapeutic systems (TTS) on Langerhan cells and skin irritation at different time ranges (6 hours, 1, 2, 4, and 7 days). Irritation was judged on morphology, histopathologic and immunofluorescence findings, and changes in the Langerhan cells system. Occlusion provoked only slight or no skin irritation. Fluhr et al.[27] evaluated the barrier damage by prolonged occlusion on the forearm for 24 to 96 h and did not find significant changes in hydration and water holding capacity. In contrast, transepidermal water loss (TEWL) increased reaching a plateau on day 2, concluding that occlusion induced barrier damage without skin dryness.

IV. EVALUATING METHODS

Various animal and human *in vivo* and *in vitro* models have been developed to study barrier function. Schaefer et al.[35] have documented these models to study skin permeability. Imokawa[36] described *in vitro* and *in vivo* models to study water-holding mechanisms of the SC. Here, we only briefly introduce the effect of occlusion on percutaneous absorption *in vivo*, both in animal and human models. Recently, this subject has been reviewed by Zhai.[37,38]

A. ANIMAL MODELS

Bronaugh et al.[39] measured the percutaneous absorption of cosmetic fragrance materials including safrole, cinnamyl anthranilate, cinnamic alcohol, and cinnamic acid, at occluded and nonoccluded application sites over a 24 hour period. They determined the absorption in the rhesus monkey *in vivo*, and also measured the absorption value through excised human skin in diffusion cells system. Each radiolabelled compound was applied, in an acetone vehicle at a concentration of $4\mu g/cm^2$. Occlusion was accomplished by taping plastic wrap to skin application site for *in vivo* experiments and by sealing the tops of the diffusion cells with Parafilm®. Occlusion of the application sites resulted in large increases in absorption, an effect consistent with the volatility of permeating molecules. When evaporation of the compounds was prevented, 75% of the applied cinnamic alcohol and 84% of the cinnamic acid were absorbed compared to 25 and 39%, respectively, without occlusion. *In vitro* experiments showed that their percutaneous absorption was increased under occlusion in comparison to nonocclusion conditions (open to the air). The greatest difference between *in vivo* and *in vitro* absorption values occurred with safrole, which was the least well absorbed and the most volatile compound.

Subsequently, they determined the percutaneous absorption of the fragrance benzyl acetate (octanol-water partition coefficient = 1.96) and five other benzyl derivatives (benzyl alcohol, octanol-water partition coefficient = 0.87; benzyl benzoate, octanol-water partition coefficient = 3.97; benzamide, octanol-water partition coefficient = 0.64; benzoin, octanol-water partition coefficient = 1.35; and benzophenone, octanol-water partition coefficient = 3.18) *in vivo* in rhesus monkeys and humans models.[40] Two occlusion methods (plastic wrap and glass chamber) were employed for 24 h. In general, absorption through occluded skin was high. Differences in absorption were observed between the methods. The low percentage (%) absorbed for benzyl acetate was noted with plastic wrap compared to the unoccluded site, whereas glass chamber occlusion resulted in the greatest bioavailability. This discrepancy might be due to compound sequestration by the plastic. No correlations were found between skin penetration of these compounds and their octanol-water partition coefficients. Under unoccluded conditions, skin penetration was reduced. There was great variability between compounds, possibly because of variations in the rates of evaporation from the application site.

Qiao et al.[41] described an *in vivo* female weanling pig model to quantify disposition (the final distribution in the organism) of parathion (PA) and its major metabolites for human dermal risk assessment following intravenous (300 μg) and topical (occluded and nonoccluded dose of 300 μg, 40 μg/cm^2 on the abdomen and back) [^{14}C]-PA. Total [^{14}C]-PA and its major metabolites in plasma, urine, blood, stratum corneum, dosed tissues, dosing device, and evaporative loss were determined. Occlusion enhanced the partition of both PA and *p*-nitrophenol (PNP) into the stratum corneum from the dosed skin surface, and also slowed down the distribution of PA and PNP in the local dosed tissues. Occlusion also altered the first pass biotransformation of PA in the epidermis. They further analyzed this data, focusing on a quantitation of the effects of application site (back vs. abdomen) and dosing method (occluded vs. nonoccluded) on *in vivo* disposition of both the parent PA and its sequential metabolites.[42] Occlusion not only increased [^{14}C] absorption and shortened the mean residence time in most compartments but also altered the systemic versus cutaneous biotransformation pattern.

They investigated the effects of anatomical site and occlusion on the percutaneous absorption and residue pattern of total [^{14}C] following topical application of PA onto four skin sites (300 μg/10 μCi; 40 μg/cm^2) in weanling pigs using occluded and nonoccluded dosing systems.[11] Urinary and fecal total excretion (% dose) was determined after 168 h dosing onto the abdomen, buttocks, back, and shoulder (n = 4/site), and the percentage (%) dose of excretion was 44, 49, 49, and 29% in the occluded system; 7, 16, 25, and 17% in the nonoccluded system, respectively. The percutaneous absorption from the shoulder was much lower than that from the other three sites under occluded conditions. However, in the nonoccluded system, absorption from the abdomen was the lowest, with shoulder and buttocks being similar, and the back the highest. They suggested that anatomic site may influence the effects of occlusion. They utilized the same model to determine the pentachlorophenol (PCP) dermal absorption and disposition from soil under occluded and nonoccluded conditions for 408 h.[43] The absorption on occluded dosed site (100.7%) was significantly enhanced (by more than 3 times, p < 0.0005) when compared to nonoccluded site (29.1%).

Mukherji et al.[44] evaluated the topical application of 2',3'-dideoxyinosine (ddI), a nucleoside analog used for treating patients with acquired immunodeficiency syndrome. A dose of ddI (approximately 180 mg/kg) dispersed in approximately 1 g ointment base was applied to the back of high follicular density (HFD) and low follicular density (LFD) rats with or without occlusion. At 24 h, the experiment was terminated and skin sections at the application site removed. Average plateau plasma levels of about 0.6 µg/ml were achieved within 1 to 2 h and maintained for 24 h. Occlusion gave a more uniform plasma profile but did not increase bioavailability. They suggest that the transfollicular absorption route for ddI did not act as an important role due to the similar bioavailability in the HFD and LFD rats.

B. HUMAN MODELS

Feldmann[45] correlated the increased pharmacological effect of hydrocortisone (HC) by occlusive conditions with the pharmacokinetics of absorption. [^{14}C]-HC in acetone was applied to the ventral forearm. The application site was either unoccluded or occluded with plastic wrap. After 24 h application, the unoccluded site was washed. At the occluded site, the wrap remained for 96 h postapplication, before washing the site. The percent of the applied dose excreted into the urine, corrected for incomplete renal elimination, was 0.46 ± 0.2 (mean ± SD) and 5.9 ± 3.5 under unoccluded and occluded conditions, respectively. The occlusive condition significantly increased (10-fold) the cumulative absorption of HC (total excretion was occluded = 4.48% versus nonoccluded = 0.46%). They noted that the difference of application duration (24 h exposure on unoccluded site versus 96-h exposure on occluded site) could influence the absorption as determined by the cumulative measurement of drug excreted into urine. However, the significant difference in percent dose at 12 and 24 h between unoccluded and occluded was not expected to be dependent upon differences in washing times. Malathion, a pesticide, was intensively studied to determine the effect of duration of occlusion.[46] In as little as 1 h (13% of absorption) there was a significant increase in penetration, and in 2 h 17%, in 4 h 24%, and in 8 h 39%.

Ryatt et al.[47] developed a human pharmacodynamic model to measure the enhanced skin penetration of hexyl nicotinate (HN) using laser Doppler velocimetry (LDV). Before applying HN, the application site was either untreated (control) or subjected to one of four 30-minute pretreatments: (a) occlusion with a polypropylene chamber; (b) occlusion (as in a) in the presence of 0.3 ml of the vehicle; (c) occlusion (as in a) in the presence of 0.3 ml of the vehicle containing 25% 2-pyrrolidone; and

(d) occlusion (as in a) in the presence of 0.3 ml of the vehicle containing 25% laurocapram (1-dodecylhexahydro-2*H*-azepin-2-one). The onset of action, time to peak, peak height, area under the curve (AUC), time-course, and magnitude of the LDV response were calculated. The onset of action and time to peak were significantly shortened, and the peak height and AUC significantly increased with pretreatments a through d (i.e., under occlusion conditions).

Ryatt et al.[33] explored the relationship between increased stratum corneum hydration by occlusion and enhanced percutaneous absorption *in vivo* in man. Percutaneous absorption of HN was monitored noninvasively by LDV following each of three randomly assigned pretreatments: untreated control, 30 minute occlusion with a polypropylene chamber, and 30 minute occlusion followed by exposure to ambient conditions for 1 h. Stratum corneum water content after the same pretreatments was measured with the dielectric probe technique. The local vasodilatory effect of the nicotinic acid ester was quantified using LDV by the onset of increased blood flow, time of maximal increase in response, magnitude of the peak response, and the area under the response-time curve. A 30 minute period of occlusion significantly shortened ($p < 0.05$) both the time of onset of the LDV-detected response to HN and the time to peak response when compared to the untreated controls. The stratum corneum water content values showed the same pattern, where the horny layer water content after 30 minute occlusion was significantly elevated ($p < 0.001$). There was a significant correlation between stratum corneum water content and area under the LDV response-time curve after 30 minute occlusion ($r = 0.8$; $p < 0.05$).

Bucks et al.[5] measured the percutaneous absorption of steroids (hydrocortisone, estradiol, testosterone, and progesterone) *in vivo* in man under occluded and "protected" (i.e. covered but nonocclusive) conditions. The [^{14}C]-labeled chemicals were applied in acetone to the ventral forearm of volunteers. After vehicle evaporation, the site was covered with a semirigid, polypropylene chamber for 24 h. The intact chambers were employed as the occlusion condition and by boring several small holes through the chamber as the "protected" conditions (i.e. the roof of chamber was covered with piece of water permeable membrane). Urine was collected for 7 days postapplication. Steroid absorption increased with increasing lipophilicity, but penetration of progesterone (the most hydrophobic) did not continue the trend. Twenty-four-hour occlusion significantly increased ($p < 0.01$) percutaneous absorption of estradiol, testosterone, and progesterone but did not effect the penetration of hydrocortisone. The more lipophilic steroids were enhanced by occlusion but not the most water-soluble (i.e. hydrocortisone).

Zhai et al.[48] defined the quantitative relationship between nicotinate ester (a model penetrant) skin permeability and hydration, as measured by water evaporation rate (WER), decay curves (at individual time points), and WER-area under the curve (WER-AUC) on human skin. They also determined the level of skin hydration and skin permeability to nicotinates following a diapering occlusion. Nine healthy Caucasian adult women were enrolled after a prescreening procedure (time to peak redness response to nicotinate). Each received three wet occlusive patches for different exposure times (10 minute, 30 minute, and 3 h) and two wet model diapers (3 h and 8 h). Prior to patching or diapering of forearms, basal values of WER, skin blood flow volume (BFV), capacitance (Cap), and redness (a*) were measured on premarked sites (a, b, c, and d). Immediately following occlusive patch or diaper removal, 20 μl of each nicotinate (methyl and hexyl nicotinate) was applied to its respective site (a or b). The WER and Cap readings were recorded at designated sites (c and d) after nicotinate applications at 0, 5, 10, 15, and 20 minutes. The a* and BFV measurements were made on each nicotinate challenged site (a and b) after nicotinate applications at 5, 10, 15, 20, 30, 40, and 60 minutes. Skin hyperhydration or WER-AUC increased with occlusive patch and diaper exposure time, but there was no statistical difference between 3 h and 8 h diaper sites. All patched sites had significantly ($p < 0.05$) increased hydration in comparison to control sites (undiapered or unpatched skin). Capacitance increased with occlusion time with patches, but not with diapers. The degree and time-course of redness from nicotinates did not vary with extent of skin hydration, but was significantly increased compared to nonhydrated skin. BFV-AUC did not show a significant increase between diapers at 3 and 8 h sites, but values varied on the patched sites, and some were significantly ($p < 0.05$) higher than control site. Wet patches and diapers increased skin hyperhydration proportional to exposure time. Permeation of nicotinates was increased for hydrated skin versus control, even after only 10 minutes of patch exposure. For these model permeants, they found no evidence of increased permeation rates with increasing hyperhydration, once a relatively low threshold of hyperhydration was achieved (e.g., that reached after a 10-minute wet patch). The data showed no meaningful differences in permeation following either diapering simulation and also suggested that the WER-AUC method was superior to capacitance for measuring the absolute extent of hyperhydration.

Animal and human models for barrier study (occlusive vs. percutaneous absorption) are summarized in Table 18.1.

V. CONCLUSIONS

Occlusion increases the percutaneous absorption of many but not all compounds. The effect of occlusion on percutaneous absorption may also be affected by the physicochemical properties (volatility, partition coefficient, and aqueous solubility), anatomical site, and vehicle. On the other hand, occlusion alone may also damage skin barrier function. Application of chemicals/drugs under occlusion conditions, increases penetration of chemicals and antigens into the skin, and therefore also increases dermatitis.[2,15,49]

Animal and human models described above have been well developed. Results from animal experiments may be used to generate kinetic data because of a closer similarity between humans and some animals (pigs and monkeys) in percutaneous absorption, and penetration for some compounds. However, no one animal will simulate penetration in humans for all compounds. Therefore, the best estimate of human percutaneous absorption is determined by *in vivo* studies in humans. We believe that to study barrier function, in particular, the effect of occlusion on percutaneous absorption, the final relevant clinical data should be derived from human models rather than animals.

TABLE 18.1
Effect of Occlusion on Percutaneous Absorption in Animal and Human *In Vivo* Models

Models			
Animal	Human	Compounds	Results
Rhesus monkey		Safrole, cinnamyl anthranilate, cinnamic alcohol, and cinnamic acid	Greater permeation of all compounds[39]
Weanling pigs		Parathion and its major metabolites	Increased absorption and shortened mean residence time; affected by anatomical site[11,41,42]
Weanling pigs		Pentachlorophenol	Absorption on occluded dosed site significantly enhanced (> 3x) compared to nonoccluded site[43]
Rhesus monkeys	Human	Benzyl acetate and five other benzyl derivatives	Increased penetration with variability between compounds[40]
Rats		2′,3′-dideoxyinosine	Provided more uniform plasma profile but no increased bioavailability[44]
	Human	Hydrocortisone	Significantly increased cumulative absorption[45]
	Human	Hexyl nicotinate	Significantly increased peak height, AUC; significantly shortened onset of action, time to peak; significant correlation between water content and area under the LDV response-time curve[33,47]
	Human	Hydrocortisone, estradiol, testosterone, and progesterone	Significantly increased percutaneous absorption of estradiol, testosterone, progesterone but did not affect the penetration of hydrocortisone[5]
	Human	Nicotinates	Nicotinates permeation increased for hydrated skin versus control even after only 10 minutes of patch exposure; no evidence of increased permeation rates with increasing hyperhydration after relatively low threshold of hyperhydration achieved (e.g., 10-min wet patch)[48]

REFERENCES

1. Kligman, A.M., Hydration injury to human skin, in *The Irritant Contact Dermatitis Syndrome,* Van der Valk, P.G.M. and Maibach, H.I., Eds., CRC Press, Boca Raton, FL, 1996, p. 187.
2. Berardesca, E. and Maibach, H.I., Skin occlusion: Treatment or drug-like device? *Skin Pharmacol.,* 1, 207, 1988.
3. Bucks, D., Guy, R., and Maibach, H.I., Effects of occlusion, in *In Vitro Percutaneous Absorption: Principles, Fundamentals, and Applications,* Bronaugh, R.L. and Maibach, H.I., Eds., CRC Press, Boca Raton, 1991, p. 85.
4. Bucks, D. and Maibach, H.I., Occlusion does not uniformly enhance penetration *in vivo,* in *Percutaneous Absorption: Drug-Cosmetics-Mechanisms-Methodology,* Bronaugh, R.L. and Maibach, H.I., Eds., Marcel Dekker, New York, 1999, p. 81.
5. Bucks, D.A. et al., Bioavailability of topically administered steroids: A "mass balance" technique, *J. Invest. Dermatol.,* 91, 29, 1988.
6. Treffel, P. et al., Effect of occlusion on *in vitro* percutaneous absorption of two compounds with different physicochemical properties, *Skin Pharmacol.,* 5, 108, 1992.
7. Cross, S.E. and Roberts, M.S., The effect of occlusion on epidermal penetration of parabens from a commercial allergy test ointment, acetone and ethanol vehicles, *J. Invest. Dermatol.,* 115, 914, 2000.
8. Wiechers, J.W., The barrier function of the skin in relation to percutaneous absorption of drugs, *Pharma. Week Sci. Edit.,* 11, 185, 1989.
9. Hostynek, J.J., Magee, P.S., and Maibach, H.I., QSAR predictive of contact allergy: Scope and limitations, in *Prevention of Contact Dermatitis: Current Problems in Dermatology,* Elsner, P. et al., Eds., Karger, Basel, 1996, p. 18.
10. Hotchkiss, S.A., Miller, J.M., and Caldwell, J., Percutaneous absorption of benzyl acetate through rat skin *in vitro* 2: Effect of vehicle and occlusion, *Food Chem. Toxicol.,* 30, 145, 1992.
11. Qiao, G.L., Chang, S.K., and Riviere, J.E., Effects of anatomical site and occlusion on the percutaneous absorption and residue pattern of 2,6-[ring-14C] parathion *in vivo* in pigs, *Toxicol. Appl. Pharmacol.,* 122, 131, 1993.
12. Graves, C.J., Edwards, C., and Marks, R., The occlusive effects of protective gloves on the barrier properties of the stratum corenum, in *Irritant Dermatitis: New Clinical and Experimental Aspects, Current Problems in Dermatology,* Elsner, P. and Maibach, H.I., Eds., Karger, Basel, 1995, p. 87.
13. Van der Valk, P.G.M. and Maibach, H.I., Post-application occlusion substantially increases the irritant response of the skin to repeated short-term sodium lauryl sulfate (SLS) exposure, *Contact Dermatitis,* 21, 335, 1989.
14. Mathias, C.G.T., Prevention of occupational contact dermatitis, *J. Am. Acad. Dermatol.,* 23, 742, 1990.
15. Estlander, T., Jolanki, R., and Kanerva, L., Rubber glove dermatitis: A significant occupational hazard-prevention, in *Prevention of Contact Dermatitis: Current Problems in Dermatology,* Elsner, P. et al., Eds., Karger, Basel, 1996, p. 170.
16. Alvarez, O.M., Mertz, P.M., and Eaglstein, W.H., The effect of occlusive dressings on collagen synthesis and re-epithelialization in superficial wounds, *J. Surg. Res.,* 35, 142, 1983.
17. Eaglstein, W.H., Effect of occlusive dressings on wound healing, *Clin. Dermatol.,* 2, 107, 1984.
18. Aly, R. et al., Effect of prolonged occlusion on the microbial flora, pH, carbon dioxide and transepidermal water loss on human skin, *J. Invest. Dermatol.,* 71, 378, 1978.

19. Rajka, G. et al., The effect of short-term occlusion on the cutaneous flora in atopic dermatitis and psoriasis, *Acta Dermatol. Venereol.,* 61, 150, 1981.

20. Faergemann, J. et al., Skin Occlusion: Effect on pityrosporum orbiculare, skin pCO_2, pH, transepidermal water loss, and water content, *Arch. Dermatol. Res.,* 275, 383, 1983.

21. Mertz, P.M. and Eaglstein, W.H., The effect of a semiocclusive dressing on the microbial population in superficial wounds, *Arch. Surg.,* 119, 287, 1984.

22. Matsumura, H. et al., Effect of occlusion on human skin, *Contact Dermatitis,* 33, 231, 1995.

23. Berardesca, E. and Maibach, H.I., The plastic occlusion stress test (POST) as a model to investigate skin barrier function, in *Dermatologic Research Techniques,* Maibach, H.I., Ed., CRC Press, Boca Raton, FL, 1996, p. 179.

24. Leow, Y.H. and Maibach, H.I., Effect of occlusion on skin, *J. Dermatol. Treat.,* 8, 139, 1997.

25. Denda, M. et al., Low humidity stimulates epidermal DNA synthesis and amplifies the hyperproliferative response to barrier disruption: implication for seasonal exacerbations of inflammatory dermatoses, *J. Invest. Dermatol.,* 111, 873, 1998.

26. Kömüves, L.G. et al., Induction of selected lipid metabolic enzymes and differentiation-linked structural proteins by air exposure in fetal rat skin explants, *J. Invest. Dermatol.,* 112, 303, 1999.

27. Fluhr, J.W. et al., Effects of prolonged occlusion on stratum corneum barrier function and water holding capacity, *Skin Pharmacol. Appl. Skin Physiol.,* 12, 193, 1999.

28. Warner, R.R. et al., Water disrupts stratum corneum lipid lamellae: Damage is similar to surfactants, *J. Invest. Dermatol.,* 113, 960, 1999.

29. Kligman, A.M., Hydration injury to human skin: A view from the horny layer, in *Handbook of Occupational Dermatology,* Kanerva, L. et al., Eds. Springer, Berlin, 2000, p. 76.

30. Baker, H., The skin as a barrier, in *Textbook of Dermatology,* Rook, A., Wilkinson, D.S., and Ebling, F.J.G., Eds., Blackwell Scientific Publications, Oxford, 1972, p. 249.

31. Haftek, M., Teillon, M.H., and Schmitt, D., Stratum corneum, corneodesmosomes and *ex vivo* percutaneous penetration, *Microscopy Res. Tech.,* 43, 242, 1998.

32. Tsai, T-F. and Maibach, H.I., How irritant is water? An overview, *Contact Dermatitis,* 41, 311, 1999.

33. Ryatt, K.S. et al., Methodology to measure the transient effect of occlusion on skin penetration and stratum corneum hydration *in vivo, Br. J. Dermatol.,* 119, 307, 1988.

34. Nieboer, C., Bruynzeel, D.P., and Boorsma, D.M., The effect of occlusion of the skin with transdermal therapeutic system on Langerhans' cells and the induction of skin irritation, *Arch. Dermatol.,* 123, 1499, 1987.

35. Schaefer, H., Zesch, A., and Stüttgen, G., Eds., *Skin Permeability,* Springer, Berlin, 1982.

36. Imokawa, G., *In vitro* and *in vivo* models, in *Bioengineering of the Skin: Water and the Stratum Corneum,* Elsner, P., Berardesca, E., and Maibach, H. I., Eds., CRC Press, Boca Raton, FL, 1994, p. 23.

37. Zhai, H. and Maibach, H. I., Effects of skin occlusion on percutaneous absorption: An overview, *Skin Pharmacol. Appl. Skin Physiol.,* 14, 1, 2001.

38. Zhai, H. and Maibach, H.I., Occlusion vs. skin barrier function, *Skin Res. Technol.,* 8, 1, 2002.

39. Bronaugh, R. L. et al., Comparison of percutaneous absorption of fragrances by humans and monkeys, *Food Chem. Toxicol.,* 23, 111, 1985.

40. Bronaugh, R. L. et al., *In vivo* percutaneous absorption of fragrance ingredients in rhesus monkeys and humans, *Food Chem. Toxicol.,* 28, 369, 1990.
41. Qiao, G. L., Williams, P. L., and Riviere, J. E., Percutaneous absorption, biotransformation, and systemic disposition of parathion *in vivo* in swine I: Comprehensive pharmacokinetic model, *Drug Metabol. Dispos.,* 22, 459, 1994.
42. Qiao, G. L. and Riviere, J. E., Significant effects of application site and occlusion on the pharmacokinetics of cutaneous penetration and biotransformation of parathion *in vivo* in swine, *J. Pharm. Sci.,* 84, 425, 1995.
43. Qiao, G. L., Brooks, J. D., and Riviere, J. E., Pentachlorophenol dermal absorption and disposition from soil in swine: Effects of occlusion and skin microorganism inhibition, *Toxicol. App. Pharmacol.,* 147, 234, 1997.
44. Mukherji, E., Millenbaugh, N. J., and Au, J. L., Percutaneous absorption of 2',3'-dideoxyinosine in rats, *Pharm. Res.,* 11, 809, 1994.
45. Feldmann, R. J. and Maibach, H. I., Penetration of ^{14}C hydrocortisone through normal skin: The effect of stripping and occlusion, *Arch. Dermatol.,* 91, 661, 1965.
46. Task group on occupational exposure to pesticides, *Occupational Exposure to Pesticides,* Federal Working Group on Pest Management, Washington, D.C., 1974.
47. Ryatt, K. S. et al., Pharmacodynamic measurement of percutaneous penetration enhancement *in vivo, J. Pharma. Sci.,* 75, 374, 1986.
48. Zhai, H. et al., Hydration vs. skin permeability to nicotinates in man, *Skin Res. Technol.,* 8, 13, 2002.
49. Zhai, H. and Maibach, H. I., Skin occlusion and irritant and allergic contact dermatitis: An overview, *Contact Dermatitis,* 44, 201, 2001.

19 Medical Glove Regulation: History and Future of Safety

Deborah D. Davis

CONTENTS

  I.   Introduction 190
 II.   Glove Regulations 190
       A. Minimum Performance and Physical Requirements 192
           1. Length 192
           2. Size 192
           3. Thickness or Gauge 192
           4. Acceptable Quality Level (AQL) 192
           5. Tensile Strength 193
           6. Ultimate Elongation 193
           7. Stress at 500% Elongation 193
III.   Donning Lubricants 193
       A. Powdered and Powder-Free 193
       B. Coatings Technologies 193
 IV.   Protein and Allergen Levels 194
       A. Labeling 194
       B. Assay Methods 194
       C. Allergen-Specific Assays 194
  V.   Storage Stability and Expiration Dating 195
 VI.   Synthetic Medical Gloves 196
       A. Polymers 196
       B. Nitrile 196
       C. Vinyl 196
       D. Neoprene 196
       E. Polyisoprene 197
       F. Material-Specific Requirements 197
VII.   Chemical Resistance 197
VIII. Appropriate Use of Gloves 199
 IX.   Glove Hydration and Conductivity 201
  X.   Glove Manufacturers 201

0-8493-1670-7/05/$0.00+$1.50
© 2005 by CRC Press LLC

XI.   Conclusions..202
References...203

I. INTRODUCTION

Medical gloves are an important part of a clinician's personal protective equipment and are highly regulated medical devices. Currently in the United States alone, an estimated 27 million surgical procedures are performed each year.[1] There are also over 22 billion examination gloves sold each year.[2] There are basic minimum requirements for medical gloves, and there are additional tests that can be performed to better understand a glove's performance. Awareness and understanding of these standards can help users make appropriate and meaningful comparisons and assessments of the many types and brands of medical gloves.

The United States' Centers for Disease Control and Prevention published a report in 1987 that emphasized the need for all healthcare workers to routinely use appropriate barrier precautions when contact with blood or other body fluids of any patient is anticipated. In 1991, the Occupational Safety and Health Administration (OSHA) enacted regulations requiring the use of work practice controls and protective clothing, including gloves, to minimize worker exposure to blood borne pathogens.

Because of the emphasis on gloves as protective barriers, the Food and Drug Administration (FDA) established regulatory requirements for patient examination gloves, surgical gloves, and some nonmedical gloves. The regulatory controls include premarket notification (or 510K) and good manufacturing practices. The 510K submission and clearance process and other regulatory controls allow FDA to monitor the introduction of these products into the U.S., and to help assure the level of public health protection they provide.

In Europe, all products which meet the definition of a medical device (as detailed in Article 1 of the Medical Devices Directive 93/42/EEC) must meet certain conditions as specified by the relevant Essential Requirements under Annex 1 of the Directive. This represents the minimum standard a manufacturer is expected to demonstrate when claiming conformity of a product with the Directive.

II. GLOVE REGULATIONS

The evolution of protective operating room attire paralleled the development of aseptic techniques in the latter half of the 19th century. Rubber surgical gloves were introduced not to protect the patient, but to protect the wearer's hands from the harsh, irritating antiseptic solutions and soaks of the 1870s and 1880s. In the late 1890s, Dr. William Halsted, chief of surgery at Johns Hopkins Hospital, popularized the use of gloves to protect patients from the bacteria present on ungloved hands.[3] Disposable latex gloves, which were first introduced around 1958, were a welcome innovation that saved countless hours of daily glove reprocessing, repairing, and sterilizing. Today, the universal use of disposable medical gloves is well established.

The FDA places medical devices into one of three regulatory classes as required by the Federal Food, Drug and Cosmetics Act. The class of a device determines the level of regulatory control that applies to it. Medical gloves currently are in Class I. The FDA is considering reclassifying medical gloves from Class I to Class II, subjecting them to additional testing and controls.[4] This would include limiting powder and protein, labeling the actual levels of powder and protein and expiration dating. For example, the standards currently state a recommended aqueous soluble protein content limit (ASTM [American Society for Testing and Materials] D5712 "Standard Test Method for Analysis of Protein in Natural Rubber and Its Products") of 200 μg/dm^2 or 10 μg/dm^2 antigenic protein (ELISA inhibition). The FDA is considering the same limit as ASTM, plus: "The FDA recommends no more than 200 μg/dm^2 total or 10 μg natural rubber latex antigenic protein per dm^2. This product contains _____ or _____."

For powder levels on powdered gloves the ASTM standard has recommended limits of not more than 10 milligrams per dm^2 for examination gloves and 15 milligrams per dm^2 for surgical gloves. The FDA is considering the same levels as ASTM, plus the labeling requirement: "FDA recommends a maximum powder level of 10 milligrams per dm^2 (15 milligrams per dm^2 for surgical gloves). This product contains _____."

Medical glove manufacturers also are required to meet the Current Good Manufacturing Practices (CGMP) regulation for medical devices (21 CFR 820), which includes establishing and maintaining control procedures to ensure that the gloves' specified design requirements are consistently met. The minimum standards for surgical and exam gloves that must be met are listed in the ASTM "Standard Specification for Rubber Surgical Gloves" (D3577) and "Standard Specification for Patient Examination Gloves" (D3578). These standards describe requirements for sterility, freedom from holes, physical dimensions and property characteristics, and recommended maximum protein and powder limits. Other optional tests can provide further information on how the gloves will perform.

This regulation requires that every manufacturer of finished medical devices establish a system for quality. This system should be set up as a continuous process for designing, producing, and distributing safe and effective medical gloves. The system must include:

- Design controls to help assure the design of gloves that are safe, effective, correctly labeled, correctly packaged, and meet user needs
- Documented design output, records, purchasing data, quality system records, production procedures and records and change controls
- Manufacturing or production controls
- Storage and distribution controls to maintain the quality of the gloves during production, storage, and distribution
- Internal system controls to collect and analyze any issues as well as prompting corrective and preventive actions

In Europe, the Comité Européen de Normalisation (CEN, European Committee for Standardization) is the organization that issues standards. The key standards for medical gloves are:

- EN 455-1 Freedom from Holes
- EN 455-2 Physical Properties
- EN 455-3 Biological Evaluation

Another European standard that has been proposed and is still in development is EN 455-4, which is intended to define aging and shelf life criteria. Additionally, individual countries may each have their own standards and requirements for medical gloves.

A. Minimum Performance and Physical Requirements

1. Length

Glove length is measured from the tip of the middle finger to the wrist cuff. For surgical gloves, length may range from 12 to 15 inches (305 to 381 mm), and for exam gloves, usually 9 to 12 inches (220 to 305 mm). The ASTM standard represents the minimum length required. Longer gloves may be needed in specific fields such as obstetrics or for special purposes. Decisions about length should be based on the type of procedure, the probability of splash and the depth of immersion. Lengths may vary among manufacturers, so users should verify that the cuffs are long enough to fit snugly over a surgical gown and provide a continuous barrier from hand to arm.

2. Size

Size is determined by the circumference of the palm at its widest point and reflects a range rather than a fixed dimension. Surgical gloves usually come in whole and half sizes, ranging from size 5.5 to 9 and may vary in fit based on the manufacturer. Exam gloves are generally sized from extra small to extra large. Correct size is essential for the glove user. If a glove is too large, dexterity can be affected; if it is too small, it can cause hand fatigue.

3. Thickness or Gauge

Surgical gloves must be at least 0.10 mm thick as measured at the finger, palm, and cuff, and exam gloves must be at least 0.08 mm thick as measured at the finger and palm. If the polymer film has not coated the glove formers evenly, greater variations in thickness may occur at different parts of the glove.

4. Acceptable Quality Level (AQL)

This typically refers to the barrier protection confidence level. A lower AQL represents a higher quality product, i.e., a manufacturing process with fewer allowable defects. For purposes of sampling inspection, the AQL is used by manufacturers to identify the maximum number of allowable defects (pinholes) per hundred units. All gloves must be statistically sampled to verify the attainment of specific AQLs. Suppliers should be asked about the average AQL for their manufacturing process.

5. Tensile Strength

Tensile strength indicates how much force, in megapascals (MPa), is required to stretch a glove sample until it breaks. Higher numbers indicate a stronger glove film.

6. Ultimate Elongation

This measures how far, as a percentage of the original sample length, the glove stretches before it breaks. For example, if a 1-inch sample stretches to 9 inches before it breaks, the elongation is 800%. Higher numbers indicate a stronger glove film.

7. Stress at 500% Elongation

Also known as modulus, this measures how much force, in megapascals (MPa), is required to stretch a glove sample to twice its length. This is a measure of comfort, and lower numbers reflect a softer, typically more comfortable glove. Medical gloves are a very personal part of protective clothing that can directly affect a clinician's ability to practice his or her craft. Comfort is dependent on proper fit, the glove materials' modulus and, to some extent, the glove's thickness.

III. DONNING LUBRICANTS

A. Powdered and Powder-Free

Powdered surgical gloves currently have an ASTM-recommended powder limit of $15mg/dm^2$. Gloves labeled as "powder-free" are required by the FDA to have 2 mg or less of total particulate per glove. New technologies in glove manufacturing are emerging, and various polymer coatings inside the gloves are eliminating or minimizing the need for powders. Historically, powder has been used to facilitate the release of gloves from formers during the manufacturing process and to aid in donning. Polymer coatings in combination with chemical lubricants are often applied to the glove surface to provide optimum wet and dry donning capabilities.

B. Coatings Technologies

A majority of the coated surgical gloves on the market are manufactured by applying polymer coatings to the inner glove surface. This is followed by postforming processes such as chlorination and lubrication. The chlorination process oxidizes the outer rubber surface to reduce the surface tackiness and also removes most of the powders deposited on the outer glove surfaces.

Polymer coatings appropriate for medical gloves must possess certain key characteristics. To provide a high-quality glove on a consistent basis, it is critical that a polymer coating is designed and engineered to meet all of these requirements:

- It must adhere to the underlying rubber latex substrate and offer durability and good donning characteristics

- It must be resistant to chlorination and the vigorous post-forming processing steps that include rinsing, extraction, and drying
- It should not degrade after sterilization

IV. PROTEIN AND ALLERGEN LEVELS

A. LABELING

In 1997, the FDA issued a ruling that medical devices containing natural rubber must be labeled with the caution statement: "This Product Contains Natural Rubber Latex Which May Cause Allergic Reactions." This ruling became effective in 1998. It also stipulated that any "hypoallergenic" claims be removed by this date, due to the potential for confusion about this claim addressing chemical or protein allergies.

Currently, the total protein level label claim for natural rubber latex gloves that manufacturers can make is using the ASTM D5712 "Standard Test Method for the Analysis of Aqueous Extractable Protein in Natural Rubber and its Products" (the modified Lowry Method). The lowest allowable claim is "These Latex Gloves Contain 50 Micrograms or Less of Total Water Extractable Protein Per Gram," due to the insensitivity of the modified Lowry assay below that level (see Chapter 5).

B. ASSAY METHODS

Immunological methods for quantifying allergen levels in rubber products are evolving rapidly (see Chapter 5 and Chapter 6). The "Standard Test Method for the Immunological Measurement of Antigenic Protein in Natural Rubber in its products" (ASTM D6499) determines the amount of antigenic protein in natural rubber and its products using rabbit antisera specific for natural rubber latex proteins. Recommended limits for antigenic protein based on this assay have been incorporated into the surgical and exam glove standards (ASTM D3577 and D3578).

C. ALLERGEN-SPECIFIC ASSAYS

Not all natural rubber latex proteins are allergens (see Chapter 2). Therefore, allergen levels may be of greater clinical significance than total protein levels. While there are no regulations requiring the use of allergen tests, the science of these assays is evolving rapidly. The RAST is an allergen-specific protein assay, a technique for detecting and quantifying IgE antibody in human serum samples. There are several FDA-approved RAST-type assays commercially available. The allergenic proteins are bound to a surface and then plasma is allowed to react with the allergens. When used with the pooled serum of known latex-allergic individuals, this assay can measure antigenic proteins from extracts of NRL-containing products. The antilatex IgE from the pooled sera binds to the antigenic latex proteins that are isolated from the latex containing product. Since the IgE is already bound to the extract proteins, it cannot bind to the allergenic proteins from the assay kit. Hence, the assay is competitive and results in a decrease in signal or color if the extract contains the allergens. However, the source of pooled allergic patient plasma can affect the test outcome and relevancy, since allergic individuals can react to different NRL proteins.[5]

Recently, immunoenzymetric assay methods have been commercialized which quantify four of the known allergenic proteins in *Hevea brasiliensis* (the natural rubber tree) latex. There are currently four separate assays, each of which involves capturing a single specificity of Hev b protein (e.g., Hev b 1, Hev b 3, Hev b 5, and Hev b 6) from a standard or unknown extract to a specific monoclonal antibody coated on a microtiter plate.

V. STORAGE STABILITY AND EXPIRATION DATING

Glove degradation is characterized by either a glove that feels too soft and tears easily or is too hard and brittle. Medical gloves must be stored appropriately to maintain their strength and barrier properties. Do not store gloves near heaters, air conditioners, sterilizers, x-ray units or in areas exposed to ultraviolet light, sunlight, or fluorescent light. Any of these factors can degrade the glove polymers. Additionally, stock should be rotated so that older gloves are used first. Factors that can compromise glove barrier properties are summarized in Table 19.1.

Only water-based lotions or moisturizers are compatible under natural rubber latex gloves. Appropriate use of lotions and moisturizers is an integral component of an effective hand care regime, but products that contain mineral oil or petroleum or lanolin are not recommended for use under natural rubber latex gloves. Users should check with the hand care product manufacturer and request compatibility testing results. There is an ASTM subcommittee that is developing a test method to assess the effects of lubricant products (such as mineral oil or petrolatum) on natural rubber latex medical products.

Because of concerns about glove degradation, the FDA also is considering requiring expiration dating on medical glove packages. A 2-year expiration date would be assigned initially based on acceptable accelerated aging resistance data (e.g., stored 7 days at 70 degrees Celsius). Longer expiration dates could be assigned

---

TABLE 19.1
Factors Compromising Barrier Properties

Stress: Simply wearing a glove places stress on it. The longer you wear a glove, the higher the probability that its barrier properties are being compromised. Consider changing surgical gloves after one hour of wearing, if not more frequently.

Storage: Do not store gloves near heaters, air conditioners, sterilizers, x-ray units, or in areas exposed to ultraviolet light, sunlight, or fluorescent light. Any of these factors can degrade the glove polymers.

Environment pollutants and extremes in temperature: Can adversely affect glove barrier properties. Gloves should be properly stored, and packaging should consist of materials that provide protection.

Exposure to chemicals and drugs: Permeation resistance varies with the glove material and the manufacturer's formulation. Gloves should be selected based on resistance to permeation to the specific drug or chemical being used. Ask the supplier for permeation test results for chemicals with which the gloves will come into contact.

Procedures: Tasks and procedures vary in the amount of stress and strain they put on a glove. In addition, there may be varying amounts of blood and other body fluids involved.

if the manufacturer has real-time aging testing data to demonstrate the continued stability of the gloves' strength and barrier properties.

VI. SYNTHETIC MEDICAL GLOVES

A. POLYMERS

A number of good synthetic polymers are used today in medical gloves. A polymer is a material composed of molecules made up of many (poly) repeats of a simpler unit, the monomer. Another term used to describe such a molecule is macromolecule, meaning big molecule. What all polymers have in common is that they are chemically constructed of repeats of the basic monomer unit, which is chemically bonded to others of its kind to form three-dimensional molecules, giving each polymer its unique physical properties. The chemical nature and length of the molecules and their orientation in relation to each other influence the properties of the polymer and the products made from them.

B. NITRILE

Nitrile exam gloves are increasing in popularity because of their excellent strength and barrier properties, puncture and tear resistance, and resistance to permeation by a wide range of chemicals. Nitrile rubbers are the polymers of acrylonitrile, butadiene, and carboxylic acid. Acrylonitrile monomer provides material hardness and permeation resistance to a wide variety of chemicals and solvents, especially to hydrocarbon oils, fats, and solvents. After vulcanization, butadiene offers softness and flexibility, and carboxylic acid provides high tensile strength and tear resistance.[6] As a plant-derived product, natural rubber latex contains proteins that act as a stabilizer. These proteins can contain allergens that may cause an allergic reaction in genetically predisposed, sensitized individuals. Nitrile synthetic lattices do not contain any proteins but instead are stabilized by chemicals such as calcium nitrate that are added to the formulation.

C. VINYL

Polyvinyl chloride (PVC) has been used for more than 50 years, since the flexible (plasticized) PVC was introduced in the mid-1930s. PVC is manufactured by polymerization of vinyl chloride monomers. Vinyl examination gloves are appropriate for short-term tasks involving minimal stress and risk of exposure to blood and other potential infectious material. They are appropriate for these tasks as long as the barrier remains intact. Users must consider the risk based on the specific procedure and the manipulations and other stresses placed on the glove film.

D. NEOPRENE

The generic term neoprene denotes rubberlike polymers and copolymers of chloroprene. Neoprenes were the first synthetic rubbers developed in the U.S. Discovered in the laboratories of the University of Notre Dame and developed by E. I. du Pont

TABLE 19.2
Exam Glove Standard Comparison by Material

Property	Requirement			
	D3578 – Type I	D3578 – Type II	D5250	D6319
Length (mm) (depending on size)	≥ 220–230	≥ 220–230	≥ 230	≥ 220–230
Width (mm) (depending on size)	70–114	70–114	76–115	75–120
Tensile strength (MPa)	≥ 18	≥ 14	≥ 9	≥ 14
Tensile Stress @ 500% (Mpa)	≤ 5.5	≤ 2.8	NA	NA
Elongation (%)	≥ 650	≥ 650	≥ 300	≥ 500
AQL (freedom from holes)	2.5	2.5	2.5	2.5

Note: Type I and II refer to different classifications based on tensile stress at 500% (modulus); NA = Not applicable; ASTM D3578 = Standard Specification for Rubber Examination Gloves; ASTM D5250 = Standard Specification for Poly (vinyl chloride) Gloves for Medical Applications; and ASTM D6319 = Standard Specification for Nitrile Examination Gloves for Medical Application.

de Nemours and Company, neoprene has inherent high tensile strength, elongation, and wear properties.

E. POLYISOPRENE

Natural rubber latex primarily consists of the polymer isoprene. Technology has finally enabled manufacturers to produce a synthetic polyisoprene with all the advantages of the natural product but without the proteins and allergens of natural rubber latex. The properties of synthetic polyisoprene are nearly identical to those of natural rubber and, often, preferred alternatives for the natural product due to their greater uniformity and consistency.

F. MATERIAL-SPECIFIC REQUIREMENTS

There are currently exam glove standards specific to natural rubber latex, poly vinyl chloride (PVC), and nitrile that specify the basic physical properties for gloves made from each of these materials (Table 19.2). Separate standards are appropriate, as each of these materials have different inherent properties. The Food and Drug Administration (FDA) requires medical gloves to meet this standard to receive clearance for marketing. As new materials are developed, consideration will need to be given to developing exam and surgical glove standards specific to each materials' unique properties.

VII. CHEMICAL RESISTANCE

When choosing a glove, the first consideration should be the barrier requirement related to the procedure or task. In addition, the level of exposure risk should be

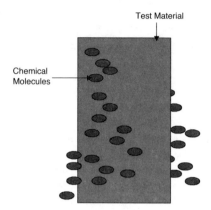

FIGURE 19.1 Chemical permeation. (From Managing Infection Control, 2003. With permission.)[7]

determined prior to selecting a glove. Many medical gloves today have clearance to be marketed as a chemotherapy glove, however, the glove used for protection from chemotherapy drug exposure must be selected specifically for the type of drugs being used. These gloves have a demonstrated resistance to permeation by specific antineoplastic agents.

Permeation is the diffusion of a chemical on a molecular basis through protective clothing such as a glove (Figure 19.1). This movement may not be readily noticed as it may occur on a molecular or microscopic level. The mass flux (rate in mass per unit area per unit time) of the chemical through the protective material once it has broken through is called the permeation rate. Penetration is defined as the bulk flow of chemical through the protective material and also may not be visible to the naked eye.[8]

Resistance of gloves to chemicals may vary significantly with the particular chemical, e.g., a glove may perform well against one chemical but poorly against another or a mixture of chemicals. A standard test method that is widely used to evaluate resistance of materials to chemical permeation is ASTM F739 "Standard Method for Determining Resistance to Chemical Permeation Under Conditions of Continuous Contact" (Figure 19.2). There are currently no standard requirements for a chemotherapy glove in terms of physical properties or required minimum permeation resistance, but there is a working group within the ASTM D11 Committee on Rubber that is developing this standard.

While nitrile and other synthetic polymers have demonstrated excellent chemical permeation resistance, it is important to verify the specific permeation resistance of a glove for the specific drug to be used. Professional groups such as the Oncology Nursing Association and the American Society of Hospital Pharmacists and the Occupational Safety and Health Administration have published guidelines and recommendations for protective clothing when using antineoplastic agents (Table 19.3).

Glove users should ask their supplier for specific permeation data for the gloves to be used, and see the MSDS sheets for the specific drug or chemical. Nitrile exam gloves are increasing in popularity because of their unique strength and

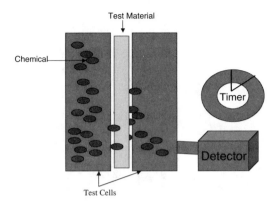

FIGURE 19.2 Permeation testing. (From Managing Infection Control, 2003. With permission.)[7]

barrier properties, durability during use, and permeation resistance to a wide variety of chemicals.

VIII. APPROPRIATE USE OF GLOVES

Scrubbing is an important first step in preparing for a surgical procedure not only from the standpoint of asepsis, but also because any foreign debris or material on your hands that comes into contact with the glove may compromise its ability to provide barrier protection. Wearing rings or any other type of jewelry may cause holes or tears and may puncture or weaken the glove. Fingernails should be short and well manicured. Even if long fingernails do not penetrate the cuff when donning the glove, they can cause significant additional stress at the fingertips, possibly compromising the barrier function.

During a surgical procedure, when the hands come into contact with instruments, sharps, and needles, it is crucial for clinicians to periodically inspect the glove for damage such as tears or pinholes. In addition, due to the "fatigue factor" of the polymer film, clinical consensus guidelines recommend changing surgical gloves every hour, and more frequently if they have contact with significant quantities of blood, fats, and other body fluids.[9]

While not a regulation, the Association of periOperating Room Nurses (AORN) "Recommended Practices for Maintaining a Sterile Field" indicates that double gloving may be needed for some procedures (according to local policies and procedures).[10] In one study involving surgeons and first assistants, the overall glove failure rate was 51% when a single pair of gloves was worn. The longer the gloves were worn, the greater the failure rate. Adding a second pair of gloves decreased the failure rate to 7%. In this study, failure was defined as blood contamination of the fingers.[11] Some surgeons chose not to participate in the study, citing loss of dexterity with two pairs of gloves and claiming the second pair was unnecessary. The results of this study demonstrate that double gloving has benefits. Based on the data obtained, the authors recommend double gloving during procedures in which a patient is known

TABLE 19.3
Summary of Recommendations Regarding Handling of Chemotheraputic Agents

Guidelines	Oncology Nursing Society (ONS) 2nd Edition, 1999	American Society of Health-Systems Pharmacists (ASHP), 1990	Occupational Safety and Health Administration (OSHA), 1995
Selection criteria	Thickness, time in contact, latex sensitivity	Fingertip thickness, fit, length, tactile sensation, and any latex sensitivity	"Thickness of the gloves... is more important than the type of material"
Ambi or hand specific?	Not Specified	Hand Specific (Surgical) for better fit and tactile sensation, particularly in drug preparation area	Not specified
Thickness (at fingertips)	0.007 inch or 0.178 mm (ASTM minimum = 0.10 mm)	Not specified, but surgical glove is recommended (ASTM minimum = 0.10 mm) Thicker fingertips are considered optimal.	Not specified, however it does state that "thickness of the gloves... is more important than the type of material"
Powder free?	Yes	Yes; however, if powder-free is unavailable, then the outside of a powdered glove should be washed before use.	Gloves with minimal or no powder are preferred since the powder may absorb any spilled hazardous material.
Glove material recommendation	Latex or Nitrile generally recommended Subject to glove manufacturing testing recommendations PVC only as a double glove beneath latex glove, if necessary for latex allergy	Latex	Latex gloves should be used for the preparation of hazardous drugs (HDs) unless the drug-product manufacturer specifically stipulates that some other glove provides better protection
Longer length?	Should be long enough to be worn under and/or over the cuffs of a gown	Should be long enough to be worn under and/or over the cuffs of a gown	Should be long enough to be worn under and/or over the cuffs of a gown
Double gloving?	Yes, reference sites variability in permeation within and between glove lots	Yes, unless evidence shows that a single glove is sufficiently protective	Yes, sites variability in permeation within and between glove lots and recommends double gloving unless it interferes with the task
Frequency recommended to change gloves	Every 60 min or when damaged or contaminated	Hourly, between batches, or when damaged or contaminated	Hourly or when damaged or contaminated
Hand washing frequency	Before and after donning	Before and after donning	Before and after donning

Note: These guidelines do not all address the use of nitrile with cytotoxic drugs since the availability of that type of glove was limited at the time of the guidelines' development. Glove users should ask manufacturers for specific permeation data for the gloves to be used, and see the MSDS sheets for the specific drug or chemical to be used.

or suspected to be infected with a transmissible virus and for major procedures lasting more than 2 hours or with a blood loss of more than 100 ml.[11]

IX. GLOVE HYDRATION AND CONDUCTIVITY

Glove hydration may be a concern for surgeons when they are using electrocautery devices. Electrocautery surgery is performed with a small probe that houses an electric current that cauterizes (burns or destroys) the tissue. Body fluids that may hydrate the glove during electrocautery surgery can act as a conduit for the flow of electricity through the gloves. While there are documented methods to measure electrical conductivity, there currently are no requirements or standard test methods for measuring the hydration rate of natural rubber latex products. As a glove hydrates, it may lose its resistivity or nonconductance of electricity, hence becoming more electrically conductive over time. Surgical gloves are not designed to insulate against electrical shock. It is extremely important that the equipment used for electrocautery surgery be properly set up to prevent burns on the patient's skin and also to protect the surgeon performing the cauterization. There are currently no standards, regulations, or standard methods concerning hydration and medical gloves.

Some research has hypothesized that as a glove hydrates, it may be more permeable to pathogens. If this were true, gloves would fail the ASTM F1671 "Standard Test Method for Resistance of Materials Used in Protective Clothing to Penetration by Bloodborne Pathogens Using Phi-x174 Bacteriophage as a Test System." This method keeps the glove film in contact with a suspension of a microbe smaller than many viruses for a total of 60 minutes. The film is then rinsed with nutrient media and the rinse tested to see if any bacteriophage penetrated the glove film (Figure 19.3a and Figure 19.3b).

X. GLOVE MANUFACTURERS

Gloves are the single most important product purchased to protect healthcare workers and their patients with a medical facility likely to be using more gloves than any other supply. Considering all the hands that need to be covered and all the possible glove choices, choosing the right gloves for the right reasons can be a complex decision. Clinical requirements need to be appropriately balanced with cost-management efforts. In addition, users should know the suppliers of their surgical gloves and other support services they could provide — for example, assessing and quantifying opportunities for improving product standardization and utilization.

While manufacturers of surgical gloves are required to comply with Current Good Manufacturing Practices (CGMP), verifying they are ISO 9001/9002 certified provides additional assurance that they have rigorous design control, documentation, and process control in place. ISO 9001/9002 have been used in the past but glove manufacturers may be moving to ISO 13485, which is more specific and appropriate to the medical device industry.

The FDA randomly inspects glove shipments coming into the U.S. and tests them for pinholes. If a manufacturer's shipment fails this test, they are put on FDA

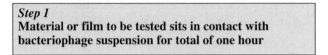

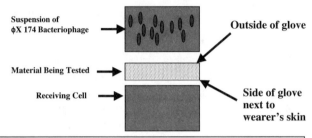

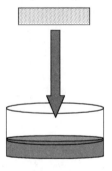

FIGURE 19.3A Step 1 and step 2 of the bacteriophage penetration test.

detention and the product cannot be sold. Purchasers should ask the manufacturer about their demonstrated track record of quality including any level of FDA detention. If this has occurred, then this questions not only the product quality (e.g., your assurance of barrier protection), but also the manufacturer's ability to consistently provide the level of service and amount of product required.

XI. CONCLUSIONS

Medical gloves are an important part of a clinician's personal protective equipment and are highly regulated medical devices. Regulations will continue to evolve to put even greater emphasis on user safety. As new materials for medical gloves are developed, standards will need to reflect the unique properties of specific materials and will help clinicians select the right gloves for the right reasons.

> **Step 3**
> **After incubation, read results:**
> **If phage have penetrated the test material the *E.coli* will not grow**

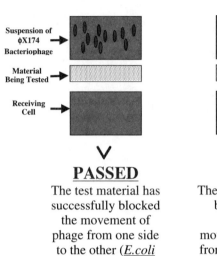

Suspension of
φX174
Bacteriophage →

Material
Being Tested →

Receiving
Cell →

∨   ∨
PASSED   **FAILED**

The test material has   The test material has
successfully blocked   been breached
the movement of   allowing the
phage from one side   movement of phage
to the other (*E.coli*   from one side to the
grows)   other (*E.coli* growth
                               inhibited)

FIGURE 19.3B Step 3 of the bacteriophage penetration test.

REFERENCES

1. Centers for Disease Control and Prevention Hospital Infections Program Advisory Committee, *Guideline for Prevention of Surgical Site Infection,* 1999.
2. IMS Health, Inc., Plymouth, PA, 2002.
3. Atkinson, L.J., *Dataview™ Analyzer Hospital Supply Index™,* Berry and Kohn's operating room technique, 7th Ed., Mosby Year Book, Inc., St. Louis, MO, 1992 .
4. FDA, Surgeons and patient examination gloves proposed rule and notice, *Federal Register,* 64 (146), 1999, 41710.
5. Kenny, D.M. and Challacombe, S.J., *ELISA and other solid phase immunoassays: Theoretical and practical aspects,* John Wiley and Sons, New York, 1996.
6. Billmey, F.W., Jr., *Textbook of Polymer Science,* John Wiley and Sons, New York, 1984.
7. Managing Infection Control, 3 (10), 2003, 30.
8. Forsberg, K. and Mansdorf, S.Z., *Quick Selection Guide to Chemical Protective Clothing,* 3rd Ed., John Wiley and Sons, New York, 1997.
9. Glove use for healthcare providers: Hand covering and barrier protection, APIC Information Brochure, 2000.
10. Recommended practices for maintaining a sterile field, *Standards, Recommended Practices and Guidelines,* Association of Operating Room Nurses, Denver, 1999.
11. Quebbeman, E.J., et al., Double gloving: Protecting surgeons from blood contamination in the operating room, *Arch. Surg.,* 127, 213, 1999.

20 Occupational Health Management of Latex Allergy

Anil Adisesh

CONTENTS

I. Introduction..205
II. Occupational Prevalence of Latex Allergy...205
III. Recognition of Cases..207
IV. Case Management...207
    A. Exposure Reduction 208
V. Advice to the Organization 209
VI. Conclusions..210
References..210

I. INTRODUCTION

Clinicians working in family or hospital practice are primarily consulted by individual patients presenting with specific symptoms. Occupational health practitioners also provide diagnostic, advisory, and to a lesser degree, treatment functions for individual patients. However, these patients are usually employees of an organization for which the practitioner is either an employee or works in a consultancy capacity. The occupational health practitioner also has a duty to advise the organization as well as the patient on matters such as recognition of existing cases, management of cases, prevention of future cases, and related medicolegal issues (Table 20.1).

II. OCCUPATIONAL PREVALENCE OF LATEX ALLERGY

Healthcare workers are the occupational group consistently reported as having the highest rates of sensitization to latex. Rates of type I sensitization in this group are reported between 2 to 17%.[1] Other groups which may be affected are domestic workers, latex rubber process workers, manufacturers of latex products, laboratory workers, and hairdressers. The most common source of occupational exposure is

TABLE 20.1
Occupational Health Actions for Latex Allergy

Policy for prevention, recognition, and management of latex allergy
Glove purchasing and usage strategy
Dissemination of information to latex exposed workers
Diagnosis of occupational latex allergy
Management and support of the latex allergic worker
Advice to management
Liason with clinicians treating employee(s)
Research

gloves made from natural rubber latex. The use of thin rubber gloves in healthcare was first introduced by William Halsted in 1889, and manufactured by the Goodyear company as a protection, for his nurse and fiancee Miss Caroline Hampton, from dermatitis caused by the then used carbolic acid disinfectant.[2] The modern recognition of type I allergy to latex is ascribed to Nutter in 1979.[3] Interestingly, this report is also consistent with a coexistent protein contact dermatitis to latex. Throughout the 1980s to date, there has been an increasing prevalence and recognition of latex allergy. The incidence of occupational asthma due to latex allergy in the U.K. from published reports has shown an increase up to 1997 (Figure 20.1).[4] It is to be hoped

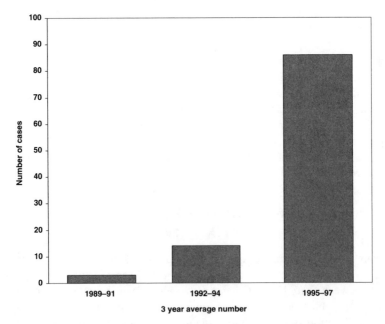

FIGURE 20.1 Occupational asthma due to latex: surveillance of work-related and occupational respiratory disease (SWORD).[4]

that a declining trend will soon emerge from these surveillance data as a result of preventive measures.

III. RECOGNITION OF CASES

Employees with symptoms may self refer to an occupational health service, however, information should also be made readily available to aid early self recognition. A program of hazard identification and training should include the common sources of workplace exposures to latex and the symptoms of latex allergy. It should be emphasized that action can be taken to support an employee with latex allergy and that this is most effective the sooner symptoms are reported. Allied to such information the organization should develop and implement a policy that outlines the action that will be taken to prevent and control latex allergy. This may be a specific "latex policy," perhaps more appropriate to healthcare facilities, or in other workplaces it could be included in a general policy for the prevention and control of sensitizing agents. An example policy is available at www.smtl.co.uk/MDRC/Latex/Latex-Allergy-Policy/latex-allergy-policy.html.[5]

At the inception of such a policy, or in areas of high latex usage, active case finding could be considered. Questionnaire surveys with follow-up of those reporting symptoms can be used but it should be recognized that there will be a high proportion of persons with symptoms who do not have type I allergy to latex. Nonetheless, as an occupational health intervention, identification of other glove/rubber associated symptoms may be useful and allow further action. Similarly supervisors or line managers could be trained in the recognition of latex allergy signs and symptoms and to make periodic inquiries of employees, so that appropriate referral to an occupational health professional occurs. Review of sickness absence reasons might ascertain cases of latex allergy with asthma, rhinitis, or skin symptoms. On employment, inquiry should be made about any known or suspected occupational or other allergies. Confirmatory testing, if not previously undertaken, can then be performed.

IV. CASE MANAGEMENT

A diagnosis of type I latex allergy should not be accepted without confirmatory immunological or other tests because of the unnecessary restrictions that may then be imposed both at work and in everyday life. Diagnosis is achieved by obtaining a full anamnesis with questions on relevant nonoccupational and occupational risk factors for latex allergy (see Chapter 1). It should be possible for any occupational health practitioner with a significant at-risk population to arrange for serum to be tested for specific IgE to latex. A positive result with a clinical history suggestive of latex allergy can be accepted as confirming latex allergy. However, a negative result should not be assumed to exclude the diagnosis, and skin prick testing should be performed with either a commercially available latex allergen preparation or an elute from the latex article responsible for work-related reactions. Skin prick tests are preferred as the initial investigation due to high sensitivity and specificity, and not least because a rapid result is available. If both of these tests are negative but the clinical history is suggestive of occupational latex allergy, a "use test" should be undertaken. In the event of all results being negative, alternative causes should be sought. If the occupational health practitioner is not trained to undertake skin prick testing, referral to an appropriate specialist will be necessary.

Employees whose presenting symptom is anaphylaxis at work should be excluded from work until the diagnosis has been established. To do otherwise may be legally difficult to defend in the event of further, possibly fatal, anaphylaxis. A *use test* must not be undertaken for subjects presenting with anaphylaxis unless immunological tests (both specific IgE and skin prick) are negative.

Latex allergy should always be considered and excluded in the differential diagnosis of occupational allergy if the possibility of exposure, even if indirect, exists. It is not sufficient to assume that the association the employee attributes is necessarily causal. Fourteen percent of nurses with work-related eye symptoms exposed to glutaraldehyde were found to have positive skin prick tests to latex in one study.[6] If concomitant sensitization is suspected to be the cause of occupational asthma, an occupational respiratory challenge study under suitable conditions conducted by competent clinicians may be justifiable. Contact dermatitis if due to irritant factors may respond to a change from powdered to nonpowdered gloves and improved skin care measures. Nonresolution with simple measures should lead to consideration of an allergic contact dermatitis to rubber chemicals and/or latex protein. Confirmation of this diagnosis will require patch tests usually by referral to a dermatologist.

A. EXPOSURE REDUCTION

Once a secure diagnosis of latex allergy (type I or IV) has been established measures need to be taken to reduce or avoid latex exposure. Exposure reduction involves firstly recognizing the major and minor sources of latex exposure in the work environment and secondly identifying alternatives. Latex glove use is the major occupational exposure, although particularly in the healthcare environment a wide range of other items contain latex. The affected employee should be provided with a ready supply of nonlatex gloves suitable for nonsterile and, where needed, sterile use. If powdered latex gloves are used, then colleagues in all work areas changing to nonpowdered low extractable protein latex gloves will usually suffice to reduce latex aeroallergen levels below those inciting asthma or rhinoconjunctivitis symptoms.[7-9] Many people who have experienced only localized contact urticaria when wearing powdered latex gloves subsequently have no symptoms with nonpowdered low protein gloves.[10] The potential for further sensitization exists with continued dermal latex exposure, and animal studies have shown that it can be sufficient to induce bronchial reactivity.[11] In view of the availability of alternatives to latex, it would seem advisable for allergic employees to use nonlatex gloves.

The vigor with which exposure reduction is pursued for an individual employee will depend upon the type and severity of their allergic symptoms. For an employee with the relatively rare presentation of a work-related anaphylactic reaction, a detailed assessment of all possible workplace exposures, both direct and indirect, with their elimination would be advisable. If this was not reasonably practicable then redeployment, retraining, ill health retirement, or, failing these, management action to terminate employment as appropriate. Anaphylaxis that has occurred to a worker when undergoing a surgical operation does not imply that all workplace exposures will cause the same effect since intraoperative exposure is usually prolonged and in contact with a serosal surface. Whether the workplace is a high usage environment for latex, e.g., hospital intensive care units, will determine how easily latex reduction and avoidance can be achieved. At least, occupational use of latex gloves must be avoided and direct contact with latex minimized.

It is essential for the management of latex allergy that the affected person is given reliable practical, preferably written, advice about latex allergy and avoidance of occupational and nonoccupational exposure appropriate to their symptoms. The psychological effects of anaphylaxis and allergy should not be underestimated. These can lead to latex allergic patients adopting an unnecessarily restricted lifestyle and erroneously believing they have acquired multiple allergies.

V. ADVICE TO THE ORGANIZATION

The employer should be advised on the basis of relevant industry and national guidance which may be specific to latex glove use, e.g., OSHA,[12] NIOSH[13] (see Chapter 19). Account must also be taken of state or national legislation, e.g., German TGRS 540.[14] A recent Court of Appeal judgement in England, *Dugmore v. Swansea NHS Trust and Another* 2002 has clarified the duty of an employer to prevent exposure to powdered latex glove use and to adequately control it where no reasonable alternatives exist. An organizational policy[5] will help managers take action within their work area to protect workers' health, thereby reducing organizational risks. The potential losses to the employer from failing to act are staff leaving post with the associated recruitment and training costs, litigation costs, increased insurance costs, and inspection by regulatory bodies, with the costs of remedial action.

Rationalization of glove use can lead to reduced costs with careful negotiation of block contracts from suppliers.[15] Additionally it might be identified that latex gloves are used unnecessarily when a more suitable and possibly cheaper glove could be used, e.g., in food handling blue vinyl gloves should be substituted for latex, which also avoids latex contamination of food items such as sandwiches. In healthcare, for protection of normal intact skin against blood or body fluid splashes, vinyl gloves are perfectly adequate if changed after soiling or each procedure, e.g., standard venipuncture. Other nonlatex alternatives such as synthetic elastomer or nitrile can be used where direct contact with blood or body fluids will be necessary in the course of the proposed procedure, e.g., rectal exam or surgery.

Occupational health professionals can also achieve preventive aims by undertaking or facilitating research in the basic science of latex allergy, its epidemiology or evaluative studies of exposure reduction. Employees working in an organization that takes preventive and timely corrective action are more likely to feel supported and to share the organizational values.

VI. CONCLUSIONS

The substitution of lower latex protein nonpowdered gloves for the previously widely used powdered natural rubber latex gloves should make the workplace more tolerable for latex allergic employees. It remains to be proven that in the long term there will be a lower proportion of exposed persons who become sensitized, as it may be that the induction period simply becomes prolonged. To this end, ongoing epidemiological studies are required alongside continued workplace vigilance. Guidance on the appropriate choice of gloves for specific tasks should be formalized by regulatory bodies perhaps with the approval of usage criteria. Employers should ensure that they have in place suitable policies to address latex allergy to inform, protect, and support employees.

REFERENCES

1. Turjanmaa, K. et al., Recent developments in latex allergy, *Curr. Opin. Allergy Clin. Immunol.*, 2, 407, 2002.
2. Porter, R., *The Greatest Benefit to Mankind,* Harper Collins, London, 1997.
3. Nutter, A.F., Contact urticaria to rubber, *Br. J. Dermatol.*, 101, 597, 1979.
4. McDonald, J.C., Keynes, H.L., and Meredith, S.K., Reported incidence of occupational asthma in the United Kingdom 1989–1997, *Occup. Environ. Med.*, 57, 823, 2000.
5. www.smtl.co.uk/MDRC/Latex/Latex-Allergy-Policy/latex-allergy-policy.html, Surgical Materials Testing Laboratory.
6. Vyas, A., Pickering, C.A.C., and Oldham, L.A., Survey of symptoms, respiratory function, and immunology and their relation to glutaraldehyde and other occupational exposures among endoscopy nursing staff, *Occup. Environ. Med.*, 57, 752, 2000.
7. Vandenplas, O. et al., Occupational asthma caused by natural rubber latex: Outcome according to cessation or reduction of exposure, *J. Allergy Clin. Immunol.*, 109, 125, 2002.
8. Allmers, H. et al., Reduction of latex aeroallergens and latex-specific IgE antibodies in sensitized workers after removal of powered natural rubber latex gloves in a hospital, *J. Allergy Clin. Immunol.*, 102, 841, 1998.
9. Hunt, L.W. et al., Management of occupational allergy to natural rubber latex in a medical center: The importance of quantitative latex allergen measurement and objective follow-up, *J. Allergy Clin. Immunol.*, 110 (2 Suppl.), S96, 2002.
10. Turjanmaa, K. et al., Long-term outcome of 160 adult patients with natural rubber latex allergy, *J. Allergy Clin. Immunol.*, 110 (Suppl.), S70, 2002.
11. Howell, M.D., Weissman, D.N., and Jean Meade, B., Latex sensitization by dermal exposure can lead to airway hyperreactivity, *Int. Arch. Allergy Immunol.*, 128, 204, 2002.
12. U.S. Department of Labor, Occupational Safety and Health Standards (1910.1030), Bloodborne pathogens.
13. DHHS (NIOSH), NIOSH Alert Preventing Allergic reactions to natural rubber latex in the workplace, DHHS (NIOSH), 1997, Publication no. 97-135.
14. Schmid, K. et al., Latex sensitization in dental students using powder-free gloves low in latex protein: A cross-sectional study, *Contact Dermatitis*, 47, 103, 2002.
15. Hunt, L.W. et al., A medical-centre-wide, multidisciplinary approach to the problem of natural rubber latex allergy, *J. O. E. M.*, 38, 765, 1996.

21 Management of Rubber-Based Allergies in Dentistry

Curtis P. Hamann, Pamela A. Rodgers, and Kim Sullivan

CONTENTS

I.   Introduction...212
II. Diagnosis and Symptom Assessment...213
     A. Health History and Risk Assessment...213
     B. Symptom Assessment...214
     C. Diagnostic Testing for Rubber-Based Allergies 214
         1. Diagnostic Testing for Type I NRL Hypersensitivity 215
         2. Diagnostic Testing for Type IV Hypersensitivity to Rubber
             Chemicals 216
III. Education of Allergic Dental Professionals 217
IV. Allergens in Natural and Synthetic Rubber 218
     A. NRL Extractable Total Protein Content..221
     B. NRL Extractable Allergenic Protein Content 222
     C. Glove Powder and NRL Protein Allergens 222
     D. Allergenic Rubber Chemicals 223
     E. Exposure Routes and Thresholds for Rubber-Based Allergens.......225
     F. Other Dental Allergens...226
V.   Mitigating Rubber Allergen Exposure 227
     A. Administrative Controls 228
     B. Dental Operatory Cleaning and NRL Remediation 228
     C. NRL Product Substitution..229
         1. Guidelines and Glove Standards..229
         2. Product Substitutions for Type I NRL Hypersensitivity 231
         3. Product Substitutions for Type IV Rubber Chemical
             Hypersensitivity..233
     D. Considerations for the Dental Patient with Rubber-Based
         Allergies...234
         1. Procedures Requiring Local Anesthesia 234
         2. Endodontic Procedures..235

0-8493-1670-7/05/$0.00+$1.50
© 2005 by CRC Press LLC

    3. Emergency Preparedness..236
    4. Psychological Issues...236
VI.   Examples of Successful Management of Rubber-Based Allergies 236
VII.   Summary and Recommendations...237
References..238

I. INTRODUCTION

Dental professionals are occupationally exposed to a plethora of rubber-based products, including medical gloves. As a result, they can be at risk for the development of type I hypersensitivity to natural rubber latex (NRL) proteins and type IV hypersensitivity to accelerators and antidegradants used in rubber manufacture. Type I reactions to NRL allergens are mediated systemically through immunoglobulin E (IgE) anti-NRL antibodies and commonly range from cutaneous symptoms of urticaria and pruritus to the rhinoconjunctival and respiratory symptoms. More serious type I systemic reactions to NRL can also include cardiovascular and gastrointestinal symptoms, and can lead to anaphylatic shock. By comparison, type IV reactions to the processing chemicals in rubber products are predominantly localized reactions generally characterized by redness, swelling, papules, or edema.

In the early 1970s, NRL gloves were not uniformly worn by dental professionals, but had been discussed for use in oral surgery.[1,2] Although recommended by the American Dental Association (ADA) and Centers for Disease Control and Prevention (CDC), exam gloves were not commonly worn by dental practitioners until the late 1980s after implementation of universal precautions to combat the rising transmission of hepatitis B and HIV.[3–5]

The first evidence of type I reactions to NRL in dentistry appeared in the mid-1980s.[6] A dental patient's immediate allergic reaction to a dental dam was described in 1984; the symptoms, which included angioedema, were suggestive of a type I NRL allergy.[7] The first clinical confirmation of a dental professional with a type I NRL hypersensitivity was reported in 1987.[8] Subsequent reports of type I NRL hypersensitivity in dentistry were not uncommon. Early research noted a prevalence of 8 to 38% in dental professionals, depending on the study population and assessment method.[9–12] In a larger cross-sectional study of over 1300 dentists conducted from 1994 to 1995, the prevalence of type I NRL hypersensitivity averaged 6%.[13] In 320 dental hygienists, the prevalence tended to be greater (~ 9%).[13] Fortunately, current research suggests a lower prevalence (~ 3%) of type I NRL hypersensitivity in dental professionals and a decreasing incidence.[14,15] These trends mirror changes in hospital workers, where the prevalence of type I NRL hypersensitivity has recently decreased due to reduced NRL allergen exposure.[16–19]

In dentistry, the prevalence of a type IV or delayed hypersensitivity to rubber processing chemicals may now be more common than a type I NRL hypersensitivity. The most common chemical allergens in natural and synthetic rubbers are thiurams, carbamates, and mercaptobenzothiazoles, which act as antidegradants and vulcanization accelerators. Recent studies report a 5 to 7% prevalence of type IV thiuram hypersensitivity in patch-tested dental personnel.[20,21] In addition, of the patch-tested individuals with a type IV hypersensitivity to carbamates, 10% worked in dentistry.[20–23]

Effective and timely management of type I and type IV rubber-based hypersensitivities are important to the health of dental personnel. Recent studies suggest that occupational skin disease of the healthcare worker can remain undiagnosed and unmanaged for an average of 3 years.[18,24] During this period, the broken skin barrier can permit pathogen or allergen penetration, as well as proliferation of resident and nonresident microflora.[25–27] As the duration of allergen exposure increases, worker's symptoms may be less likely to improve following diagnosis.[28] Therefore, recurring and chronic skin reactions from unmanaged occupational allergies are likely to result in increased time away from work and, in severe cases, temporary or permanent disability due to occupational asthma, anaphylaxis, or severe skin disease.

To date there is no curative treatment for type I and type IV rubber-based allergies. Although research continues, immunotherapy and desensitization regimens for type I NRL allergy are not yet sufficiently safe and effective.[29] Therefore, management of both types of allergies is based primarily on obtaining an accurate diagnosis, and minimizing exposure to the identified allergen(s). Allergic dental workers must be educated about proper skin care, potential sources and routes of exposure, and management options for controlling exposure to the allergens in rubber and nonrubber products. Within dental and medical environments, eliminating exposure to NRL gloves with a high allergen content has been shown to be the most successful strategy to reduce allergic worker symptoms and IgE levels, as well as the apparent rate of sensitization.[17,19,30,31]

II. DIAGNOSIS AND SYMPTOM ASSESSMENT

A. Health History and Risk Assessment

Consistent with National Institute of Occupational Safety and Health (NIOSH) recommendations, dental workers (and patients) should be screened for their risk of type I NRL protein or type IV rubber chemical hypersensitivity. This can be accomplished through a comprehensive health history or allergy screening questionnaire. Risk factors common to both types of hypersensitivities include an atopic history (seasonal rhinitis, asthma, food allergy, eczema), healthcare occupation, recurring occupational or recreational exposure to rubber products, and a history of skin or systemic reactions to rubber products. In addition, dental workers with a medical history of multiple childhood surgeries, spina bifida, myelomeningocele, or urogenital anomalies are at increased risk for type I NRL hypersensitivity.

Between 20 and 40% of dental workers self-report NRL glove-related symptoms with dermatitis and could be considered history-positive.[13,32–34] But physicians should interpret information from self-administered questionnaires carefully. Patient perceptions of symptoms, skin disease, allergies, and general health problems vary greatly and may be different from that of healthcare providers.[35] In fact, patient-provided information on specific medical conditions may match their physician's diagnosis only 50% of the time.[36] The accuracy of recalled information can be influenced by a patient's age, education, and psychosocial factors.[37] Allergic reactions may be recalled after testing: individuals with an initial negative history may remember relevant symptoms after subsequent testing for type I or type IV hypersensitivity.[34,38]

B. Symptom Assessment

A key issue that should be emphasized in examinations and interviews is an accurate assessment of a patient's allergic symptoms, both localized and systemic. Although more than 20% of dental professionals report symptoms of glove intolerance, few dental workers also test positive. For example, of those with glove-related symptoms, only 6 to 11% were diagnosed with a type I NRL hypersensitivity.[13,33] Conversely, patients may not recognize symptoms: at least 25% of purported history-negative dentists tested positive for type I NRL hypersensitivity.[13] Patients may exhibit localized or systemic reactions after exposure to rubber products during dental or medical procedures, but may not comprehend the significance of the reaction. Allergic or unpleasant reactions to certain foods (e.g., bananas, kiwis, avocados, tomatoes, and chestnuts) or plants (e.g., ficus, timothy grass) may not be immediately identified, but are consistent with a type I NRL hypersensitivity due to the presence of IgE antibodies to cross-reacting panallergens.[39] Because the positive predictive value of self-reported dermatitis symptoms is low for many allergens, dental worker symptoms are best confirmed through direct visual assessment or at least detailed patient interviews.[40,41]

Recurring symptoms can be useful in differentiating between type I NRL protein and type IV rubber chemical hypersensitivities. Dental workers suspected to have one (or both) of these occupationally based allergies should be encouraged to extensively document for their physician the occurrence, duration and degree of any skin lesions or systemic reactions such as conjunctivitis, rhinitis, urticaria, and asthmalike symptoms. For individuals with skin symptoms consistent with type IV delayed hypersensitivity, collecting product content information (e.g., Material Safety Data Sheets, product inserts, box and product labels) from the dental office and home can help identify potential allergens.

C. Diagnostic Testing for Rubber-Based Allergies

Individuals suspected to be at risk on the basis of history or symptom assessment should be further tested for type I NRL hypersensitivity, type IV hypersensitivity to rubber-processing chemicals, or both. This is usually accomplished by skin prick or serologic testing combined with patch testing but can be supplemented with provocation testing (also known as "use" or "challenge" testing). Although recommended by CDC, NIOSH and several professional organizations, it can be difficult for dental professionals to obtain all relevant tests for a definitive diagnosis.[42,43] Of those allergists and dermatologists who evaluate patients for rubber-based allergies, not all perform skin prick, serologic, patch, and provocation or use tests.

According to surveys, allergists are reportedly at least 5 times more likely to evaluate patients for "latex allergy" than dermatologists (95 vs. 17%, respectively).[44,45] The majority of allergists commonly use serologic and skin prick testing to diagnose a "latex allergy." However, half of surveyed allergists (53%) reportedly do not perform patch testing, and one quarter do not perform skin prick testing.[45,46]

By comparison, of those dermatologists who evaluate patients for "latex allergy," most use a diagnostic method based on serologic and use testing.[44] Although dermatologists were more likely to perform patch testing, only 3.5% performed skin prick testing in evaluating patients for "latex allergy."[44] However, dermatologists who were members of the American Contact Dermatitis Society, and likely to have a professional interest and greater training in occupational dermatitis, were 4 to 5 times more likely to evaluate for latex allergy and to skin prick test.[44]

1. Diagnostic Testing for Type I NRL Hypersensitivity

The most clinically relevant tests used to date include skin prick, serologic, and provocation or challenge testing, while *in vitro* basophil activation (histamine release) measurements are more commonly utilized in research protocols.[47–49] Of the methods used clinically, problems with sensitivity and specificity have been reported, which can lead to unacceptably high rates of false-negatives and false-positives as well as distorted prevalence estimates.[50] Comparison between studies is often difficult due to differences in the populations investigated, as well as the methods utilized. Future skin prick reagents may utilize purified recombinant NRL allergens or monoclonal antibodies based on these purified allergens.[51,52] These reagents may help clarify symptom elicitation thresholds and provide better diagnostic tools.

Skin prick testing can be performed using nonammoniated NRL reagent (e.g., prepared by Stallergenes, Antony, France and Greer Laboratories, Lenoir NC) or physician-prepared aqueous extracts of NRL gloves as the source of NRL antigens. While nonammoniated commercial NRL reagents are available in Europe and Canada, they are not yet sold in the U.S. When used to diagnose type I NRL hypersensitivity, the sensitivity of commercial nonammoniated NRL reagents ranges from 90 to 98%.[53–57] The specificity of these reagents is reported at or near 100%, depending upon the population. The corresponding false-negative rate would be less than 10% and false-positive rate would be nearly zero. As a result, many investigators consider skin prick testing for type I NRL hypersensitivity the more reliable and accurate diagnostic tool, particularly when combined with a positive history. Despite earlier concerns about anaphylatic reactions, skin prick testing is now considered a safe and very effective diagnostic method when these standardized reagents are used.[58]

The overwhelming majority of dermatologists (87.5%) and allergists (74%) in the U.S. who use skin prick testing in the evaluation of type I NRL hypersensitivity use solutions prepared from gloves.[44,45] Unfortunately, these glove extracts are rarely standardized with respect to NRL allergen or protein content. Moreover, as the NRL allergen content of commercial gloves decreases due to manufacturing changes, modern gloves become a poor source of NRL allergens. Therefore it is not surprising that skin prick testing with glove extracts has a more variable sensitivity of 64 to 96%, and a potentially high false-negative rate, depending upon the glove source and population tested.[56]

Serologic testing for the presence of anti-NRL IgE antibodies (e.g., Pharmacia CAP™, DPC AlaSTAT™, DPC AlaBLOT, and Hycor HyTECH™) is available in the U.S. and elsewhere. The semiquantitative Allergodip-Latex has also been developed for screening purposes.[59] Numerous investigations have shown that the sensitivity and specificity of serologic methods can be lower than that of skin prick testing. For the CAP assay, sensitivity has been reported to range from 75 to 97% with a specificity of 76 to 97%.[53,55,59–61] By comparison, AlaSTAT assay sensitivity has been reported to be in the range of 73 to 100%, with a specificity of 33 to 97%, depending upon assay threshold values.[53,55,59–61] While the HyTECH assay reportedly has a high sensitivity (90 to 92%), its low specificity (~ 70%) and associated high false-positive rate is problematic.[61] Based on these sensitivity and specificity values, higher rates of false negatives (10 to 25%) and false positives (at least 10 to 15%) are likely with serologic assays. These problems appear to be more pronounced when levels of anti-NRL IgE antibodies are near low-positive test thresholds.[48]

Although physicians have access to diverse diagnostic modalities, they can be faced with a clinically-based judgement call, particularly in the U.S. where commercial skin prick reagents are not yet available. If the conservative diagnostic path based on serologic testing and patient history yields discordant results, some physicians select provocation testing. But these methods vary widely with regard to exposure route (respiratory or skin exposure) and choice of endpoint.[48] In addition, the quality and quantity of NRL glove allergens used for exposure can vary markedly. Again, because NRL glove protein and allergen content has decreased over the last several years, it is difficult to find gloves that provide sufficiently high NRL allergen content to be dependably diagnostic. Moreover, the test is difficult to blind to patient perceptions.[45] Because of the lack of control of these variables, provocation testing has a high rate of adverse patient reactions.[45] Therefore, until these test methods improve, utilization of combined skin prick and serologic, or multiple serologic tests using different methods may be most appropriate for dental workers with a complex allergic history and equivocal symptoms.[48,62]

2. Diagnostic Testing for Type IV Hypersensitivity to Rubber Chemicals

In addition to other standard allergens, patch testing for a contact allergy to rubber processing chemicals uses the more common sensitizers found in rubber products. These include: (1) 3% carba mix (diphenylguanidine, zinc dibutyldithiocarbamate, zinc diethyldithiocarbamate), (2) 1% thiuram mix (tetramethylthiuram monosulfide, tetramethylthiuram disulfide, disulfiram, dipentamethylenethiuram disulfide), (3) 1% mercapto mix (N-cyclohexylbenzothiazyl-sulfenamide, dibenzothiazyl disulfide, morpholinylmercaptobenzothiazole), and (4) 2% mercaptobenzothiazole.[63] Of these, thiurams and carbamates are among the twelve most common contact allergens according to data published by the North American Contact Dermatitis Group.[63,64] Thiurams and carbamates are also more commonly used in the manufacture of natural and synthetic rubber gloves.[65]

Patch testing is invaluable in diagnosing type IV rubber-based allergies, as well as differentiating between allergic and irritant responses. But there are limitations: the accuracy of patch test results is known to vary with the allergen and patch test system, as well as duration of exposure and evaluation times.[66] Skin condition can also influence the accuracy of patch test results. Ideally, patients to be patch tested should not be using systemic steroids and the skin to be tested should be free from topical steroids, dermatitis, skin damage, sunburn, or significant tanning.[67] False negative results may increase with low allergen concentration, poor skin contact, single readings, and short evaluation times (3 to 4 days).[67] False positives can be created by elevated allergen concentrations or mechanical pressure reactions.

Overall, the diagnosis of type IV hypersensitivity to one or more chemicals in a standard tray is estimated to have a sensitivity of 70 to 80%, with a corresponding false-negative rate of less than 30%.[68] With respect to rubber-based allergens, Shertz et al. reported a 76 and 75% sensitivity for thiuram and carba mix, respectively, using Finn chambers.[69] By comparison, T.R.U.E. test panels were less sensitive, yielding a 46 and 64% sensitivity for thiuram and carba mixes, respectively.[69,70] Geier et al. reported 77% sensitivity for the combined use of mercapto mix and mercaptobenzothiazole using Finn chambers, with a 99.7% specificity.[71]

As with other clinical test methods, the presence of clinically relevant symptoms, a positive history, and a high likelihood of a type IV hypersensitivity (i.e., a high-risk population) will increase the predictive value of patch testing and lower the possibility of diagnostic errors.[72]

Certain positive patch test reactions are strongly and significantly associated, especially thiuram mix with zinc diethylcarbamate.[73,74] It may be necessary to retest allergens that gave equivocal or suspicious responses and increase allergen concentrations, as allergens that test negative with an initial patch test can retest positive.[69] In general, patch testing performed per the guidelines of the North American Contact Dermatitis Group using a 48-hour exposure time, coupled with multiple readings for up to a week after patch removal, and minimization of interference from poor skin condition will maximize the predictive value of administered patch tests.[63]

III. EDUCATION OF ALLERGIC DENTAL PROFESSIONALS

In addition to learning to recognize sources of rubber allergens and ways to avoid them, dental workers must be educated about the importance of skin health, type I and type IV allergy symptoms, and the chemical content of other products to which they are exposed. In general, the importance of patient education is frequently overlooked and underemphasized by both medical and dental professionals. As a result, NIOSH and the ADA — as well as other professional healthcare worker organizations — strongly recommend instructing dental workers about the symptoms and sources of rubber-based allergies.[42,75]

Success in reducing the prevalence of type I NRL protein hypersensitivity has been linked in part to educational programs and awareness campaigns.[16,76] In general, atopic dental professionals should have sufficient understanding of the problem to be aware of any new symptoms. With respect to type IV hypersensitivity, investigators have shown that patch test-positive patients who were educated about their allergy, and received product chemical information were more likely to have resolved dermatitis.[77,78] Like other patients, dental workers may require instruction about reading product labels and recognizing alternative brand or chemical names for allergen sources. Patients who do not receive sufficient education about their patch test results are more likely to have persistent and severe dermatitis.[79] These studies underscore the need for comprehensive patient education programs regarding both type I NRL hypersensitivity and type IV hypersensitivity to rubber processing chemicals.

Communication of risk is an important feature of education about rubber-based allergies. Several guidelines can be particularly useful in responding to the concerns of a dental worker with type I NRL hypersensitivity. First, involve the dental worker in managing their allergy as an equal partner, as one healthcare professional to another. Second, plan and evaluate efforts carefully, coordinating and collaborating with other credible resources. Third, listen to the dental worker's concerns and fears openly and compassionately. Fourth, assist in finding a management solution that meets the needs of both the dental worker as well as their employer.[80]

Instruction about skin biology, proper hand washing, and appropriate use of hand care products is a vital element of managing rubber-based allergies. Healthy skin is an essential barrier to damage from abrasion, chemicals, and infectious agents, and cannot be replaced by gloves or other barriers. Constant hand washing and chemical exposure can adversely affect the skin health and resident microbial flora of the hands of healthcare workers.[27,81] Although a progressive link between type IV and type I rubber-based hypersensitivity has never been established, animal studies have shown that skin absorption of NRL protein allergens occurs more readily through abraded or damaged skin.[82]

Misinformation can also be a significant obstacle. Erroneous or incomplete information on type I and type IV hypersensitivity has been published in reputable dental journals.[83,84] Widely read consumer print media generally suffers from similar problems of quality and accuracy.[85] A recent review of health information on the Internet found overall quality to be a significant problem.[86] Therefore, physicians must continue to provide accurate information and resources for their patients on these occupational health topics.

From a broader perspective, dermatologists and allergists should challenge atopic dental professionals to become aware of the chemical content of all products to which they are exposed. Physicians should assist and encourage patients in soliciting chemical content information from manufacturers in Material Safety Data Sheets (MSDS), ingredient lists, and technical information sheets, or by specific request. Dental workers may not be aware of the resources readily available from professional organizations, NRL allergy awareness groups, journal articles, and credible Internet sites (Table 21.1).

IV. ALLERGENS IN NATURAL AND SYNTHETIC RUBBER

To assist dental professionals in managing their allergies, physicians must understand rubber-based allergens, including sources and levels of exposure in dentistry. Commonly used rubber products in dentistry include NRL exam and surgical gloves,

TABLE 21.1
Educational Resources Concerning NRL Allergies and Occupational Skin Diseases

Internet Sites

Spina Bifida Association: www.sbaa.org

Latex Allergy Links: http://latexallergylinks.tripod.com/

FDA Center for Devices and Radiological Health (CDRH): www.fda.gov/cdrh/index.html

American Academy of Allergy, Asthma and Immunology: www.aaaai.org

Allergy, Asthma and Immunology Online: http://allergy.mcg.edu/physicians/ltxhome.html

U.S. OSHA latex allergy site: www.osha-slc.gov/SLTC/latexallergy/index.html

Allergen Patch Test (T.R.U.E. Test): www.truetest.com

Center for Disease Control and Prevention: www.cdc.gov/niosh/98-113.html

National Library of Medicine: www.nlm.nih.gov/

Toxicology Data Network: http://toxnet.nlm.nih.gov/

On-Line Courses

www.cll.purdue.edu/extendeduniversity/selfdirected/correspondencecourses/iahcsmm/pdfs/lesson43.pdf

www.phcg.com/library/pdfs/ltcn/apr2001/314-0102.pdf

www.duj.com/Patriarca.html

dental dams, prophy cups, orthodontic bands, elastic bands on masks, vial stoppers, bandages, tubing, and others (Table 21.2). NRL proteins, and occasionally NRL allergens, have been extracted from both dental and consumer rubber products.[19,87–89] The common chemical allergens — rubber accelerators and antidegradants — are found in natural and synthetic rubber products used at home and in dentistry. However, of these products, NRL gloves are likely to be the primary source of allergenic NRL proteins and rubber processing chemicals for dental workers.

The glove manufacturing process has recently been reviewed in detail by Yip and Cacioli.[90] However, a few key points should be addressed. Crude NRL, obtained by tapping the *Hevea brasiliensis* tree, is processed into either a liquid latex concentrate or a coagulated latex. The coagulated latex is more extensively processed with heat, water, and/or solvents before being used in the manufacture of dry-rubber goods such as tires, hoses, and shoes. The extractable total protein content of dry-rubber products is usually very low, i.e., less than 50 µg protein/g (some less than 20 µg protein/g) and the NRL allergen content negligible. Therefore, dry-rubber goods are not considered an important source of exposure for NRL protein allergens.[90]

The liquid latex concentrate is further refined for use in thin-film products (e.g., gloves, dental dams, catheters, and condoms), foam products, molded or extruded products. Ammonia preservation, centrifugation, leaching, and chlorination processes reduce the level of extractable total protein 200-fold from 8-10 mg/g in crude NRL to 0.05 mg/g extractable total protein, as found in many NRL gloves.[65,90] Only a fraction of the extractable total protein in finished products is allergenic, and includes several quantifiable allergens to date: Hev b 1, Hev b 3, Hev b 5 and Hev b 6.02, and Hev b 8.[51,91–94] The surface availability of these NRL allergens in thin-film products can be affected by manufacturing techniques such as leaching, wash-

TABLE 21.2
Potential Sources of NRL in Medical, Dental, and Consumer Rubber Products

Medical and Dental Products		Consumer Products	
Adhesives	Anesthesia equipment	Adhesives and glues	Balls
Anesthetic cartridges	Bandaids	Balloons	Bathing caps
Bite blocks	Blood pressure cuff	Bathing suits	Bungee cords
Bulb syringe and droppers	Catheters and tubing	Carpet backing	Condoms
Dental dams	Dressings and closures	Contraceptive diaphragm	Crutch pads, tips, grips
Ear plugs	Electrode grounding pads	Diapers, pads, and rubber pants	Elastic in socks and underwear
Elastic wraps	Enema tips	Erasers	Feeding nipples
Endotracheal tubes	Elastic bands from masks, hats, shoe covers	Fabric and art paint	Gum massagers
Exercise bands for physical therapy	Finger cots	Gloves, kitchen and garden	Handles on tools, racquets, clubs, bicycles
Gloves, medical	G tubes	Newsprint	Rubber bands
Irrigator tubing	IV access: injection ports, bags, pumps, adaptors	Rubber toys	Scuba gear: masks, goggles, fins, wetsuit
Orthodontic rubber bands	Oxygen face masks	Shoes: sneakers, sandals, beach thongs	Wheelchair cushions and tires
Penrose drain	Dental polishing disc	Zippered plastic storage bags	
Prophy cups	Pulse oximeter		
Respirators	Reflex hammer		
Rubber mixing bowls	Resuscitators		
Rubber sheeting	Rubber mattresses and pillows		
Suction tubing and tips	Stethoscope		
Stoppers, medication vial	Syringes, disposable		
Tourniquets	Tape		
	Vascular stockings		

ing, and chlorination.[65,90] As the surface availability of NRL allergens changes on thin-film products, so does the opportunity for absorption by the skin of dental workers, and the potential for sensitization or symptom elicitation.

Before crude NRL or a similar raw synthetic rubber is further processed, it is amended with chemicals that influence its physical properties through a process known as compounding. As many as 200 organic and inorganic chemicals can be added to natural and synthetic rubbers in various combinations. The two major categories that account for 90% of rubber compounding chemicals are antidegradants and vulcanization accelerators. Chemicals such as mercaptobenzothiazoles, thiurams, and carbamates are used to increase the vulcanization rate of rubber and decrease cure time. They also may be added to reduce age and environment-dependent oxidation and deterioration in nonvulcanized elastomers and vulcanized synthetic or natural rubbers. Unfortunately, these compounds are frequently sensitizing in healthcare workers. As with NRL protein allergens, the chemical allergen content of finished glove products can depend on the amount of chemical added initially, as well as the leaching, washing, and chlorination processes.

A. NRL EXTRACTABLE TOTAL PROTEIN CONTENT

The extractable total protein content of NRL medical gloves is determined by a modified Lowry method.[95] This method has several problems including interference by rubber processing chemicals and casein additives, reproducibility problems, marked variability at lower protein levels, limited linearity over a broad protein range, and poor correlation with HPLC data, which is considered the "gold standard" of protein analysis.[51,96–98] As a result, the American Society for Testing and Materials (ASTM) protein standard sets a detection limit of 50 μg protein per gram and the ASTM glove standards recommend "reasonable allowances" for Lowry assay results.[95,99,100]

The extractable protein content of NRL gloves can vary significantly due to changes in rubber agricultural, harvesting, and manufacturing practices.[65] Because each lot of NRL gloves is not usually tested for extractable protein content, the actual glove protein content can be substantially different than that reported by the manufacturer. To add to the complexity of this issue, the extractable total protein content of NRL gloves can be expressed in at least three different units: (1) per unit mass as μg protein/g glove (often used by manufacturers), (2) per unit surface area as μg protein/dm^2 or square decimeter (ASTM standards), or (3) per glove as total μg protein (guidelines of the Food and Drug Adminstration (FDA). These different numbers can be interconverted using values of 6–13 dm^2 total surface area per glove (based on nominal width and length) or a total weight of 6–10 g per glove.[95] The mix of assay problems, values, and units makes it difficult for manufacturers and healthcare professionals alike to evaluate the total protein content of gloves with confidence.

For NRL medical grade gloves commercially available in the U.S. and Europe, the extractable total protein content has decreased over the last 5 to 7 years.[101] In nearly 40 different NRL exam gloves, the extractable total protein content ranged from 20 to nearly 200 μg protein/g glove for powder-free NRL gloves and from 34 to over 1100 μg protein/g glove for powdered NRL gloves by modified Lowry analysis (unpublished data on 1999 commercially available gloves). Similar levels of NRL glove extractable total protein have been reported by other investigators.[97,102] For NRL surgical gloves, recently reported extractable total protein values range from 3 to 114 μg protein/g glove for powder-free gloves, and 0 to 182 μg protein/g glove for powdered gloves.[96]

B. NRL Extractable Allergenic Protein Content

Glove NRL allergenic protein content is assessed by immunological assays of aqueous glove extracts.[97,103,104] Common methods include RAST inhibition and ELISA inhibition assays that utilize pooled human sera with anti-NRL antibodies developed in response to product allergens. The ASTM antigenic protein assay uses rabbit anti-NRL antibodies developed to crude ammoniated NRL proteins. The most recently developed assay is the FITkit™ (FIT Biotech) which uses monoclonal antibodies to determine the levels of four NRL allergens (Hev b 1, Hev b 3, Heb 5, and Hev b 6.02).[51] Less commonly used are skin-prick and basophil histamine release testing of glove extracts.[49] The accuracy the commonly used assays for NRL allergenic protein content is limited by variability, differences in antibody sources, and the use of different NRL standards.[96,97,104] Due to differences in immunological methods, NRL allergenic protein content can be expressed in different units (i.e., arbitrary units or μg allergen per gram glove, or μg antigen per dm^2 surface area) making cross-study comparisons of product NRL allergen levels difficult if not impossible. The recent use of multiple monoclonal antibodies to specific NRL allergens present in gloves may ultimately prove more useful in evaluating product allergenicity.[51]

Nearly a 1000-fold range in NRL allergenic protein levels has been previously reported, and NRL allergenic protein levels do not always correlate to corresponding total protein content.[96,97,105] For powdered NRL exam gloves, Beezhold has previously reported NRL antigenic protein levels of 0 to 2800 μg allergen/g but substantially lower levels (< 100 μg allergen/g) for powder-free NRL gloves according to the LEAP antigenic protein assay.[97] More recent studies suggest NRL extractable allergen content is decreasing in gloves, as with total protein content.[51,96] Palosuo et al. reported on the concentration of specific allergens in the extract from NRL gloves. Hev b 6.02 allergen content exceeded that of Hev b 1, 3, and 5, and ranged from 0 to 111 μg allergen/g glove; the sum of all four allergens ranged from 0 to 150 μg allergen/g glove.[51] Interestingly, skin prick testing with these extracts indicated that when the NRL allergen content exceeded 10 μg allergen/g glove, 100% of type I hypersensitive patients responded.

C. Glove Powder and NRL Protein Allergens

Many dental workers still believe that glove powder is the source of their allergic reactions. They are unaware that the powder on medical gloves usually consists of absorbable cornstarch, but may also include oatstarch, casein, or calcium carbonate.[106] And while uncommon instances of cornstarch powder allergy have been reported in the literature, bound NRL proteins are the more likely source of allergic reactions.[107–109]

Glove powder is applied during NRL glove manufacture, principally by dipping gloves through a wet slurry consisting of cornstarch, magnesium oxide, surfactants, biocides, and other ingredients.[106] Variations in glove manufacturing can affect the NRL total and allergenic protein level in the slurry, as well as in the glove.[90,108,110] Because cornstarch binds NRL proteins, powder-bound NRL allergen levels can equal or exceed that of the nascent glove material.[108,109] Animal studies have also suggested that cornstarch powder, and possibly lipopolysaccharide from powder-associated endotoxin, may act an as immunoadjuvant, enhancing the immune response to relatively small amounts of NRL allergens.[111–113]

Glove powder content is determined by gravimetric analysis and is reported as mg per dm^2 surface area (ASTM) or as total mg per glove (FDA).[114,115] ASTM reported glove powder levels on 1999 available powdered gloves ranged from 10 to 38 mg/dm^2 for exam gloves, and 8 to 52 mg/dm^2 for surgical gloves.[106] Similarly, the 1997 FDA Medical Glove Powder Report noted that a medium-sized powdered glove was likely to contain between 120 mg and 400 mg of powder and debris, which is equivalent to 13 to 44 mg/dm^2 based on nominal size measurements.[116] New ASTM glove standards and FDA recommendations for glove powder levels aim to reduce the glove powder content substantially.

D. ALLERGENIC RUBBER CHEMICALS

Of the 200 or more chemical additives in natural and synthetic rubber products, those that are most likely to sensitize dental workers are thiurams, carbamates, and mercaptobenzothiazoles. Collectively known as accelerators and antidegradants, they are essential to the efficient control of vulcanization during oven curing and may also be added to reduce oxidation-dependent aging. All vulcanized rubbers (synthetic and natural), including those made of NRL, chloroprene (Neoprene®), nitrile, and synthetic polyisoprene contain some type of accelerator or antidegradant. These chemicals can also be found in a diverse range of consumer goods including rubber-based products, skin and hair care products, adhesives, fungicides and insecticides, as well as veterinary medications (Table 21.3 and Table 21.4). Their presence in products at work and at home can increase exposure and exacerbate symptoms.

TABLE 21.3
Common Dental Products Containing Specific Rubber Chemical Allergens

Products	Vulcanizing/Antidegradant Chemical		
	Carbamates	Thiurams	Mercaptobenzothiazoles
Adhesives, tapes, and glues	X		
Disinfectants	X		
Hand care products: soaps, lotions, creams, and moisturizers	X		
Rubber dental equipment: dental dams, prophy cups, mixing bowls, handles, aprons, tubing	X	X	X
Rubber emergency equipment: gas mask, tourniquet, stethoscope	X	X	X
Rubber gloves: medical and utility	X	X	X
Rubber office equipment: earphones, rubber bands, electrical cords, erasers	X	X	X

TABLE 21.4
Consumer Products Containing Specific Rubber Chemical Allergens

Products	Vulcanizing/Antidegradant Chemical		
	Carbamates	Thiurams	Mercaptobenzothiazole
Adhesives, tapes, and glues	X		
Fungicides, herbicides	X	X	X
Insecticides	X	X	
Rubber consumer products: tires, condoms, diaphragms, hoses, earplugs, balloons, cables, cords, goggles, handles on golf clubs, racquets, tools	X	X	X
Rubber in fabric: elastic waist bands, socks, underwear, swimwear	X	X	X
Rubber in shoes, slippers, boots, insoles, soles	X	X	X
Skin care products: soaps, lotions, moisturizers, creams, sunscreens	X		
Shampoos and conditioners	X		

Few investigators have attempted to quantify the levels of allergenic chemicals in rubber products. Methods have varied and glove chemicals have been extracted into acetone or an aqueous synthetic sweat solution prior to analysis. Chemical content has been assessed using gas chromatography, gas chromatography-mass spectroscopy, and high performance thin layer chromatography.[96,117,118]

Over the years, chemical content has apparently changed with a decreased use of mercaptobenzothiazoles, and a reduction in elutable thiuram glove levels. In 1993, Knudsen et al. reported that 1.6 to 6.5 mg of thiurams and carbamates were eluted from the interior surface of NRL surgical gloves, an amount that was reportedly similar to patch test concentrations.[118] In 2000, Knudsen et al. reported thiurams in only one glove brand studied.[117] Brehler et al. also demonstrated undetectable levels of thiurams, but found significant levels (up to 10,000 $\mu g/g$) of carbamates and mercaptobenzothiazoles in acetone extracts of selected surgical gloves. Unfortunately, a clear correlation between patient reactions and glove chemical content has not yet been established with these methods.

Identifying all chemicals added throughout natural and synthetic rubber product manufacture can be challenging. Formulations and processing methods may be proprietary or otherwise protected. Product manufacturers may be aware of the chemicals they add, but not of all chemicals in the raw material. For example, thiurams are frequently used in the preservation of raw NRL after harvesting.[119] Without specific testing, manufacturers may not be aware of chemical changes that may occur during manufacturing: carbamates can be transformed into thiurams, yielding a cross-reactive product. Manufacturers may also change source suppliers, alternate between multiple facilities, or make subtle manufacturing changes that can affect the potential allergenicity of the finished product. Identifying these changes can be difficult and may not be noted on product labels. Moreover, distributors may change product manufacturers without an identifying brand name or label change.

E. EXPOSURE ROUTES AND THRESHOLDS FOR RUBBER-BASED ALLERGENS

Like other healthcare workers, dental professionals are most likely to be occupationally exposed to NRL protein allergens via the skin, mucous membranes of the nose, eyes, oral cavity, and the upper and lower respiratory tract.[120,121] In sensitized individuals this exposure can result in the manifestation of symptoms. Percutaneous, gastrointestinal, or urogenital exposure during medical procedures may also provoke symptoms. Occupationally related sensitization routes are probably those associated with repeated and/or lengthy exposure, such as the skin and respiratory tract. However, this pathway has not yet been fully elucidated in humans. Recent research has shown that skin, nasal, or intratracheal NRL exposure can sensitize animals, and is associated with symptom elicitation.[122,123]

In the dental operatory as in other healthcare institutions, NRL allergens in the powder and on glove surfaces can become aerosolized through glove handling, donning, and removal.[31,124] In hospital areas where powdered gloves with a high NRL allergenic protein content were used frequently, aerosolized NRL allergenic protein levels in room air exceeded 600 ng/m^3.[124,125] This is several fold greater than the 15 ng/m^3 or less airborne levels observed when powder-free NRL gloves were used.[31,124,126] A similar trend was observed in a dental clinic where NRL aeroallergen levels ranged as high as 90 ng/m^3 where powdered high-allergen (~ 1600 µg/g) NRL gloves were used. These levels decreased to less than 10 ng/m^3 when powder-free and low-powder low allergen NRL gloves were used.[31]

Elevated levels of airborne NRL generally increase worker respiratory exposure. Mitakakis et al. showed that the nasal mucosa of healthcare workers can be exposed to at least 10 to 24 times more NRL allergen while wearing powdered gloves.[127] Swanson et al. reported that personal respiratory exposures approached 1000 ng/m^3 where powdered gloves were frequently used.[124] Respiratory exposure is consistent with the small size of some (~ 20%) of airborne NRL-laden particles.[19,128]

The majority of airborne NRL-laden particles are relatively large (7–14 µ, mass median aerodynamic diameter) and likely to settle within 24 hours. These NRL-laden particles contaminate clothing, skin, operatory surfaces, and existing dust, and can be reintroduced into the air with dental worker activity.[19,124] Charous et al. reported levels of NRL allergenic protein ranging from 15 to 84 µg/g in dust obtained from dental operatory carpet and upholstery.[31] In addition, vigorous dusting of furniture cushions raised NRL aeroallergen levels to nearly 400 ng/m^3. Reiter reported significant NRL allergen contamination (over 4000 ng/in^2) of an infrequently cleaned area in a dental operatory, as well as moderate contamination of suspended ceiling tiles.[129]

Skin and respiratory thresholds for NRL allergens are difficult to establish due to the multiplicity of NRL protein allergens in finished rubber products, their apparent differential allergenicity and bioavailability, as well as variations in sensitized patient responsiveness.[120] From clinical studies of other allergens, it is known that submicrogram quantities may elicit an allergic response in a sensitized individual.[130] Although dose-response relationships have not yet been established for each exposure route or for each NRL protein and chemical allergen, guidelines have been proposed. Baur et al. has suggested that aerosolized NRL allergen levels remain below 0.6 ng/m^3 to prevent symptom elicitation in healthcare workers.[30,126] However, investigators at Mayo Clinic suggest a more practical lower limit of 10 ng/m^3 to minimize symptoms in type I NRL hypersensitive workers.[19] They also suggest that airborne NRL allergen levels greater than 50 ng/m^3 have a high probability of symptom elicitation.

Dental practitioners are exposed to accelerators and antidegradants such as thiurams, carbamates, and mercaptobenzothiazoles primarily through direct skin or mucosal contact. The same is true for those chemicals added to synthetic nonvulcanized elastomers, including plasticizers, stabilizers, antioxidants, bacteriocides, and colorants. These potential chemical allergens may be released from the surface of the thin-film products when they become wet (e.g., water, sweat, or saliva) or solubilized from the product if exposed to dental solvents.[117,118] While effective levels for diagnostic testing with many rubber processing chemicals have been developed, thresholds for sensitization or symptom elicitation, and correlation to product levels have not yet been established.

F. OTHER DENTAL ALLERGENS

Diagnosis and management of glove-related allergies is complicated by the plethora of irritating and allergenic chemicals to which a dental worker's hands are exposed. Because symptoms of these allergies are often confined to their hands, dental professionals (and physicians) may misinterpret them as glove-related.[131] Chemicals that are increasingly associated with type IV delayed hypersensitivity include the disinfectants glutaraldehyde and glyoxal, and the methacrylates in dental bonding agents.[20,131–134] At the 2 to 4% concentration found in disinfectants and sterilants, glutaraldehyde is a skin irritant and potential sensitizer according to animal studies.[135,136] Methacrylates (e.g., 2-hydroxyethyl methacrylate) can be potent sensitizers and are found at 50 to 90% concentrations in uncured preparations in adhesives, glues, and artificial fingernail preparations.[137] Cross-sensitization to other related methacrylates can also occur.[132,138] Unfortunately, dental professionals are frequently unaware of chemical hazards in the operatory. Moreover, they often do not use sufficient personal protective equipment (e.g., aprons, eyeshields, or face shields) or gloves with adequate chemical resistance. Workers commonly wear medical grade gloves while using these chemicals, which provide little or no skin protection.[139–143]

To further confound diagnosis in dental professionals, recent studies have shown that airborne glutaraldehyde and methacrylates may elicit asthmalike symptoms in healthcare workers.[14,132,144,145] These symptoms can be due to both allergic and irritant responses to these chemicals.[146,147] Vapor pressures and evaporation rates of concentrated glutaraldehyde solutions and uncured methacrylate monomers are sufficient for vaporization and subsequent perfusion of room air. In rooms without adequate ventilation, dental workers may be exposed to glutaraldehyde or methacrylate vapor above recommended limits.[148] Because these chemicals can induce respiratory symptoms similar to those of a type I NRL protein hypersensitivity, this underscores the need for a thorough diagnosis in symptomatic dental professionals with exposure to both NRL and these chemicals.

Dental workers may apply moisturizing hand lotions and creams to relieve symptoms of irritant and allergic dermatitis and hydrate skin.[149] These products may assist in restoring the epidermal barrier, but evidence of their clinical and physiological efficacy is somewhat equivocal in controlled trials.[150,151] Hand care products are also likely to contain antimicrobials and preservatives, including thimerosal or methylchloroisothiazolinone — two of the more common allergens in dental workers.[22,152] Through regular application of these allergens to broken skin on their hands, dental professionals may unknowingly exacerbate an existing allergy, or facilitate sensitization to new allergens.[153]

Barrier or skin protection creams are marketed to healthcare workers to prevent or diminish exposure to the allergens in gloves. While many barrier creams have little effect, a few have modestly reduced skin irritation and improved epidermal barrier status, although blinded, randomized, controlled clinical trials are rare.[154–156] As with hand lotions, some barrier creams may contain irritants and allergens that can worsen the skin condition, or facilitate transfer of protein and chemical allergens to the skin.[153] Because some barrier and skin protection products are made with a mineral oil or petroleum base, they can also accelerate the failure of NRL gloves during use and are specifically contraindicated by the Occupational Safety and Health Administration (OSHA) and the CDC for this reason.[157]

V. MITIGATING RUBBER ALLERGEN EXPOSURE

The overall goal is to reduce the frequency and severity of NRL allergy symptoms in allergic individuals, as well as minimize future development of NRL allergies in exposed workers. NIOSH, CDC, and several professional organizations have made recommendations for accomplishing this goal in the healthcare environment. For dentistry, effective strategies include administrative controls such as NRL management protocols and guidelines, and remediation of residual environmental NRL from dental operatories. Special considerations for type I NRL hypersensitive patients should also be addressed, including preparedness for anaphylatic-type reactions, appropriate modifications to dental procedures, and mitigating patient fears of adverse reactions. At present, lowering exposure levels of NRL allergens appears dependent upon elimination of NRL glove products with high allergen content. The success of intervention programs to date has been based on substitution of these high allergen NRL gloves with one of the following: (1) powdered NRL gloves with a very low allergen content (i.e., incapable of eliciting a skin prick response in a sensitized individual, per the Finnish experience), (2) powder-free NRL gloves with low allergen content, and (3) synthetic rubber products, powdered or powder-free.[17,19,30,31,158]

A. ADMINISTRATIVE CONTROLS

Per recommendations by the ADA, NIOSH, and CDC, NRL allergy management protocols should be developed for the dental office that are applicable to both workers and patients.[42,43,75] These protocols should discuss key topics such as: (1) evaluation of patients and staff for the risk of type I or type IV rubber-based allergies, including diagnostic measures; (2) measures for identifying, substituting, and isolating products that contain NRL and rubber allergens; (3) special dental patient treatment and management regimens; (4) education about type I and type IV rubber-based allergies; and (5) emergency preparedness for adverse patient or dental worker reactions, should they occur.[159] These essential points can be accomplished through the use of standardized questionnaires for risk assessment, rubber product checklists, professional continuing education coursework, and emergency treatment training and drills.

Dental and medical practitioners alike must determine criteria for implementing NRL allergy patient management protocols. For example, is the criteria based solely on a patient's history, with or without concurrent symptoms? If not, will diagnostic testing be required prior to dental treatment? While the most conservative strategy is to "assume" some type of NRL allergy based on history alone, case reports in the literature demonstrate the failure of this approach long-term. The personal and economic costs of "assumed" diagnoses can be significant.[38]

B. DENTAL OPERATORY CLEANING AND NRL REMEDIATION

The ultimate goal is to create a workspace that contains little to no NRL allergens in the air or on environmental surfaces. Per NIOSH recommendations issued in 1997, good housekeeping procedures should be implemented to remove dust and debris that might contain NRL residue.[42] Areas that may be contaminated with NRL-containing dust should be targeted for frequent and thorough cleanings. Based on observations in hospital environments, NIOSH also recommended that ventilation filters and vacuum bags used in areas where NRL glove use is high should be changed frequently.[160] Research suggests that aerosolized NRL allergenic protein concentration should be less than 10 ng/m^3 to minimize symptom elicitation in sensitized workers in the healthcare environment.[30,124,126]

Recent studies have shown that aerosolized NRL particles can settle in the dental operatory and contaminate countertops, shelving, drawers, carpeting, suspended ceiling tiles, and spaces behind cabinetry.[31,129] If not removed by cleaning, these settled NRL particles can be agitated and reintroduced into the air with activity or air movement. Because ventilation and work flow patterns of offices, reception areas, laboratory spaces, and operatories are often contiguous, it is important to thoroughly clean all work spaces. For effective remediation of NRL particles, Reiter recommends a combination of thorough vacuuming of spaces with a HEPA-filtered vacuum and wet-wiping all surfaces with isopropyl alcohol.[129] More than one cleaning may be required, depending upon the degree of existing contamination and degree of sensitization of the dental worker or patient. Although hospital ventilation filters have been shown to contain significant NRL allergen levels, similar levels have not been found in the ventilation ducts of dental operatories.[31,160] While this may be related to air sampling limitations, it may be more appropriate to change ventilation filters frequently, and reserve extensive duct cleaning for institutional environments or areas with significant NRL aeroallergen levels.

C. NRL PRODUCT SUBSTITUTION

The most conservative strategy for dental professionals diagnosed with a type I NRL hypersensitivity is to avoid contact with and exposure to NRL products. To establish a latex-safe environment, dental professionals should identify all products at home and at work that contain NRL and to which they are exposed. This can be a daunting task, as there are approximately 40,000 consumer products that are reported to contain NRL.[161] Product manufacturers, healthcare professional organizations, and nonprofit organizations such as the Spina Bifida Organization (Table 21.1) can help identify medical and consumer products that contain NRL, and recommend potential substitutes.

Beyond the limits dictated by a type I NRL or type IV rubber-based hypersensitivity, the choice of dental gloves should include consideration of the glove user needs and preferences (Table 21.5). This may include chemical resistance to biocides, solvents, resins, and adhesives, and puncture resistance to dental sharps such as needles, dental burs, curettes, metal bands, sharp instruments, and rough bony surfaces. User preferences can include dexterity and flexibility, as well as comfort and fit. When powder-free gloves are needed, alternative donning or sweat-absorbing agents may become important criteria. Potential alternative agents include other glove powders (i.e., oatstarch), glove chlorination, or polymer coatings (silicone, polyacrylate, or polyurethane) to reduce internal tackiness. A good match between allergy considerations, material characteristics, and user preferences for dental professionals ensures a more likely acceptance of new gloves as well as better compliance with hand care and gloving guidelines.

1. Guidelines and Glove Standards

Professional medical and dental organizations and NIOSH have recommended various glove options for reducing NRL exposure levels overall for healthcare workers.[42,75,162,163] These recommendations have included (1) eliminating the routine use of NRL gloves by food preparation workers, housekeeping staff, and maintenance workers; (2) using NRL gloves with a low allergen or low protein content; and (3) eliminating powdered NRL gloves. While some states and organizations have urged the elimination of all NRL gloves or all powdered gloves regardless of material, neither of these extreme options is feasible nor prudent.[116] Moreover, the success of substitution with powder-free NRL gloves of low-allergen or low-protein content indicates that these extreme elimination measures are unnecessary to reduce airborne NRL levels, symptom elicitation, and the prevalence of type I NRL hypersensitivity.[15–19,31,164,165]

Dental professionals should be aware that OSHA's Bloodborne Pathogen Standard requires employers to provide alternative gloves and personal protective equipment for allergic employees. Section 1910.1030 (d)(3)(iii) states that employers will

TABLE 21.5
Medical Grade Gloves Available to Dental Professionals

Glove Type	Commercially Available Glove Materials *	Contains NRL Protein?	Contains Rubber Chemicals?
Examination Gloves:			
Nonsterile and sterile	Natural-rubber latex (NRL)	Y	Y
single-use disposable.	Nitrile[1]	N	Y
	Nitrile and chloroprene (Neoprene®) blends[1]	N	Y
	Nitrile and NRL blends[1]	Y	Y
	Butadiene methyl methacrylate[1]	N	Y
	Polyvinyl chloride (PVC, vinyl)	N	N
	Polyurethane (Intacta®)	N	N
	Styrene-based copolymer (Elastylon®)[2]	N	N
Surgical Gloves:			
Sterile single-use	NRL	Y	Y
disposable.	Nitrile	N	Y
Orthopedic surgical gloves	Chloroprene (Neoprene®)	N	Y
may be thicker.	NRL and nitrile or chloroprene blends	Y	Y
	Synthetic polyisoprene	N	Y
	Styrene-based copolymer (Elastylon®)[2]	N	N
	Polyurethane (Intacta®)	N	N

* Material Comment Codes:
[1] Likely to have enhanced chemical and/or puncture resistance.
[2] Deteriorates when used with methyl methacrylates in dental bonding agents and cements.

provide alternative personal protective equipment including glove liners, powder-free gloves, or "similar alternatives."[166] While NIOSH and the CDC have recommended reducing the use of powdered NRL gloves, the Bloodborne Pathogen Standard does not specifically require the elimination or substitution of powdered NRL gloves or other NRL products in the healthcare environment where sensitized individuals work.

New guidelines and recommendations for NRL glove protein and allergen content have been developed by the U.S. FDA and ASTM in collaboration with the Malaysian Rubber Research Institute to reflect research developments and concerns about the increased prevalence of type I NRL hypersensitivity.[90,101,167] Therefore the goal of the FDA and ASTM is to reduce the NRL allergen content of medical gloves in order to lower the severity and frequency of symptoms in individuals with type I NRL hypersensitivity, as well as reduce the incidence of this allergy. ASTM standards recommend that NRL gloves contain no more than 200 µg extractable total protein per dm[2] surface area.[99,100] FDA guidelines recommend that NRL gloves contain less than 1200 µg extractable total protein per glove, which is a somewhat more conservative value and is roughly equivalent to 100 μg to 200 μg extractable total protein per dm² surface area depending on glove size.[115] While the FDA has not yet issued guidelines regarding antigenic protein levels, ASTM standards recommend that NRL gloves contain no more than 10 μg antigenic protein per dm² surface area.[99,100] This value is similar to the lowest NRL allergen protein level (~ 10 μg/g glove) observed by Palosuo et al. associated with 100% skin prick reactivity in type I NRL sensitized individuals.[51]

To diminish the potential for airborne NRL allergens, endotoxin contamination, and postsurgical adhesions, regulatory agencies have encouraged glove powder reductions. Current ASTM medical glove standards (irrespective of material) set a glove powder limit of 10 mg per dm² surface area for powdered exam gloves and 15 mg per dm² for powdered surgical gloves.[99,100] The FDA has proposed a slightly less conservative upper limit for all medical grade gloves of 120 mg powder per glove, which is equivalent to roughly 10 mg to 20 mg per dm² surface area.

The FDA has proposed — but not yet implemented — new regulations that would change medical grade gloves from a Class I to a Class II medical device, which would require more stringent manufacturing quality control requirements.[115] In their draft glove guidance manual, the FDA also outlined new label requirements for all powdered medical gloves that would include warning statements about potential adverse reactions associated with glove powder.[115,168] The FDA would add more label requirements for NRL gloves, including protein content information to expand existing label requirements for warnings about possible allergic reactions. Finally, the FDA has proposed new guidelines requiring skin allergy and irritancy testing in humans for NRL gloves (or other medical devices) sold with any claim related to its low "chemical content" or "dermatitis potential."[169,170] Overall, these outlined regulatory changes are intended to improve manufacturing quality control, and clarify product labeling so as not to misrepresent the allergenicity of gloves and NRL products to healthcare workers.

With respect to individual glove products, it is important to understand that regulatory agencies impose protein and powder content limits during the manufacturer's initial application for permission to sell a product (known in the U.S. as the 510k application).[168] Whether the manufacturer continues to meet these control limits is evaluated during random audits of imported goods. Neither glove manufacturers nor regulatory agencies are required to monitor NRL glove protein or powder levels on a regular basis.

2. Product Substitutions for Type I NRL Hypersensitivity

For dental professionals diagnosed with a type I NRL hypersensitivity, the most conservative strategy is to avoid contact with and exposure to products that contain NRL, particularly those likely to have a high allergen content. Type I NRL allergic dental workers should avoid the use of any NRL-based glove including "hypoallergenic" gloves, low-allergen NRL gloves, blends of NRL with nitrile or chloroprene, or polymer-coated NRL gloves.

It is important to note that powdered and powder-free NRL gloves with a very low allergen content have been successfully worn by sensitized healthcare workers in Finland. These gloves have been selected for their negative skin prick test result as well as a very low glove allergen level by immunoassay and are used throughout the hospital.[17] This selection process is critical to prevent use of gloves (powdered or powder-free) that potentially contain significant NRL allergens, even if the total protein content is negligible.[171] In addition, even when total allergen content is low, the concentrations of select NRL allergens (e.g., Hev b 5 and Hev b 6.02) may cross elicitation thresholds.[171] Because absolute and widely applicable clinical thresholds for symptom elicitation have yet to be established regarding product NRL allergen content or airborne NRL allergens, use of NRL gloves by type I NRL hypersensitive dental workers is not recommended.

With respect to medical gloves, alternatives for dental workers with type I NRL hypersensitivity should be made of synthetic rubber (e.g., nitrile, neoprene, or synthetic polyisoprene), PVC, polyurethane, or styrene-based copolymers (Table 21.5). Each glove material can have unique attributes. For example, for increased chemical or puncture resistance, nitrile or neoprene (or blends thereof) gloves may be chosen. For routine short-term dental work, PVC or polyurethane blends may be cost-effective choices.

Most commonly handled dental products can also be found manufactured in synthetic materials. For example, dental dams can be found in polyurethane, bite blocks in silicone rubber, prophy cups in plastic, and tubing in silicone rubber. For those products where substitution may be impractical, such as natural rubber pieces on equipment, NRL-allergic dental workers can insulate themselves from direct contact using fabric, plastic film, or synthetic glove material. Fortunately, most hard-rubber products are not likely to contribute significant levels of allergenic NRL proteins. Therefore, it is usually unnecessary to remove and replace rubber components, equipment parts, and carpet backing simply because it contains NRL.

In addition to providing synthetic rubber glove alternatives to type I allergic workers, dental offices should reduce overall NRL aeroallergen levels. Based on current knowledge, powdered NRL gloves with a high protein or high allergen content are probably the greatest source of surface and aerosolized NRL allergens in the dental operatory.[31,124,129] Unfortunately there is no clear understanding yet of the roles of glove powder and NRL allergens in provoking a type I NRL allergy. While cornstarch is an established carrier of NRL allergens, it may directly or indirectly facilitate the development of immune reactions to those NRL allergens.[111–113] Although protein concentrations, allergen levels, and powder content generally trend together, the variances in each are large, and exceptions can be found in every study. Therefore, NRL powdered gloves can be found with negligible NRL allergen content. Similarly, low or no powder does not guarantee a low-allergen glove.

Given current regulatory requirements, assay methods, and the limited information from manufacturers, the most conservative approach is to use either powder-free low protein (or low allergen) NRL gloves or powdered synthetic rubber gloves. To reduce overall NRL protein allergen levels in the dental operatory where allergic workers or patients can be exposed, current recommendations are to select powder-free gloves with a total protein content less than 50 µg/g (or 200 µg/dm^2) and an allergenic NRL protein content of less than 10 µg/dm^2. As discussed above, due to the total protein and immunological protein assay limitations, these protein values should be interpreted cautiously. When the level of airborne NRL allergens is reduced through these glove substitution strategies, multiple studies have shown improvements in skin and respiratory symptoms, as well as reduced anti-NRL IgE levels in healthcare workers with type I NRL hypersensitivity.[19,30,127,172]

Cost-driven dental workers may prefer to select the least expensive gloves, and appropriate glove choices may be deterred by the perception of increased costs. Certainly, the increased leaching, washing, chlorination, and quality control used to lower protein and chemical allergen content can raise the cost of any glove. But in reality, the cost of gloves has diminished remarkably over the last few years. Many powder-free NRL exam glove options are available to dentists in the cost range of $5 to $10 per box, similar to the cost of powdered NRL gloves. Moreover, nitrile glove and PVC exam gloves can now be obtained for the same, if not lower, costs. An exception to this exists when a dental worker is allergic to NRL proteins and rubber processing chemicals and also reacts to PVC or polyurethane gloves. In this case, styrene-based copolymer exam gloves may be required and can cost significantly more. This caveat also generally applies to surgical gloves used by oral surgeons, which are more expensive overall due to manufacturing and sterilization requirements. Because fewer synthetic surgical glove options are commercially available, they are likely to be more expensive than powder-free NRL surgical gloves.

3. Product Substitutions for Type IV Rubber Chemical Hypersensitivity

Dental professionals diagnosed with type IV hypersensitivity to one or more of the accelerators or antidegradants should avoid rubber and nonrubber products that contain those chemicals both at work and home (Table 21.3 and Table 21.4). Glove products that contain either natural or synthetic vulcanized rubber, including NRL, nitrile, chloroprene, butadiene methyl methacrylate, or synthetic polyisoprene, also contain rubber accelerators or antidegradants, most often thiurams or carbamates. As a result, dental workers allergic to the cross-reactive carbamates and thiurams are unlikely to remedy their problem by changing from NRL to nitrile or chloroprene gloves. Even synthetic and natural rubber gloves with reportedly nondetectable residual chemical content may elicit reactions in some sensitized individuals due to sensitivity differences between patient thresholds and analytical methods. One exception may be for workers with a type IV hypersensitivity to only mercaptobenzothiazoles or mercapto mix. Because mercaptobenzothiazoles are now less frequently used in gloves, and do not cross-react with other accelerators, an alternative natural or synthetic rubber glove may be found that is manufactured with carbamates or thiurams.[173] However, this approach should be used cautiously due to the potential for patients to develop multiple allergies to the chemicals used in manufacturing rubber gloves.[73]

Dental professionals with a type IV hypersensitivity to thiurams, or carbamates (and to a lesser extent mercaptobenzothiazoles) should choose medical gloves made of polyvinyl chloride (PVC or vinyl), polyurethane (polyisocyanates), or styrene-based copolymers, which are not vulcanized. Gloves made of PVC elastomers are created by heat-dependent fusion of the plastisol polymer.[119,174] Similarly, polyurethane and polyurethane-PVC elastomeric blends such as the Intacta® polymer (Dow Chemical) are created by heat-dependent processes.[175] By comparison, styrene-based rubber elastomers such as the styrene-butadiene-styrene (SBS) and styrene-isoprene-styrene (SIS) blend in the Elastylon® copolymer (ECI Medical Technologies) are created by solvent evaporation.[176] These nonvulcanized synthetic elastomers are unlikely to contain accelerators and the base polymers are not common cutaneous sensitizers. However, PVC, polyurethane, polyolefin, and styrene-based products may contain plasticizers (e.g., phthalates), epoxy resins, stabilizers (e.g., epoxidized soybean oil), antioxidants (e.g., butylhydroxytoluene), lubricants, UV absorbers, fungicides, bacteriocides, and colorants.[119] Although little information is available on the bioavailability of these chemicals in finished products, they can be the source of irritant and allergic reactions to PVC, polyurethane, and styrene-based rubber products.[119,177–181]

D. CONSIDERATIONS FOR THE DENTAL PATIENT WITH RUBBER-BASED ALLERGIES

Special treatment procedures may be required for those patients with a type I NRL hypersensitivity or a type IV hypersensitivity to rubber processing chemicals. Relevant modification to standard dental office procedures should be identified in a dental office's latex allergy management protocol. If no protocol is available, these special considerations should be extensively reviewed with the patient's dental care practitioner(s). They may include simple administrative controls such as prominent identification of the allergy in the patient's dental record. For type I NRL hypersensitive patients, dental treatment may require operatory cleaning and early morning scheduling, particularly if the office has regularly used powdered high protein NRL gloves without remediation. In cases with an extensive allergic history, dentists may also need to consider alternative methods of administering dental anesthesia, emergency preparedness, and mitigating patient anxiety. For patients with either type I NRL hypersensitivity or type IV hypersensitivity to rubber chemicals, dental professionals and their patients should be aware of possible complications from unsuspected allergens.

1. Procedures Requiring Local Anesthesia

Dental anesthesia cartridges represent a unique replacement challenge. Designed to fit into a specialized aspirating syringe, the cartridge contains a stopper and diaphragm with natural rubber components. The degree to which NRL antigens are solubilized from these components and contaminate the anesthetic is not well quantified, but is believed to be low. Thomsen and Burke reported no quantifiable NRL allergen in medication vials containing rubber stoppers.[182] However, Primeau et al. detected very low levels of NRL allergens extracted from medication vials with rubber stoppers using CAP inhibition analysis.[183] These same extracts also elicited positive intradermal skin reactions in type I allergic individuals. Rubber septa have previously been implicated in systemic reactions in type I NRL allergic individuals.[182–184] Therefore, the current consensus is that NRL allergens can be leached from rubber septa, stoppers, and other components and contaminate vial contents. This is consistent with data from extracts of dry rubber demonstrating very low but detectable NRL protein and allergen content.[90] But because the amount and character of these NRL allergens can vary, as can the sensitivity of the allergic individual, the risk of an adverse reaction is difficult to predict.

The most conservative approach that is usually recommended is to administer dental anesthetics to type I NRL allergic individuals from glass ampules. However, there are few suppliers of small glass ampules (5 to 20 mL) of lidocaine, bupivacaine, mepivacaine, prilocaine, and articaine anesthetics.[105] Even more rarely are these manufactured in the appropriate concentration or with epinephrine, per dental anesthesia protocols.[105] A new polypropylene vial system (Polyamp Duofit™ by Astra-Zeneca) may provide a solution in the future, but is currently of limited availability. Those dental professionals that need to provide anesthesia without possible NRL contamination should contact their anesthetic distributor or manufacturer directly for assistance.

2. Endodontic Procedures

Although over a hundred years have passed since its introduction, endodontic points made of gutta-percha are still considered the material of choice for filling or obturating root canals. Because gutta-percha is a natural rubber of botanical origin, the possibility of NRL cross-reactivity exists. Previously, Boxer et al. reported diffuse urticaria (hives) and swelling in a type I NRL-allergic dental hygienist during root canal surgery.[185] Symptoms persisted until the gutta-percha was removed 1 month later, but a type I reaction to gutta-percha points could not be confirmed. Gazelius et al. recorded a similar case of a long-term reaction to gutta-percha in a nurse with a type IV allergy to rubber compounding chemicals.[186] By comparison, other clinicians have described successful root canal placement in type I NRL-allergic patients.[187,188] Despite isolated case reports, no clinician has demonstrated a type I reaction to gutta-percha points to date. Moreover, Hamann et al. showed that no detectable cross-reactivity existed between NRL and 19 brands of commercial gutta-percha points when tested with RAST inhibition, direct ELISA, and ELISA inhibition.[189] In vivo SPT results confirmed that a type I NRL-allergic patient is unlikely to react to commercial gutta-percha points. These results are similar to the findings of Costa et al. who also noted that gutta-percha proteins are probably denatured during manufacture, minimizing the allergenic character of gutta-percha points.[190]

While more endodontic points are now made with synthetic rubber instead of gutta-percha, concerns regarding their content should be addressed with the respective manufacturer prior to patient treatment. Other chemicals used during endodontic procedures can be potent allergens, including eugenol (in fragrances and root canal sealers), disinfectants such as glutaraldehyde and chlorhexidine, methacrylates in bonding agents, and formaldehyde derivatives (in root canal sealers and resins).[20,191,192] Patients with an allergic history should be informed about the dental materials used and their potential to cause allergenic or irritant reactions.

3. Emergency Preparedness

Dental professionals should be instructed in emergency procedures for patients or staff with a type I NRL allergy who experience an adverse reaction. In the 2002 guidelines published by the American Dental Association, dental offices should have injectable epinephrine, injectable antihistamines, and a bronchodilator in their emergency drug kit.[193] All medicines and supplies should be current and readily accessible, and dentists should be familiar with their administration. Dental staff should review office emergency procedures, be certified in basic life support, and complete training drills using mock emergency situations.[193] Although rarely required, the phone numbers of critical emergency services should be readily available as it is important that medical assistance be quickly obtained when needed.

4. Psychological Issues

Patients with type I NRL hypersensitivity may exhibit anxiety-related symptoms such as light-headedness, shortness of breath, difficulty breathing, and an apparent tightness in the chest. For patients who have experienced previous anaphylatic episodes or have an extensive allergic history, this anxiety may be understandable. However, because these symptoms can mimic type I systemic reactions, dental practitioners may misinterpret this response and make unnecessary adjustments in patient care.[121] Assessing a patient's anxiety and discussing it with them can be helpful in reducing patient fear.[194] Other available options to reduce anxiety during dental treatment include behavioral management, relaxation programs, distraction techniques, hypnosis, and medication.[195]

VI. EXAMPLES OF SUCCESSFUL MANAGEMENT OF RUBBER-BASED ALLERGIES

Several studies have been published highlighting the success of NRL management strategies in both dentistry and medicine. In general these have focused principally on intervention with low protein powder-free NRL gloves and appropriate management policies. Hermesch et al. reported a decrease in airborne particulate counts during use of powder-free NRL gloves in a dental school clinic, but NRL aeroallergen levels were not determined.[196] Saary et al. reported a significant decrease over a 6-year period in the number of dental school students and staff with type I NRL allergy.[15] Although this decrease was coincident with a change to low protein powder-free NRL gloves, NRL allergen exposure levels and product content was not reported. In 1999, Charous et al. first reported details on the relationship of NRL glove allergen content and airborne NRL in dental operatories.[31] NRL aeroallergens often exceeded 10 ng/m^3, and were dispersed throughout the clinic, including waiting rooms and laboratory facilities. Powdered NRL glove allergen content ranged from 570 to 1624 µg/g, as determined by immunoassay and was associated with elevated NRL aeroallergen levels (> 50 ng/m^3). Use of low allergen powder-free NRL gloves (19 µg allergen/g glove) in most areas and a lightly powdered NRL glove (126 µg allergen/g glove) in one operatory still reduced NRL aeroallergen levels from 90 ng/m^3 to below detection.

Charous et al. also observed that upholstery, carpeting, and environmental surfaces were significant reservoirs of NRL allergens in the dental clinic. [31] This allowed dispersion and reintroduction of NRL allergens, contaminating other areas irrespective of airflow. Remediation efforts (i.e., thorough cleanings of the operatory and office areas) resulted in significant decreases in surface contamination. Similarly, Reiter reported that several thorough cleanings of the dental operatory were required to lower airborne NRL allergens to below 10 ng/m^3, even after replacement of NRL products with synthetic materials. [129]

Recent studies in hospital environments have reported similar successful outcomes of NRL product substitution and remediation efforts. Turjanmaa et al. reported that all type I NRL allergic healthcare workers were able to return to work after switching Finnish hospitals to NRL gloves with a low allergen content (powdered and powder-free). [17] No healthcare worker reportedly retired or changed their work as a result of their allergy, with most even wearing low allergen NRL gloves. It should be noted that glove allergen content had been determined through extensive testing of glove extracts by *in vitro* immunologic analyses and *in vivo* skin prick testing of type I NRL allergic patients. [197] The positive outcome was no doubt possible because of the extensive glove testing and selection process established by the Finnish government, as well as the strong diagnostic paradigm established for healthcare workers. Unfortunately, an equivalent process in the U.S., U.K., and other countries is not commonly available.

Research at the Mayo Clinic charted institutional changes in airborne NRL allergen levels vs. healthcare type I NRL symptoms with changes in NRL glove allergen content. [19] In 1993, airborne NRL allergen levels varied between 14 and 200 ng/m^3 while personal NRL allergen exposures ranged from 10 to nearly 900 ng/m^3. [124] When powder free NRL gloves with a low allergen content were substituted, airborne NRL allergen levels dropped to below 10 ng/m^3. [19] Coincident with this change, the number of reported symptoms and new cases of NRL type I allergy decreased.

Overall successful interventions have included worker education, voluntary health history assessment, and skin prick testing, coinciding with use of low protein powder-free NRL exam gloves and lower protein reduced-powder NRL surgical gloves, in addition to synthetic rubber gloves. As a result of the decreased NRL exposure, healthcare worker serum anti-NRL IgE levels also diminish. [30,158] Similarly, reductions in allergy-related symptoms, asthma-like symptoms, and type I NRL allergy diagnoses occur after global glove changes are implemented. [16,18,164,165]

VII. SUMMARY AND RECOMMENDATIONS

Assuming approximately 550,000 individuals working in dentistry in the U.S. (Bureau of Labor statistics), there may be 16,500 dental professionals with a potential type I NRL hypersensitivity based on an estimated 3% prevalence. By comparison, the estimated prevalence in dentistry of a type IV hypersensitivity to one of the two more common rubber processing chemicals — thiurams or carbamates — is at least

5 to 7%. Therefore, there may be twice as many dental workers with a type IV delayed hypersensitivity to rubber processing chemicals, as compared to a type I NRL protein hypersensitivity.

Dental workers with a suspected allergic reaction to rubber products should be screened for their risk of type I NRL protein and type IV rubber chemical hypersensitivities. Risk factors include an atopic history, occupation, recurring exposure to rubber products, history of reactions to rubber products, multiple childhood surgeries, and congenital anomalies such as spina bifida. Diagnostic paradigms should include at a minimum skin prick testing or serological testing for IgE antibodies to NRL allergens, as well as patch testing for delayed skin reactions to thiurams, carbamates, and mercaptobenzothiazoles. Physicians should understand the limitations of test methods and appropriately address potential false-negative results.

In the healthcare environment a three-pronged approach is applied in the management of rubber-based allergies, both protein and chemically derived. First, dental professionals must be educated about relevant allergy symptoms, potential rubber allergen sources, and appropriate measures to avoid exposure. In addition they should become aware of the myriad of dental chemicals that are also allergenic. Second, product and environmental sources of the offending allergen (NRL protein or rubber processing chemicals) should be identified and substitute products obtained. In cases where alternatives are not readily available, isolation of the allergen is desirable. Third, the dental operatory, clinic, and laboratory should be extensively cleaned to remediate environmental levels of NRL allergens, and particularly of NRL protein allergens.

Because NRL gloves are the largest source of NRL protein allergens, and certainly a major source of rubber processing chemicals, several guidelines have been adopted by regulatory agencies and professional organizations. Briefly, dental professionals with a type I NRL hypersensitivity should wear synthetic rubber gloves (with or without powder) composed of a material (e.g., nitrile, PVC, polyurethane) suitable to their needs and preferences. It is just as important for coworkers working in the same environment to change to low protein, low allergen, NRL gloves (< 50 $\mu g/g$ glove, or 40 to 80 $\mu g/dm^2$) with reduced or no powder, or alternatively, synthetic rubber gloves (with or without powder) to lower the overall aerosolized NRL allergen levels to less than 10 ng/m^3.

Due to the complexity of the issue, there are no established thresholds for the development of or symptom elicitation in type I NRL sensitivity. However, new guidelines are being formulated based on practical exposure and clinical experiences. While still imperfect, these guidelines appear to be reducing the prevalence of type I NRL protein hypersensitivity in healthcare. Certainly, when disability costs, lost work time and productivity are considered, providing guidelines and appropriate alternatives is a reasonable and economical strategy.

REFERENCES

1. Crawford, J.J., Parker, W.D., and Parker, N.H., Asepsis in periodontal surgery, *J. Dent. Res.*, 53, 99, 1974.

2. Centers for Disease Control & Prevention, Outbreak of hepatitis B associated with an oral surgeon — New Hampshire, *MMWR Morb. Mortal. Wkly. Rep.,* 36, 132, 1987.

3. Verrusio, A.C. et al., The dentists and infectious diseases: A national survey of attitudes and behavior, *J. Am. Dent. Assoc.,* 118, 553, 1989.

4. Council on Dental Material and Devices, Council on Dental Therapeutics and American Dental Association, Infection control in the dental office, *J. Am. Dent. Assoc.,* 97, 673, 1978.

5. Centers for Disease Control & Prevention, Recommended infection-control practices for dentistry, *MMWR Morb. Mortal. Wkly. Rep.,* 35, 237, 1986.

6. Nutter, A.F., Contact urticaria to rubber, *Br. J. Dermatol.,* 101, 597, 1979.

7. Blinkhorn, A.S. and Leggate, E.M., An allergic reaction to rubber dam, *Br. Dent. J.,* 156, 402, 1984.

8. Axelsson, J.G.K., Johansson, S.G.O., and Wrangsjo, K., IgE-mediated anaphylactoid reactions to rubber, *Allergy,* 42, 46, 1987.

9. Berky, Z.T., Luciano, W.J., and James, W.D., Latex glove allergy: A survey of the U.S. Army Dental Corps, *J. Am. Med. Assoc.,* 268, 2695, 1992.

10. Yassin, M.S. et al., Latex allergy in hospital employees, *Ann. Allergy,* 72, 245, 1994.

11. Katelaris, C.H., Widmer, R.P., and Lazarus, R.M., Prevalence of latex allergy in a dental school, *Med. J. Aust.* 164, 711, 1996.

12. Safadi, G.S. et al., Latex hypersensitivity: Its prevalence among dental professionals, *J. Am. Dent. Assoc.,* 127, 83, 1996.

13. Hamann, C.P. et al., Natural rubber latex hypersensitivity: Incidence and prevalence of type 1 allergy in the dental professional, *J. Am. Dent. Assoc.,* 129, 43, 1998.

14. Piirila, P. et al., Occupational respiratory hypersensitivity in dental personnel, *Int. Arch. Occup. Environ. Health,* 75, 209, 2002.

15. Saary, M.J. et al., Changes in rates of natural rubber latex sensitivity among dental school students and staff members after changes in latex gloves, *J. Allergy Clin. Immunol.,* 109, 131, 2002.

16. Allmers, H., Schmengler, J., and Skudlik, C., Primary prevention of natural rubber latex allergy in the German health care system through education and intervention, *J. Allergy Clin. Immunol.,* 110, 318, 2002.

17. Turjanmaa, K. et al., Long-term outcome of 160 adult patients with natural rubber latex allergy, *J. Allergy Clin. Immunol.,* 110, S70–S74, 2002.

18. Tarlo, S.M. et al., Outcomes of a natural rubber latex control program in an Ontario teaching hospital, *J. Allergy Clin. Immunol.,* 108, 628, 2001.

19. Hunt, L.W. et al., Management of occupational allergy to natural rubber latex in a medical center: The importance of quantitative latex allergen measurement and objective follow-up, *J. Allergy Clin. Immunol.,* 110, S96, 2002.

20. Wrangsjo, K., Swartling, C., and Meding, B., Occupational dermatitis in dental personnel: Contact dermatitis with special reference to (meth)acrylates in 174 patients, *Contact Dermatitis,* 45, 158, 2001.

21. Wallenhammar, L.M. et al., Contact allergy and hand eczema in Swedish dentists, *Contact Dermatitis,* 43, 192, 2000.

22. Schnuch, A. et al., Contact allergies in healthcare workers: Results from the IVDK, *Acta Derm. Venereol.,* 78, 358, 1998.

23. Gibbon, K.L. et al., Changing frequency of thiuram allergy in healthcare workers with hand dermatitis, *Br. J. Dermatol.,* 144, 347, 2001.

24. Holness, D.L. and Mace, S.R., Results of evaluating health care workers with prick and patch testing, *Am. J. Contact Dermal.,* 12, 88, 2001.

25. McNeil, S.A. et al., Outbreak of sternal surgical site infections due to Pseudomonas aeruginosa traced to a scrub nurse with onychomycosis, *Clin. Infect. Dis.,* 33, 317, 2001.

26. Manzella, J.P. et al., An outbreak of herpes simplex virus type I gingivostomatitis in a dental hygiene practice, *J. Am. Med. Assoc.,* 252, 2019, 1984.

27. Larson, E.L. et al., Changes in bacterial flora associated with skin damage on hands of health care personnel, *Am. J. Infect. Control,* 26, 513, 1998.

28. Adisesh, A., Meyer, J.D., and Cherry, N.M., Prognosis and work absence due to occupational contact dermatitis, *Contact Dermatitis,* 46, 273, 2002.

29. Suphioglu, C., Rolland, J.M., and O'Hehir, R.E., Latex allergy: Towards immunotherapy for health care workers, *Clin. Exp. Allergy,* 32, 667, 2002.

30. Allmers, H. et al., Reduction of latex aeroallergens and latex-specific IgE antibodies in sensitized workers after removal of powdered natural rubber latex gloves in a hospital, *J. Allergy Clin. Immunol.,* 102, 841, 1998.

31. Charous, B.L., Schuenemann, P.J., and Swanson, M.C., Passive dispersion of latex aeroallergen in a healthcare facility, *Ann. Allergy Asthma Immunol.,* 85, 285, 2000.

32. Kerosuo, E., Kerosuo, H., and Kanerva, L., Self-reported health complaints among general dental practitioners, orthodontists, and office employees, *Acta Odontol. Scand.,* 58, 207, 2000.

33. Wrangsjo, K. et al., Protective gloves in Swedish dentistry: Use and side-effects, *Br. J. Dermatol.,* 145, 32, 2001.

34. Bollinger, M.E. et al., A hospital-based screening program for natural rubber latex allergy, *Ann. Allergy Asthma Immunol.,* 88, 560, 2002.

35. Vermeulen, R. et al., Ascertainment of hand dermatitis using a symptom-based questionnaire: Applicability in an industrial population, *Contact Dermatitis,* 42, 202, 2000.

36. Levy, S.M. and Jakobsen, J.R., A comparison of medical histories reported by dental patients and their physicians, *Spec. Care Dentist.,* 11, 26, 1991.

37. Gordon, M.M., Capell, H.A., and Madhok, R., The use of the Internet as a resource for health information among patients attending a rheumatology clinic, *Rheumatology,* 41, 1402, 2002.

38. Hamann, C.P., Rodgers, P.A., and Sullivan, K., Allergic contact dermatitis in dental professionals: Effective diagnosis and treatment, *J. Am. Dent. Assoc.,* 134, 185, 2003.

39. Wagner, S. and Breiteneder, H., The latex-fruit syndrome, *Biochem. Soc. Trans.,* 30, 935, 2001.

40. Fleming, C.J., Burden, A.D., and Forsyth, A., Accuracy of questions related to allergic contact dermatitis, *Am. J. Contact Dermatitis,* 11, 218, 2000.

41. Katelaris, C.H. et al., Screening for latex allergy with a questionnaire: Comparison with latex skin testing in a group of dental professionals, *Aust. Dent. J.,* 47, 152, 2002.

42. NIOSH. Latex allergy: A prevention guide. 1998. NIOSH.

43. Centers for Disease Control & Prevention and Dept.of Health & Human Services, Draft recommended infection control practices for dentistry, *Federal Register,* 68, 6488, 2003.

44. Warshaw, E.M. and Nelson, D., Prevalence of evaluation for latex allergy and association with practice characteristics in United States dermatologists: Results of a cross-sectional survey, *Am. J. Contact Dermatitis,* 12, 139, 2001.

45. Farrell, A.L. et al., Prevalence and methodology of evaluation for latex allergy among allergists in the United States: Results of a cross-sectional survey, *Am. J. Contact Dermatitis,* 13, 183, 2002.

46. Farrell, A.L. et al., Prevalence and methodology of patch testing by allergists in the United States: Results of a cross-sectional survey, *Am. J. Contact Dermatitis,* 13, 157, 2002.

47. Hamilton, R.G., Peterson, E.L., and Ownby, D.R., Clinical and laboratory-based methods in the diagnosis of natural rubber latex allergy, *J. Allergy Clin. Immunol.,* 110, S47–S56, 2002.
48. Hamilton, R.G., Diagnosis of natural rubber latex allergy, *Methods,* 27, 22, 2002.
49. Mahler, V. et al., Prevention of latex allergy by selection of low-allergen gloves, *Clin. Exp. Allergy,* 30, 509, 2000.
50. Yeang, H.Y., Prevalence of latex allergy may be vastly overestimated when determined by *in vitro* assays, *Ann. Allergy Asthma Immunol.,* 84, 628, 2000.
51. Palosuo, T., Alenius, H., and Turjanmaa, K., Quantitation of latex allergens, *Methods,* 27, 52, 2002.
52. Yip, L. et al., Skin prick test reactivity to recombinant latex allergens, *Int. Arch. Allergy Immunol.,* 121, 292, 2000.
53. Turjanmaa, K. et al., Latex allergy diagnosis: *In vivo* and *in vitro* standardization of a natural rubber latex extract, *Allergy,* 52, 41, 1997.
54. Hamilton, R.G. and Adkinson, N.F., Jr., Diagnosis of natural rubber latex allergy: multicenter latex skin testing efficacy study, *J. Allergy Clin. Immunol.,* 102, 482, 1998.
55. Ebo, D.G. et al., Latex-specific IgE, skin testing, and lymphocyte transformation to latex in latex allergy, *J. Allergy Clin. Immunol.,* 100, 618, 1997.
56. Blanco, C. et al., Comparison of skin-prick test and specific serum IgE determination for the diagnosis of latex allergy, *Clin. Exp. Allergy,* 28, 971, 1998.
57. Gruber, C. et al., Is there a role for immunoblots in the diagnosis of latex allergy? Intermethod comparison of *in vitro* and *in vivo* IgE assays in spina bifida patients, *Allergy,* 55, 476, 2000.
58. Shojaei, A.R. and Haas, D.A., Local anesthetic cartridges and latex allergy: A literature review, *J. Can. Dent. Assoc.,* 68, 622, 2002.
59. Kutting, B., Weber, B., and Brehler, R., Evaluation of a dipstick test (Allergodip-Latex) for *in vitro* diagnosis of natural rubber latex allergy, *Int. Arch. Allergy Immunol.,* 126, 226, 2001.
60. Ownby, D.R., Magera, B., and Williams, P.B., A blinded, multi-center evaluation of two commercial *in vitro* tests for latex-specific IgE antibodies, *Ann. Allergy Asthma Immunol.,* 84, 193, 2000.
61. Hamilton, R.G., Biagini, R.E., and Krieg, E.F., Diagnostic performance of Food and Drug Administration-cleared serologic assays for natural rubber latex-specific IgE antibody, *J. Allergy Clin. Immunol.,* 103, 925, 1999.
62. Kim, K.T., Safadi, G.S., and Sheikh, K.M., Diagnostic evaluation of type I latex allergy, *Ann. Allergy Asthma Immunol.,* 80, 66, 1998.
63. Marks, J.G. et al., North American Contact Dermatitis Group patch test results for the detection of delayed-type hypersensitivity to topical allergens, *J. Am. Acad. Dermatol.,* 38, 911, 1998.
64. Marks, J.G., Jr. et al., North American Contact Dermatitis Group patch-test results, 1996–1998, *Arch. Dermatol.,* 136, 272, 2000.
65. Guin, J.D., Hamann, C., and Sullivan, K., Natural and synthetic rubber, in *Occupational Skin Disease,* Adams, R.M., Ed., W.B. Saunders Company, Philadelphia, 1999, chap. 29.
66. Uter, W.J., Geier, J., and Schnuch, A., Good clinical practice in patch testing: Readings beyond day 2 are necessary: A confirmatory analysis., *Am. J. Contact Dermatitis,* 7, 231, 1996.
67. Elston, D. et al., Pitfalls in patch testing, *Am. J. Contact Dermatitis,* 11, 184, 2000.

68. Nethercott, J.R., Sensitivity and specificity of patch tests, *Am. J. Contact Dermatitis,* 5, 136, 1994.

69. Sherertz, E.F. et al., Patch testing discordance alert: False-negative findings with rubber additives and fragrances, *J. Am. Acad. Dermatol.,* 45, 313, 2001.

70. Vozmediano, J.M.F. and Hita, J.C.A., Concordance and discordance between TRUE Test and Finn Chamber, *Contact Dermatitis,* 42, 182, 2000.

71. Geier, J. et al., Diagnostic screening for contact allergy to mercaptobenzothiazole derivatives, *Am. J. Contact Dermatitis,* 13, 66, 2002.

72. Diepgen, T.L. and Coenraads, P.J., Sensitivity, specificity and positive predictive value of patch testing: The more you test, the more you get? *Contact Dermatitis,* 42, 315, 2000.

73. Brasch, J. et al., Associated positive patch test reactions to standard contact allergens, *Am. J. Contact Dermatitis,* 12, 197, 2001.

74. Knudsen, B.B. and Menne, T., Contact allergy and exposure patterns to thiurams and carbamates in consecutive patients, *Contact Dermatitis,* 35, 97, 1996.

75. American Dental Association, The dental team and latex hypersensitivity, *J. Am. Dent. Assoc.,* 130, 257, 1999.

76. Trape, M., Schenck, P., and Warren, A., Latex gloves use and symptoms in health care workers 1 year after implementation of a policy restricting the use of powdered gloves, *Am. J. Infect. Control,* 28, 352, 2000.

77. Paul, M.A., Fleischer, A.B., and Sherertz, E.F., Patient's benefit from contact dermatitis evaluation: Results of a follow-up study, *Am. J. Contact Dermatitis,* 6, 63, 1995.

78. Edman, B., The usefulness of detailed information to patients with contact allergy, *Contact Dermatitis,* 19, 43, 1988.

79. Holness, D.L. and Nethercott, J.R., Is a worker's understanding of their diagnosis an important determinant of outcome in occupational contact dermatitis? *Contact Dermatitis,* 25, 296, 1991.

80. Tyler, D., Disability and medical management of natural latex sensitivity claims, *J. Allergy Clin. Immunol.,* 110, S129–S136, 2002.

81. Larson, E., Prevalence and correlates of skin damage on the hands of nurses, *Heart & Lung,* 26, 404, 1997.

82. Hayes, B.B. et al., Evaluation of percutaneous penetration of natural rubber latex proteins, *Toxicol. Sci.,* 56, 262, 2000.

83. Academy of General Dentistry, Latex allergy, *Acad. Gen. Dent. Impact,* 3, 17, 2001.

84. Lassiter, T.E. and Panagakos, F.S., Latex allergies: How they affect the dental profession, *J. Pract. Hyg.,* 11, 51, 1998.

85. Rochon, P.A. et al., Comparison of review articles published in peer-reviewed and throwaway journals, *J. Am. Med. Assoc.,* 287, 2853, 2002.

86. Eysenbach, G. et al., Empirical studies assessing the quality of health information for consumers on the world wide web: A systematic review, *J. Am. Med. Assoc.,* 287, 2691, 2002.

87. Jones, R.T. et al., Latex allergen contents of rubber gloves packaged in sterile medical kits and trays, *J. Allergy Clin. Immunol.,* 102, 694, 1998.

88. Martin, K.M. et al., The protein content of dental rubber dams, *J. Dent.,* 25, 347, 1997.

89. Turjanmaa, K. and Reunala, T., Condoms as a source of latex allergen and cause of contact urticaria, *Contact Dermatitis,* 20, 360, 1989.

90. Yip, E. and Cacioli, P., The manufacture of gloves from natural rubber latex, *J. Allergy Clin. Immunol.,* 110, S3, 2002.

91. Vallier, P. et al., Identification of profilin as an IgE-binding component in latex from *Hevea brasiliensis, Clin. Exp. Allergy,* 25, 332, 1995.

92. Chardin, H. et al., Interest of two-dimensional electrophoretic analysis for the characterization of the individual sensitization to latex allergens, *Int. Arch. Allergy Immunol.*, 128, 195, 2002.

93. Sutherland, M.F. et al., Specific monoclonal antibodies and human immunoglobulin E show that Hev b 5 is an abundant allergen in high protein powdered latex gloves, *Clin. Exp. Allergy*, 32, 583, 2002.

94. Poulos, L.M. et al., Inhaled latex allergen (Hev b 1), *J. Allergy Clin. Immunol.*, 109, 701, 2002.

95. American Society for Testing and Materials, D5712-99 Standard Test Method for The Analysis of Aqueous Extractable Protein in Natural Rubber and Its Products Using the Modified Lowry Method, in *Annual Book of ASTM Standards*, ASTM. Philadelphia, 1999.

96. Brehler, R., Rutter, A., and Kutting, B., Allergenicity of natural rubber latex gloves, *Contact Dermatitis*, 46, 65, 2002.

97. Beezhold, D.H., Kostyal, D.A., and Tomazic-Jezic, V.J., Measurement of latex proteins and assessment of latex protein exposure, *Methods*, 27, 46, 2002.

98. Chen, S.F., Teoh, S.C., and Porter, M., A false-positive result with the American Society for Testing and Materials D5712-95 test method for protein given by a common vulcanization accelerator, *J. Allergy Clin. Immunol.*, 100, 713, 1997.

99. American Society for Testing and Materials, D3578-01a^{e2}. Standard Specification for Rubber Examination Gloves, in *Annual Book of ASTM Standards*, ASTM, Philadelphia, 2001.

100. American Society for Testing and Materials, D3577-01a^{e2}. Standard Specification for Rubber Surgical Gloves, in *Annual Book of ASTM Standards*, ASTM, Philadelphia, 2001.

101. Yeang, H.Y. et al., Allergenic proteins of natural rubber latex, *Methods*, 27, 32, 2002.

102. Yip, E. et al., Correlation between total extractable proteins and allergen levels of natural rubber latex gloves, *J. Natural Rubber Res.*, 12, 120, 1997.

103. American Society for Testing and Materials, D6499-00 Standard Test Method for The Immunological Measurement of Antigenic Protein in Natural Rubber and its Products, in *Annual Book of ASTM Standards*, ASTM, Philadelphia, 2000.

104. Palosuo, T. et al., Measurement of natural rubber latex allergen levels in medical gloves by allergen-specific IgE-ELISA inhibition, RAST inhibition, and skin prick test, *Allergy*, 53, 59, 1999.

105. Haas, D.A., An update on local anesthetics in dentistry, *J. Can. Dent. Assoc.*, 68, 546, 2002.

106. Truscott, W., Glove powder reduction and alternative approaches, *Methods*, 27, 69, 2002.

107. Crippa, M. and Pasolini, G., Allergic reactions due to glove-lubricant-powder in health-care workers, *Int. Arch. Occup. Environ. Health*, 70, 399, 1997.

108. Lundberg, M., Wrangsjo, K., and Johansson, S.G., Latex allergens in glove-powdering slurries, *Allergy*, 50, 378, 1995.

109. Tomazic, V.J. et al., Cornstarch powder on latex products is an allergen carrier, *J. Allergy Clin. Immunol.*, 93, 751, 1994.

110. Swanson, M.C. and Ramalingam, M., Starch and natural rubber allergen interaction in the production of latex gloves: A hand-held aerosol, *J. Allergy Clin. Immunol.*, 110, S15-S20, 2002.

111. Barbara, J. et al., Immunoadjuvant properties of glove cornstarch powder in latex-induced hypersensitivity, *Clin. Exp. Allergy*, 33, 106, 2003.

112. Slater, J.E. et al., Lipopolysaccharide augments IgG and IgE responses of mice to the latex allergen Hev b 5, *J. Allergy Clin. Immunol.*, 102, 977, 1998.

113. Williams, P.B. and Halsey, J.F., Endotoxin as a factor in adverse reactions to latex gloves, *Ann. Allergy Asthma Immunol.,* 79, 303, 1997.

114. American Society for Testing and Materials, D6124-00 Standard Test Method for Residual Powder on Medical Gloves, in *Annual Book of ASTM Standards,* ASTM, Philadelphia, 2000.

115. Food and Drug Administration, Medical glove guidance manual: Draft document, FDA CDRH, 1999, pp. 1-1–12-2.

116. Food and Drug Administration, Medical Glove Powder Report. 1-21, Dept. of Health and Human Services, Rockville MD, 1997, p. 1–21.

117. Knudsen, B.B. et al., Allergologically relevant rubber accelerators in single-use medical gloves, *Contact Dermatitis,* 43, 9, 2000.

118. Knudsen, B.B. et al., Release of thiurams and carbamates from rubber gloves, *Contact Dermatitis,* 28, 63, 1993.

119. Hamann, C.P. and Kick, S.A., Allergies associated with medical gloves: Manufacturing issues, *Dermatol. Clin.,* 12, 547, 1994.

120. Ebo, D.G. and Stevens, W.J., IgE-mediated natural rubber latex allergy: Practical considerations for health care workers, *Ann. Allergy Asthma Immunol.,* 88, 568, 2002.

121. Charous, B.L. et al., Natural rubber latex allergy in the occupational setting, *Methods,* 27, 15, 2002.

122. Woolhiser, M.R., Munson, A.E., and Meade, B.J., Immunological responses of mice following administration of natural rubber latex proteins by different routes of exposure, *Toxicol. Sci.,* 55, 343, 2000.

123. Howell, M.D., Weissman, D.N., and Jean, M.B., Latex sensitization by dermal exposure can lead to airway hyperreactivity, *Int. Arch. Allergy Immunol.,* 128, 204, 2002.

124. Swanson, M.C. et al., Quantification of occupational latex aeroallergens in a medical center, *J. Allergy Clin. Immunol.,* 94, 445, 1994.

125. Sussman, G.L. et al., Incidence of latex sensitization among latex glove users, *J. Allergy Clin. Immunol.,* 101, 171, 1998.

126. Baur, X., Measurement of airborne latex allergens, *Methods,* 27, 59, 2002.

127. Mitakakis, T.Z. et al., Particulate masks and non-powdered gloves reduce latex allergen inhaled by healthcare workers, *Clin. Exp. Allergy,* 32, 1166, 2002.

128. Phillips, M.L., Meagher, C.C., and Johnson, D.L., What is "powder free?" Characterisation of powder aerosol produced during simulated use of powdered and powder free latex gloves, *Occup. Environ. Med.,* 58, 479, 2001.

129. Reiter, J.E., Latex sensitivity: An industrial hygiene perspective, *J. Allergy Clin. Immunol.,* 110, S121, 2002.

130. Bindslev-Jensen, C., Briggs, D., and Osterballe, M., Can we determine a threshold level for allergenic foods by statistical analysis of published data in the literature? *Allergy,* 57, 741, 2002.

131. Kanerva, L. et al., A multicenter study of patch test reactions with dental screening series, *Am. J. Contact Dermatitis,* 12, 83, 2001.

132. Kanerva, L., Cross-reactions of multifunctional methacrylates and acrylates, *Acta Odontol. Scand.,* 59, 320, 2001.

133. Kucenic, M.J. and Belsito, D.V., Occupational allergic contact dermatitis is more prevalent than irritant contact dermatitis: A 5-year study, *J. Am. Acad. Dermatol.,* 46, 695, 2002.

134. Shaffer, M.P. and Belsito, D.V., Allergic contact dermatitis from glutaraldehyde in health-care workers, *Contact Dermatitis,* 43, 150, 2000.

135. Ballantyne, B. and Jordan, S.L., Toxicological, medical and industrial hygiene aspects of glutaraldehyde with particular reference to its biocidal use in cold sterilization procedures, *J. Appl. Toxicol.,* 21, 131, 2001.

136. Ballantyne, B., Myers, R.C., and Blaszcak, D.L., Influence of alkalinization of glutaraldehyde biocidal solutions on acute toxicity, primary irritancy, and skin sensitization, *Vet. Hum. Toxicol.,* 39, 340, 1997.

137. Kanerva, L. et al., Statistics on allergic patch test reactions caused by acrylate compounds, including data on ethyl methacrylate, *Am. J. Contact Dermatitis,* 6, 75, 1995.

138. Rustemeyer, T. et al., Cross-reactivity patterns of contact-sensitizing methacrylates, *Toxicol. Appl. Pharmacol.,* 148, 83, 1998.

139. Munksgaard, E.C., Permeability of protective gloves by HEMA and TEGDMA in the presence of solvents, *Acta Odontol. Scand.,* 58, 57, 2000.

140. Munksgaard, E.C., Permeability of protective gloves to (di)methacrylates in resinous dental materials, *Scand. J. Dent. Res.,* 100, 189, 1992.

141. Andersson, T. and Bruze, M., *In vivo* testing of the protective efficacy of gloves against allergen-containing products using an open chamber system, *Contact Dermatitis,* 41, 260, 1999.

142. Lehman, P.A., Franz, T.J., and Guin, J.D., Penetration of glutaraldehyde through glove material: Tactylon versus natural rubber latex, *Contact Dermatitis,* 30, 176, 1994.

143. Jordan, S.L.P. et al., Glutaraldehyde permeation: Choosing the proper glove, *Am. J. Infect. Control,* 24, 67, 1996.

144. Di Stefano, F. et al., Glutaraldehyde: An occupational hazard in the hospital setting, *Allergy,* 54, 1105, 1999.

145. Lindstrom, M. et al., Dentist's occupational asthma, rhinoconjunctivitis, and allergic contact dermatitis from methacrylates, *Allergy,* 57, 543, 2002.

146. Vyas, A. et al., Survey of symptoms, respiratory function, and immunology and their relation to glutaraldehyde and other occupational exposures among endoscopy nursing staff, *Occup. Environ. Med.,* 57, 752, 2000.

147. Palczynski, C. et al., Occupational asthma and rhinitis due to glutaraldehyde: Changes in nasal lavage fluid after specific inhalatory challenge test, *Allergy,* 56, 1186, 2001.

148. Nishiwaki, Y. et al., Cross-sectional study of health effects of methyl methacrylate monomer among dental laboratory technicians, *J. Occup. Health,* 43, 375, 2003.

149. Goh, C.L. and Gan, S.L., Efficacies of a barrier cream and an afterwork emollient cream against cutting fluid dermatitis in metalworkers: A prospective study, *Contact Dermatitis,* 31, 176, 1994.

150. Loden, M., Barrier recovery and influence of irritant stimuli in skin treated with a moisturizing cream, *Contact Dermatitis,* 36, 256, 1997.

151. Jemec, G.B. and Na, R., Hydration and plasticity following long-term use of a moisturizer: A single-blind study, *Acta Derm. Venereol.,* 82, 322, 2002.

152. Schnuch, A. et al., Patch testing with preservatives, antimicrobials and industrial biocides: Results from a multicentre study, *Br. J. Dermatol.,* 138, 467, 1998.

153. Allmers, H., Wearing test with 2 different types of latex gloves with and without the use of a skin protection cream, *Contact Dermatitis,* 44, 30, 2001.

154. Frosch, P.J. et al., Efficacy of skin barrier creams (II): Ineffectiveness of a popular "skin protector" against various irritants in the repetitive irritation test in the guinea pig, *Contact Dermatitis,* 29, 74, 1993.

155. Berndt, U. et al., Efficacy of a barrier cream and its vehicle as protective measures against occupational irritant contact dermatitis, *Contact Dermatitis,* 42, 77, 2000.

156. McCormick, R.D., Buchman, T.L., and Maki, D.G., Double-blind, randomized trial of scheduled use of a novel barrier cream and an oil-containing lotion for protecting the hands of health care workers, *Am. J. Infect. Control,* 28, 302, 2000.

157. Voeller, B., et al., Mineral oil lubricants cause rapid deterioration of latex condoms, *Contraception,* 39, 95, 1989.

158. Hamilton, R.G. and Brown, R.H., Impact of personal avoidance practices on health care workers sensitized to natural rubber latex, *J. Allergy Clin. Immunol.,* 105, 839, 2000.

159. Hamann, C.P., Rodgers, P.A., and Sullivan, K., Management of dental patients with allergies to natural rubber latex, *Gen. Dentistry,* 50, 526, 2002.

160. Page, E.H. et al., Natural rubber latex: Glove use, sensitization, and airborne and latent dust concentrations at a Denver hospital, *J. Occup. Environ. Med.,* 42, 613, 2000.

161. Condemi, J.J., Allergic reactions to natural rubber latex at home, to rubber products, and to cross-reacting foods, *J. Allergy Clin. Immunol.,* 110, S107–S110, 2002.

162. AAAAI and ACAAI joint statement concerning the use of powdered and non-powdered natural rubber latex gloves, *Ann. Allergy Asthma Immunol.,* 79, 487, 1997.

163. Bain, E.I., ANA position statement on latex allergy, *Massachusetts Nurse,* 1, 13, 1998.

164. Liss, G.M. and Tarlo, S.M., Natural rubber latex-related occupational asthma: Association with interventions and glove changes over time, *Am. J. Ind. Med.,* 40, 347, 2001.

165. Vandenplas, O. et al., Occupational asthma caused by natural rubber latex: outcome according to cessation or reduction of exposure, *J. Allergy Clin. Immunol.,* 109, 125, 2002.

166. Occupational Safety and Health Administration, OSHA bloodborne pathogens standard, *Federal Register,* 56(235), 64175, 1991.

167. Farnham, J.J., Tomazic-Jezic, V.J., and Stratmeyer, M.E., Regulatory initiatives for natural latex allergy: U.S. perspectives, *Methods,* 27, 87, 2002.

168. Food and Drug Administration, Guidance for medical gloves: A workshop manual, FDA Publication #97-4257, U.S. Department of Health and Human Services, Rockville, MD, 1996.

169. Food and Drug Administration, Premarket Notification [510(k)] submissions for Testing for Skin Sensitization to Chemicals in Natural Rubber Products, U.S. Department of Health and Human Services, Rockville, MD, 1999.

170. Food and Drug Administration, Testing for Skin Sensitization to Chemicals in Latex Products; Draft Guidance, *Federal Register,* 63, No. 85, 24559, 1998.

171. Kujala, V. et al., Extractable latex allergens in airborne glove powder and in cut glove pieces, *Clin. Exp. Allergy,* 32, 1077, 2002.

172. Baur, X., Chen, Z., and Allmers, H., Can a threshold limit value for natural rubber latex airborne allergens be defined? *J. Allergy Clin. Immunol.,* 101, 24, 1998.

173. Fisher, A.A., Rietschel, R.L., and Fowler, J.F., Jr., Allergy to rubber, in *Fisher's Contact Dermatitis,* Rietschel, R.L. and Fowler, J.F., Jr., Eds., Lippincott, Williams, Wilkins, Philadelphia, 2000, chap. 31.

174. Daniels, C.A. and Gardner, K.L., Rubber-related polymers, part I: Poly (vinyl chloride), in *Rubber Technology,* Morton, M., Ed., Van Nostrand Reinhold, New York, 1987, chap. 20.

175. Schollenberger, C.S., Polyurethane elastomers, in *Rubber Technology,* Morton, M., Ed., Van Nostrand Reinhold, New York, 1987, chap. 15.

176. Holden, G., Thermoplastic elastomers, in *Rubber Technology,* Morton, M., Ed., Van Nostrand Reinhold, New York, 1987, chap. 16.

177. Sugiura, K. et al., Di(2-ethylhexyl) phthalate (DOP) in the dotted polyvinyl-chloride grip of cotton gloves as a cause of contact urticaria syndrome, *Contact Dermatitis,* 43, 237, 2000.

178. Walker, S.L. et al., Occupational contact dermatitis from headphones containing diethylhexyl phthalate, *Contact Dermatitis,* 42, 164, 2000.

179. Lee, H.N. et al., Cross-reactivity among epoxy acrylates and bisphenol F epoxy resins in patients with bisphenol A epoxy resin sensitivity, *Am. J. Contact Dermatitits,* 13, 108, 2002.

180. Sugiura, K. et al., Contact urticaria due to polyethylene gloves, *Contact Dermatitis,* 46, 262, 2002.

181. Sugiura, K. et al., A case of contact urticaria syndrome due to di(2-ethylhexyl) phthalate (DOP) in work clothes, *Contact Dermatitis,* 46, 13, 2002.

182. Thomsen, D.J. and Burke, T.G., Lack of latex allergen contamination of solutions withdrawn from vials with natural rubber stoppers, *Am. J. Health Syst. Pharm.,* 57, 44, 2000.

183. Primeau, M.N., Adkinson, N.F., Jr., and Hamilton,R.G., Natural rubber pharmaceutical vial closures release latex allergens that produce skin reactions, *J. Allergy Clin. Immunol.,* 107, 958, 2001.

184. Terrados, S. et al., The presence of latex can induce false-positive skin tests in subjects tested with penicillin determinants, *Allergy,* 52, 200, 1997.

185. Boxer, M.B., Grammer, L.C., and Orfan, N., Gutta-percha allergy in a health care worker with latex allergy, *J. Allergy Clin. Immunol.,* 93, 943, 1994.

186. Gazelius, B., Olgart, I., and Wrangsjo, K., Unexpected symptoms to root filling with gutta-percha: A case report, *Int. Endodontic J.,* 19, 202, 1986.

187. Kleier, D.J.S.K., Management of the latex hypersensitive patient in the endodontic office, *J. Endod.,* 25, 825, 1999.

188. Knowles, K.I. et al., Rubber latex allergy and the endodontic patient, *J. Endod.,* 24, 760, 1998.

189. Hamann, C.P. et al., Cross-reactivity between gutta-percha and natural rubber latex: Assumptions vs. reality, *J. Am. Dent. Assoc.,* 133, 1357, 2002.

190. Costa, G.E., Johnson, J.D., and Hamilton, R.G., Cross-reactivity studies of gutta-percha, gutta-balata and natural rubber latex (*Hevea brasiliensis*), *J. Endod.,* 29, 584, 2001.

191. Grade, A.C. and Martens, B.P., Chronic urticaria due to dental eugenol, *Dermatologica,* 178, 217, 1989.

192. Haikel, Y. et al., Anaphylactic shock during endodontic treatment due to allergy to formaldehyde in a root canal sealant, *J. Endod.,* 26, 529, 2000.

193. ADA Council On Scientific Affairs, Office emergencies and emergency kits, *J. Am. Dent. Assoc.,* 133, 364, 2002.

194. Dailey, Y.M., Humphris, G.M., and Lennon, M.A., Reducing patients' state anxiety in general dental practice: A randomized controlled trial, *J. Dent. Res.,* 81, 319, 2002.

195. King, D.M. et al., Behavioral management instruction of anxious clients in the dental hygiene curricula, *J. Dent. Hyg.,* 74, 280, 2000.

196. Hermesch, C.B. et al., Effect of powder-free latex examination glove use on airborne powder levels in a dental school clinic, *J. Dent. Educ.,* 63, 814, 1999.

197. Palosuo, T., Turjanmaa, K., and Reinikka-Railo, H. Allergen content of latex gloves: A market surveillance study of medical gloves used in Finland in 1997, National Agency for Medicines Medical Devices Centre, Finland, 1997.

22 Management of Latex Allergy: Allergist's Perspective

Ignatius C. Chua, Alison J. Owen, and Paul E. Williams

CONTENTS

I. Introduction...249
II. Management of NRL Allergy...250
    A. Principles Underlying Drug Management......................................250
        1. Increasing Patient Awareness of NRL allergy..........................250
        2. Treatment of Local Symptoms..251
        3. Treatment of Systemic Symptoms..252
        4. Emergency Rescue Medication for Patient Self-Medication.....252
        5. Training Patients to Deal with Severe Allergic Reactions.........254
III. Planned Clinical Management of NRL Allergic Patients.........................256
    A. Spina Bifida Patients...256
    B. Patients with Symptoms/Confirmatory Evidence of NRL
        Allergy...256
    C. NRL-Free Environments 256
IV. Latex Immunotherapy...256
V. Prognosis...257
VI. Useful Addresses 258
References...258

I. INTRODUCTION

All physicians including medical, surgical, and dental practitioners must be aware of the impact of natural rubber latex (NRL) allergy on clinical practice, both in terms of prevention and also emergency management. It is important to appreciate that NRL allergy may initially present with local symptoms only and develop more serious systemic manifestations with subsequent exposure. The group of patients for whom this is most pertinent are those who present skin manifestations only, who should be carefully observed for the possible development of other more serious symptoms.

II. MANAGEMENT OF NRL ALLERGY

A. PRINCIPLES UNDERLYING DRUG MANAGEMENT

Allergic reactions occurring by IgE-mediated activation of mast cells may affect many organs and many types of drugs are available to treat them. Mast cells are present in the mucosa throughout the respiratory, gastrointestinal, and genital tracts, and in the skin. They contain preformed granules comprising various protein enzymes and chemical mediators, including histamine. They bear IgE receptor molecules on their cell surface which bind avidly to the IgE Fcε chains. These receptors' intracytoplasmic chains extend into the mast cell and the close apposition of a critical number of such intracytoplasmic chains enables a threshold of biochemical activity to be exceeded. This results in activation of the mast cell via various serial protein phosphorylation and biochemical events.

When an allergen is encountered, for example on nasal or lung mucosa, mast cell activation occurs with two main consequences. First, the granules are extruded from the mast cell into the surrounding tissues. Second, biologically active mediators are synthesised from precursor lipids in the surface membrane of the cell via stimulation of the arachidonic acid/leukotriene pathway. The mediators formed *de novo* include leukotriene C4 (LTC4) and platelet activating factor (PAF). The molecules released from mast cells upon activation by allergen (histamine, LTC4 and others) act on many types of adjacent cells nearby to produce itching, swelling, and the other symptoms of allergy. Histamine acts instantly via H_1 histamine receptors to cause pruritus, contraction of nonvascular smooth muscle (including bronchial, intestinal), and relaxation of vascular smooth muscle. LTC4 and PAF have a more delayed action via recruitment of other immune cells and inflammatory mechanisms. The allergen-specific IgE/high affinity IgE receptor/mast cell system thus acts as an elaborate coupling mechanism serving to couple exposure to allergen with the occurrence of immediate and delayed inflammation at the site of exposure. The symptoms experienced will depend on where the allergen is encountered, and also will determine what treatment is most appropriate, as summarized in Table 22.1.

1. Increasing Patient Awareness of NRL allergy

The most effective strategy regarding NRL reactions is to prevent them occurring, and this is the cornerstone of management. Fundamental to this is active engagement of the patient in the process. Time spent at the point of diagnosis, explaining the mechanisms and impact of exposure to NRL to the patient is crucial. Subjects covered at this time should include:

- NRL avoidance in daily life
- How to recognize and manage both mild and severe allergic reactions
- The carriage of emergency rescue medication at all times

TABLE 22.1
Suggested Treatment of Symptoms with Varied Routes of Allergen Exposure

Organ	Precipitating allergens	Disease	Symptoms	Treatments
Lungs	House dust mite (HDM), pollens, NRL	Asthma	Wheeze, cough	β-Agonists, steroids
URT	Pollens, NRL, various	Allergic rhinitis	Runny/itchy nose, sneeze	Antihistamines (AH)
Eyes	HDM, pollen, cat, NRL	Allergic conjunctivitis	Itching, lacrimation	AH
CVS/RS	Nuts, fish, NRL, others	Anaphylaxis	Collapse, wheezing, angiedema	Adrenaline, hydrocortisone IV, AH
GIT	Various	Food allergy	Abdominal pain, vomiting, diarrhea	Avoidance
Skin	HDM, NRL, others	Dermatitis, urticaria	Itchy excoriated skin ± 2° infection	Emollients, steroids, AH

Note: URT: upper respiratory tract; GIT: gastrointestinal tract; CVS: cardiovascular system; RS: respiratory system; and IV: intravenous.

- The wearing of a MedicAlert bracelet or other similar such identification
- The carriage of NRL free gloves in case emergency resuscitation may be required
- Discussion of scenarios where NRL exposure is likely, e.g., dental visits, gynacological examinations, and other investigative procedures
- Alerting healthcare professionals early about their NRL allergy so as to facilitate the use of NRL-free protocols for any treatment

Discussions with the patient should be reinforced by giving written material to take home. A recent meta-analysis has shown that the use of a combination of teaching strategies (verbal ± written ± video) improves patients' retention of knowledge over a prolonged period, compared to verbal instruction alone.[1] In our experience, an effective way of supplementing this education is to copy all outpatient clinic correspondence concerning their NRL allergy to the patient. If carried by the patient, the latter can also provide information early on to anyone who may need to assist in an emergency.

2. Treatment of Local Symptoms

Histamine is an important chemical mediator in type I hypersensitivity reactions, acting via H_1 histamine receptors on mast cells to produce pruritus, contraction of nonvascular smooth muscle and relaxation of vascular smooth muscle. Antihistamines binding to the H_1 histamine receptors thus prevent these histamine-induced consequences. The first generation antihistamines (e.g., chlorpheniramine) cross the blood-brain barrier, thus additionally acting at central H_1 receptors, causing drowsiness and impaired cognitive and motor performance.[2] The second generation antihistamines, e.g., Cetirizine, cross the blood brain barrier to a lesser degree and are therefore less sedating. Antihistamines are well absorbed after oral administration with peak plasma concentrations often being achieved within 2 hours, although symptom improvement is often experienced earlier than this.

No reported studies have looked at the effectiveness of relieving or reducing the nonsystemic symptoms of NRL allergy. Management of local symptoms occurring as a result of food allergy may be informative in that symptoms may range from mild and localized to severe systemic reactions. In one recent study using predetermined management plans, 15% of patients (88 out of 567) experienced a reaction to nuts during a follow-up period of 12 months. Sixty-two of these were mild reactions (localized edema, pruritus, or generalized urticaria) and settled after administration of oral antihistamines.[3] Oral antihistamines may thus effectively treat mild, localized symptoms of NRL allergy, and this is reflected commonly in clinical practice.

3. Treatment of Systemic Symptoms

The principles of management should follow the current Resuscitation Council algorithm.[4] Epinephrine remains the drug of choice in the immediate treatment of anaphylaxis and should be administered intramuscularly. Its α-receptor agonist activity causes vasoconstriction. Its β-receptor agonist activity dilates airway smooth muscle and stimulates myocardial contractility. This algorithm is reproduced in Figure 22.1.

4. Emergency Rescue Medication for Patient Self-Medication

Which patient should carry which type of rescue medication will depend upon the type of allergic reaction experienced after NRL exposure. The American Academy of Asthma Allergy and Immunology Task Force Report in 1993,[5] supplemented by the position statement on anaphylaxis in 1998,[6] remains the authoritative guide. It recommends that patients with a history of anaphylaxis should carry self-injectable epinephrine if they also have either clinical reactivity to NRL or if they test positive for NRL allergy in laboratory tests.[5,6] Patients who have not had any episodes of anaphylaxis should carry oral antihistamine tablets. Patients who have coexistent asthma should also carry an inhaled salbutamol device. Anaphylaxis is difficult to define, but a good working definition is that it involves one or both of two severe features: respiratory difficulty (possibly due to laryngeal edema or asthma) and hypotension (presenting as fainting, collapse, or loss of consciousness).[7]

The management of patients who have experienced generalized urticaria and few other clinically significant symptoms remains more contentious, as is the case for patients who had true IgE-mediated food allergy. In one large study of deaths from anaphylaxis, patients who had died from anaphylactic reactions following exposure to foods and nuts commonly had coexistent asthma that was poorly con-

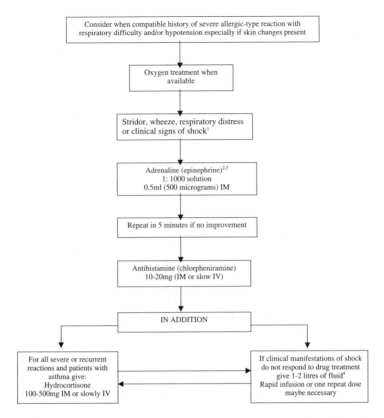

FIGURE 22.1 Treatment algorithm for adults by first medical responders. (From Resuscitation Council, 2001. With permission.)[4]

trolled in the period prior to the fatal episode. In view of this, and in the absence of contrary evidence, it would seem reasonable to recommend for patients who have NRL allergy and coexistent asthma, that the asthma should be well controlled at all times, especially when entering a situation where they may become exposed to NRL.[8,9] Due consideration should also be paid to the views of the patients and whether carriage of self-injectable epinephrine would in this situation give the patient greater peace of mind in the management of their NRL allergy.

An essential responsibility of the prescribing clinician is to ensure that the patient knows how to use the self-injectable epinephrine device correctly and safely in an emergency. Most studies on this have focused on children rather than adults, but their findings are highly relevant to adults. A retrospective investigation of parental knowledge and first aid management of anaphylaxis, and the use of epinephrine auto-injector device had highly revealing findings. Less than 25% of parents were able to describe the symptoms of airway breathing or circulatory impairment in an allergic reaction 20 months after the initial consultation, and only 24% were able to use the epinephrine device correctly.[10] Parents whose child had experienced more than two anaphylactic reactions scored higher than those whose child had had fewer than two reactions. This would suggest that knowledge of the signs, symptoms, and management of anaphylaxis gained through personal experience correlates with appropriate emergency self-management. The correct use of the epinephrine auto-injector device is a skill that diminishes with time, unless reiterated through personal experience or further tuition.

Patients who have experienced local symptoms only after NRL exposure may manage their symptoms satisfactorily if they carry oral antihistamine tablets, and inhaled salbutamol if they have asthma, both to be used promptly at the earliest relevant symptom. The importance of carrying rescue mediation at all times, together with a MedicAlert bracelet indicating where the medication is to be found about their person, should be emphasized to every patient.

5. Training Patients to Deal with Severe Allergic Reactions

Patients should be trained to self-administer epinephrine with a trainer device. This allows demonstration of its mode of action. It also provides a crucial opportunity for the patient to demonstrate the action drill back to the trainer, which is a vital step to promote skill retention. At each outpatient follow-up visit, this should be repeated as it is a skill that diminishes with time. The patient should be tested and observed while performing the action drill using a trainer device. Confidence to self-administer epinephrine does not equate with competence at doing so. The most vital steps in the action drill that patients most commonly get wrong are the removal of the safety cap (the grey cap) and selecting the correct end of the device for injection into the thigh.[11]

Two self-injectable epinephrine devices are currently available, the Epipen and the Anapen. Both have a similar mode of action and both contain a single dose of epinephrine, 0.3 mg for adults and 0.15 mg for children respectively. In order to give patients the opportunity to practice the action drill safely, and to enable them to make others around them more familiar with the epinephrine device, a trainer device should be made available for them to take away at the end of the training session. As an integral part of the training process, written material on the epinephrine device and NRL avoidance strategies should be given to the patient. It is often useful to supplement training with audio-visual aids such as videos produced by the Anaphylaxis Campaign. Figure 22.2 and Figure 22.3 show the Epipen and Anapen devices, and the action drill is detailed below:

To Administer an Epipen the Patient Should Be Instructed To:

- Telephone emergency medical services for help
- Remove the grey safety cap
- Grasp the EPIPEN firmly, placing the black tip at right angles to the outside of the thigh (through clothing if necessary) and press hard until the device functions (it should click)
- Hold in place for 10 seconds for the device to inject all of the epinephrine
- Remove the EPIPEN and massage the area for a few seconds

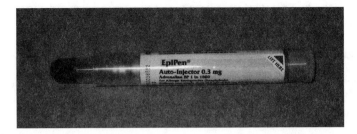

FIGURE 22.2 (See color insert following page 112.) Epipen device. (Photo courtesy of ALK-Abelló, U.K.)

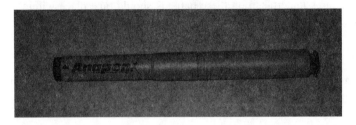

FIGURE 22.3 (See color insert following page 112.) Anapen device. (Photo courtesy of Celltech Pharmaceuticals, Ltd., U.K.)

- Note the time the injection was given
- Replace the Epipen in the plastic packaging, taking care to avoid pricking others with the needle, and give it to emergency medical personnel who will dispose of it safely

A useful mnemonic we have employed in our training package:

If you experience:
Airway
Breathing or
Circulatory symptoms you should
Dial 999/911 and use your
Epipen then go for
Follow-up at hospital

Follow-up arrangements for patients who have NRL allergy should to be tailored to individual needs. Patients who do not experience further allergic reactions may not need regular follow-up, but could be discharged with fast-track access in the event of another severe allergic reaction. Some patients will require close follow-up, for example, to repeat their Epipen training and manage any coexistent asthma. For patients who are not otherwise under review, a nurse practitioner–led clinic to provide practical support and repeat annual training is useful.

III. PLANNED CLINICAL MANAGEMENT OF NRL ALLERGIC PATIENTS

A. Spina Bifida Patients

Evidence would suggest that the risk of sensitization in this group of patients may be as high as 34% during invasive procedures.[12] Surgery and other invasive procedures should thus be carried out within a NRL-free environment.[5]

B. Patients with Symptoms/Confirmatory Evidence of NRL Allergy

Any procedures undertaken on these patients should take place within a NRL-free environment with readily available facilities for resuscitation.

C. NRL-Free Environments

Although low-powder latex gloves are now routinely used in clinical environments, the extent to which they are used results in significant levels of NRL exposure. Therefore procedures undertaken on NRL-allergic patients should ideally take place within a predesignated room which remains NRL-free at all times. However, this in reality is not always a practical or feasible arrangement. Such patients should thus have their procedures scheduled to occur in the morning, first on the list of procedures, when the NRL load is at its lowest. Only NRL-free gloves and equipment should come into direct contact with the patient.[13]

Figure 22.4 shows a summary algorithm for the overall management of NRL allergy.

IV. LATEX IMMUNOTHERAPY

Desensitization immunotherapy is an effective treatment for some types of allergy (e.g., venom anaphylaxis and seasonal allergic rhinitis) with excellent treatment outcomes and symptom reduction.[14–20] It is hypothesized to act by changing the bias of immune responses from humoral to cell-mediated. Such therapy reduces the level of IgE-mediated mast cell activation following natural encounter with the trigger allergen. The therapy is not without clinical risk and possible serious adverse events include anaphylaxis. It is thus performed in specialist centers by appropriately trained personnel.

Trials of immunotherapy for the management of NRL allergy indicate further investigation is required prior to this becoming a viable therapeutic option to offer patients. In one randomized double-blind placebo-controlled study of such desensitization immunotherapy in 17 healthcare workers, there was a reduction in allergic symptoms after 12 months of treatment, but 4 out of 9 subjects in the active treatment group experienced angiedema following desensitization injections.[14] Sublingual administration of NRL immunotherapy has been reported to improve symptoms with fewer systemic allergic reactions.[15] At present this type of therapeutic approach cannot be recommended outside the clinical trial setting.

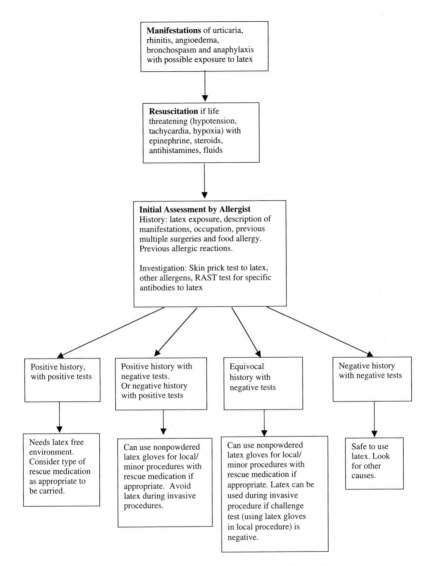

FIGURE 22.4 Algorithm for management of natural rubber latex allergy.

V. PROGNOSIS

Following diagnosis of NRL allergy, patients should be vigilant for possible NRL exposure at all times. NRL is present in many articles associated with daily living, thus making complete avoidance virtually impossible. The natural history of NRL allergy has not been delineated in detail, but two studies have encouraging findings.[21,22] In these two studies, 32 children and 160 adults with a history of mild, moderate, and severe symptoms after NRL exposure were given advice regarding NRL avoidance and oral antihistamines to take as required. Twenty-two children and 24 adults became accidentally exposed to NRL during follow-up for 2.8 years and 3 years respectively. Local symptoms only ensued, with no cases experiencing severe symptoms requiring hospital attention.[21,22] This would seem to suggest that stringent avoidance in association with prompt administration of rescue medication successfully deals with NRL exposure in daily life.

VI. USEFUL ADDRESSES

MedicAlert Foundation International	**MedicAlert Foundation**
2323 Colorado Avenue	1 Bridge Wharf
Turlock	156 Caledonian Avenue
CA 95382	London N1 9UU
U.S.	U.K.
www.medicalert.org	

Epipen Distributors
Dey LP   Alk-Abello (UK) Ltd
2751 Napa Valley Corporate Drive   2 Tealgate
Napa   Hungerford
CA 94558   Berkshire RG17 0YT
U.S.   U.K.

Anapen Distributors
CellTech Manufacturing Inc.   CellTech Pharmaceuticals
P.O. Box 31710   208 Bath Road
Rochester   Slough
New York   Berkshire
14603   SL1 3WE
U.S.   U.K.

The Anaphylaxis Campaign
www.anaphylaxiscampaign.org.uk

American Latex Allergy Association
www.latexallergyresources.org

Latex Allergy Support Group
www.lasg.co.uk

REFERENCES

1. Theis, S.L. and Johnson, J.H., Strategies for teaching patients: A meta-analysis, *Clin. Nurse Specialist,* 9, 100, 1995.
2. Oral antihistamines for allergic disorders, *Drug Therapeutics Bull.,* 40, 59, 2002.
3. Ewan, P.W. and Clark, A.T., Long term prospective observational study of patients with peanut and nut allergy after participation in a management plan, *Lancet,* 357, 111, 2001.

4. Resuscitation Council (U.K.): Update on the Emergency Medical Treatment of Anaphylactic Reactions for first medical responders and for community nurses, *J. Accident Emergency Med.,* 18, 393, 2001.

5. Committee Report Task Force on allergic reactions to latex, *J. Allergy Clin. Immunol.,* 92, 16, 1993.

6. American Academy of Asthma, Allergy and Immunology, Diagnosis and management of anaphylaxis, *J. Allergy Clin. Immunol.,* 2, 101, S465, 1998.

7. Ewan, P.W., Anaphylaxis, *Br. Med. J.,* 316, 1442, 1998.

8. Pumphrey, R.S., Lessons for management of anaphylaxis from a study of fatal reactions, *Clin. Exp. Allergy,* 30, 1144, 2000.

9. Pumphrey, R.S.H., Duddridge, M., and Norton, J., Fatal latex allergy, *J. Allergy Clin. Immunol.,* 107, 558, 2001.

10. Gold, M.S. and Sainsbury, R., First Aid Management in children who were prescribed an epinephrine autoinjector (Epipen), *J. Allergy Clin. Immunol.,* 106, 171, 2000.

11. Sicherer, S.H., Forman, J.A., and Noone S.A., Use assessment of self administered epinephrine amongst food-allergic children and paediatricians, *Paediatrics,* 105, 359, 2000.

12. Slater, J.E., Mostello, L.A., and Shaer, C., Rubber specific IgE in children with spina bifida, *J. Urology,* 146, 578, 1991.

13. Ownby, D., Latex allergy, in *Allergy in primary care,* 1st Ed., Altman, L.C., Becker, J.W., and Williams, P.V., Eds., W. B. Saunders, Philadelphia, 2000.

14. Leynadier, F. et al., Specific immunotherapy with a standardised latex extract versus placebo in allergic healthcare workers, *J. Allergy Clin. Immunol.,* 106, 585, 2000.

15. Patriarca, G. et al., Sublingual desensitisation: A new approach to latex allergy problem, *Anaes. Analogues,* 95, 956, 2002.

16. Frankland, A.W. and Augustin, R., Prophylaxis of summer hayfever and asthma: A controlled trial comparing crude grass pollen extracts with the isolated main protein component, *Lancet,* 1, 1055, 1954.

17. Varney, V.A. et al., Usefulness of immunotherapy in patients with severe summer hayfever uncontrolled by antiallergic drugs, *Br. Med. J.,* 302, 265, 1991.

18. Walker, S.M. et al., Grass pollen immunotherapy for seasonal rhinitis and asthma: a randomised, controlled trial, *J. Allergy Clin. Immunol.,* 107, 87, 2001.

19. Hunt, K.J. et al., A controlled trial of immunotherapy in insect hypersensitivity, *New Engl. J. Med.,* 299, 157, 1978.

20. Muller, U. et al., Immunotherapy in bee sting hypersensitivity. Bee venom versus whole body extract, *J. Allergy Clin. Immunol.,* 34, 369, 1979.

21. Ylitalo, L. et al., Natural rubber latex allergy in children: A follow up study, *Clin. Exp. Allergy,* 30, 1611, 2000.

22. Turjanmaa, K. et al., Long term outcome of 160 adult patients with natural rubber latex allergy, *J. Allergy Clin. Immunol.,* 110, S70, 2002.

Index

A

A. alternata, 20
Acceptable quality level (AQL), 192
ACD, *see* Allergic contact dermatitis
Acetone, 48
Acidic NRL protein, 18
Active barrier creams, 154
ADA, *see* American Dental Association
AL, *see* Ammoniated raw latex
AlaSTAT assay, 70, 216
Albuterol inhaler, 61
Alcohol consumption, 135
Allergenic proteins, 15–26
    acidic NRL protein, 18–19
    allergenic NRL proteins, 16–21
    allergens in NRL products, 23–24
    class 1 chitinase, 20
    enolase, 20
    future aspects, 24
    1,3-β-glucanase, 16–18
    Hev b 12, 20
    Hev b 13, 20–21
    IgE-binding epitopes of NRL allergens, 21–22
    manganese superoxide dismutase, 20
    microhelix protein complex, 18
    other NRL allergens, 21
    patatin-like protein, 19
    profilin, 19–20
    prohevein, hevein, and prohevein C-domain, 19
    rubber elongation factor, 16
    rubber particle protein, 18
    T-cell epitopes of NRL allergens, 22–23
Allergens, measurement in natural rubber latex products, 87–96
    methods for measuring natural rubber latex allergens, 89–94
        qualitative, 89–90
        quantitative, 91–94
        semiquantitative, 90–91
    NRL allergens in source material and in manufactured products, 88–89
Allergen-specific assays, 194
Allergic contact dermatitis (ACD), 119–125, 165
    eczematous variants, 121
    latex gloves and, 147

natural rubber latex, 122–123
    prognosis for, 133–134
    rubber depigmentation, 121–122
    rubber purpura, 121
    sites involved, 120–121
    tests for, 127–132
        other rubber additives, 130
        patch testing with natural rubber latex, 130–131
        rubber additives, 127–128
        rubber mixes, 128–130
    unusual delayed-type reactions, 122
Allergist, perspective of latex allergy, 249–259
    latex immunotherapy, 256
    management of NRL allergy, 250–255
        emergency rescue medication for patient self-medication, 252–254
        increasing patient awareness of NRL allergy, 250–251
        training patients to deal with severe allergic reactions, 254–55
        treatment of local symptoms, 251–252
        treatment of systemic symptoms, 252
    planned clinical management of NRL allergic patients, 256
        NRL-free environments, 256
        patients with symptoms/confirmatory evidence of NRL allergy, 256
        spina bifida patients, 256
    prognosis, 257–258
    useful addresses, 258
Allergy
    IgE-mediated, 68
    induction, proteins responsible for, 72
    prevalence, 1, 2
Amaranthus caudatus, 22
American Academy of Asthma Allergy and Immunology Task Force Report, 252
American Contact Dermatitis Society, 215
American Dental Association (ADA), 212, 217, 228
American Society of Hospital Pharmacists, 198
American Society for Testing and Materials (ASTM), 191, 221, 223
Amine antioxidant, 121
Ammoniated raw latex (AL), 70, 77

AMP, *see* Antimicrobial protein
Anaphylaxis, 3, 59, 100
   definition of, 252
   fatal, 60
   management of, 254
   repeated episodes of, 114
Anesthesia, local, 234
Anesthetists, 57
Angiedema, 62
Antabuse®, 49
Antibiotics, 159
Antibodies
   anti-TMA-IgE, 109
   IgE, 24, 59, 68, 69, 88, 214
   rabbit, 74
Antidegradants, 41, 45, 49, 51, 212, 226
Antihistamines, 252
Antimicrobial protein (AMP), 22
Antimicrobials, 227
Antioxidants, 31, 121, 226
Antioxonants, 31, 44, 46
Anti-TMA-IgE antibodies, 109
Anxiety, 236
AORN, *see* Association of periOperating Room
     Nurses
AQL, *see* Acceptable quality level
Aqueous Cream BP, 154, 157
Arachidonic acid metabolites, 99
Association of periOperating Room Nurses
     (AORN), 199
Asthma, 3, 102
ASTM, *see* American Society for Testing and
     Materials
Atopic dermatitis, 111
Atopic diathesis, 5
Azathioprine, 160

B

Bacterial endotoxin, 142
Bacteriocides, 226
Baculovirus expression system, 22
Balata, 36
Barrier creams (BC), 165, 166
Barrier creams/moisturizers, 165–176
   barrier creams, 154, 166–167
     active, 154
     application methods and efficacy, 167
     definition and terms, 166
     mechanism of action and duration,
       166–167
     reasons to use, 166
     U.S. Food and Drug Administration
       monograph skin protectants, 167

moisturizers, 167–171
   definitions and terms, 167
   effect of moisturizers on skin, 168
   moisturizers in preventing irritant contact
     dermatitis, 168–171
BC, *see* Barrier creams
Benzyl acetate, 180
Betnovate®, 158
BFV, *see* Blood flow volume
BHT, *see* Butyl hydroxytoluene
Biocides, 222, 229
Bioengineering instruments, 149
Bleached rubber syndrome, 120
Blood
   donations, 2
   flow volume (BFV), 182–183
Blooming, 120
Bronchoconstriction, 58, 59
Bronchospasm, 102
Bronopol, 155
Butyl hydroxytoluene (BHT), 130, 234
Butyl rubber, 40

C

Calamine, 167
CAP assay, 215
CAP System FEIA, 70
Capture enzyme immunoassay, 91, 92
Carbamates, 29, 129, 212, 224
Carboxylic acid, 196
Cardiovascular collapse, 58
Carpet, rubber-backed, 120
Casein powder, 50
CD, *see* Contact dermatitis
CDC, *see* Centers for Disease Control and
     Prevention
CD4+ T cells, 59
Centers for Disease Control and Prevention
     (CDC), 212, 227, 228, 230
Cetirizine, 252
CGMP, *see* Current Good Manufacturing
     Practices
Challenge testing, 214
Chemical additives, 27–56
   antidegradants, 44
   future developments, 50–51
   manufacture of rubber, 28–40
     history of rubber manufacturing, 28–29
     manufacturing processes, 29–34
     rubber and rubberlike elastomers, 34–40
   pigments, fragrances, and flavorants, 46
   processing aids, 47
   releasing agents and lubricants, 47

rubber compounding, 40–50
    allergenicity of rubber additives, 47–50
    chemical additives, 41–47
    vulcanizing agents, 41
Chemical partition coefficient, 177
Chemical penetration, 153
C. herbarum, 20
Chicle, 36
Childhood atopy, 7
Chitinases, 137
Chlorination, 33
Chlorpheniramine, 60, 252
Chronic dyshidrotic palmar eczema, 160
Class 1 chitinase, 20
Cocoa butter, 167
Colorants, 226
Compounding, 31, 40
Condoms, latex, 62
Confirmatory testing, 207
Contact dermatitis (CD), 127, 141, 165
Contact urticaria, 97–105
    classification, 98–100
        immunological, 98–100
        nonimmunological, 98
        undetermined mechanisms, 100
    clinical features of, 100–103
Contact urticaria syndrome, 100, 101,
        107–112
    immunologic contact urticaria, 108–109
        contact chemical allergy as animal
            model, 109
        mechanisms, 108
        protein allergy as animal model, 109
        respiratory chemical allergy as animal
            model, 108–109
    nonimmunologic contact urticaria, 110
        animal models, 110
        mechanisms, 110
    predictive testing, 110–111
        agents causing ICU or NICU, 110–111
        medicaments for ICU or NICU, 111
    prognosis for, 113–118
        follow-up studies, 113–115
        patients with spina bifida, 116–117
        primary prevention, 115–116
Copolymers, 36, 232, 233
Corticoderm® cream, 158
Corticosteroids
    systemic, 159
    topical, 158
Cotton gloves, 153
Counterirritants, 97
Crepe rubber, 30
Cross-reactivity, 135, 224
Cumulative irritation assay, 149

Current Good Manufacturing Practices (CGMP),
        191, 201
Cutaneous erythema, 97
Cutting oils, 166
Cyclosporin, 160

D

Delayed-type hypersensitivity reactions, 119
Dental hygiene technicians, latex allergy
        among, 8
Dental students, latex sensitivity among, 10
Dental workers, cost-driven, 233
Dentistry, management of rubber-based allergies
        in, 212–247
    allergens in natural and synthetic rubber,
        218–227
        allergenic rubber chemicals, 223–225
        exposure routes and thresholds for rubber-
            based allergens, 225–226
        glove powder and NRL protein allergens,
            222– 223
        NRL extractable allergenic protein
            content, 222
        NRL extractable total protein content, 221
        other dental allergens, 226–227
    diagnosis and symptom assessment, 213–217
        diagnostic testing for rubber-based
            allergies, 214–217
        health history and risk assessment,
            213–214
        symptom assessment, 214
    education of allergic dental professionals,
        217–218
    examples of successful management of
        rubber-based allergies, 236–237
    mitigating rubber allergen exposure, 227–236
        administrative controls, 228
        considerations for dental patient with
            rubber-based allergies, 234–236
        dental operatory cleaning and NRL
            remediation, 228–229
        NRL product substitution, 229–234
    recommendations, 237–238
Deoxycholic acid (DOC), 72
Dermatitis
    hydration, 179
    potential, 231
Desensitization immunotherapy, 256
Diagnostic tests, strengths and weaknesses of, 3
Dialkydithiocarbamates, 37
Dibenzylcarbamyl chloride, 120
Dielectric probe, 182
Diethyl dithiocarbamate, 49

Dimethicone, 167
Dinitrofluorobenzene (DNFB), 109
Diphenylguanidine (DPG), 129
Dipping technology, 31
Dishpan hands, 155
Disinfectants, 141
2,2-Dithio-bis-benzothiazole (MBTS), 143, 144
DNA synthesis, 178
DOC, *see* Deoxycholic acid
DPG, *see* Diphenylguanidine
Dry film leaching, 33
D-Squames®, 169
D5712 test, 78

E

Eczema, 133
Edema, 58
Educational resources, 219
EIA, *see* Enzyme immunoassay
Elastomers, styrene-based, 39
Electrical capacitance, 143
Electrocautery surgery, 201
Electrolyte flux, 147
Elimination diets, 138
ELISA, 19, 69, 74, 77, 90
Emergency
    preparedness, 236
    self-management, 254
Emulsifying Ointment BP, 154, 157
Emulsion treated hands, 171
Endotoxins, 142, 231
Enolase, 20
Enzyme immunoassays (EIA), 88
Eosinophil chemotactic factor, 99
EPA Clean Air Act, 46
Epinephrine, 61, 252, 253
Epipen, 63, 254, 255
Erythema
    index, 143
    multiforme-type rashes, 122
Evaporimeter, 147
Exaggerated use studies, 149
Exam glove standard comparison, 197
Exposure reduction, 208
Eyelash curlers, rubber-containing, 120

F

Fatigue factor, 199
FCA, *see* Freund's Complete Adjuvant
FDA, *see* U.S. Food and Drug Administration
Federal Food, Drug and Cosmetics Act, 190

Fingertip dermatitis, 120
FITkit®, 76, 92, 93, 95, 222
Flame retarders, 130
Flavorants, 31, 46
Food
    allergy, 7, 62, 214, 252
    cross-reaction with latex, 137, 138
Fragrances, 31, 46
Freund's Complete Adjuvant (FCA), 110
Fungicides, 223, 234

G

Gas chromatography-mass spectroscopy, 224
Glove(s), 152
    appropriate use of, 199
    cotton, 153
    expiration dating, 195
    hydration, 201
    invisible, 154, 166
    manufacture, 114, 201
    occlusion, 171
    powder, 222
    powder-free, 193
    protection afforded by, 153
    -related symptoms, 3
    use, excessive, 101
1,3-β-Glucanase, 16–18, 137
Glutaraldehyde, eye symptoms related to, 208
Glycerine, 153
Glycine max, 20
Goodyear, Charles, 29
Gutta-percha, 36, 235

H

Hair care products, 223
Hand care products, 227
Hand dermatitis, management of, 151–164
    important issues, 152–157
        avoidance of irritants, 155–156
        hand protection with gloves, 152–153
        prognosis and ongoing management,
            156–157
        use of soap substitutes and moisturizers,
            153–155
    information sheet for patients with hand
        dermatitis, 163–164
    treatment of, 157–160
        corticosteroids, 158–159
        emollients, 157–158
        other modalities, 160
        photochemotherapy, 159

systemic immunosuppressives, 160
topical immunosuppressives, 160
topical and systemic antibiotics, 159
Hand dermatoses, rubber-based, 28
Handwashing, frequent, 28
HC, *see* Hydrocortisone
HCW, *see* Healthcare workers
Healthcare workers (HCW), 57, 59, 62
latex-allergic, 114, 115
latex sensitivity of, 205
NRL allergy among, 97
Hev b 13, 20–21
Hevea brasiliensis, 15, 20, 29, 30, 36, 88, 136,
195, 219
Hevein, 137
Hexyl nicotinate (HN), 181, 182
HFD, *see* High follicular density
High follicular density (HFD), 181
High performance thin layer chromatography, 224
Histamine, 100, 108, 250, 251
HIV, 28
HN, *see* Hexyl nicotinate
Horseradish peroxidase (HRP), 92
Hospital intensive care units, 209
Housewife's eczema, 155
HPLC amino acid analysis, 73, 78
HRP, *see* Horseradish peroxidase
Humectants, 168
Hycor HYTECH, 70
Hydration dermatitis, 179
Hydrocortisone (HC), 181
Hydroquinone-type compounds, 122
Hypersensitivity, allergy versus, 1
Hypoallergenic claims, 194
Hypotension, 59
HyTECH assay, 216

I

ICD, *see* Irritant contact dermatitis
ICU, *see* Immunologic contact urticaria
IgE
antibodies, 24, 59, 68, 69, 214
-based immunological inhibition assays, 88
-binding epitopes, 21, 89
-immunoblotting analysis, 89
levels, strategy to reduce, 213
-mediated allergy, 68
receptor molecules, 250
test, 122
Immunoblotting, 69, 89, 90
Immunologic contact urticaria (ICU), 98, 107,
108, 141, 147
Immunotherapy, 24, 256

Indwelling latex, 6
Infectious agents, 218
Insecticides, 223
International Union of Pure and Applied
Chemistry (IUPAC), 48
Intralesional steroids, 159
Invisible gloves, 154, 166
In vitro testing, 68, 75, 77, 237
IPPD, see *N*-Isopropyl-*N*-phenyl-*p*-
phenylenediamine
Irgalite Orange F2G, 49
Irritant contact dermatitis (ICD), 165
definition of, 142
prevention of, 168, 171, 172
Irritants, example, 156
N-Isopropyl-*N*-phenyl-*p*-phenylenediamine
(IPPD), 49, 121, 129, 133
IUPAC, *see* International Union of Pure and
Applied Chemistry

J

Jelutong, 37

K

Kallikrein-generating factors, 100

L

Lactic acid, 153
Langerhans cells stresses, 178
Lanolin, 155
Laser Doppler velocimetry (LDV), 147, 181,
182
Latex
ammonia treated raw, 69
condoms, 62
policy, 207
protein content of fresh liquid, 15
pure, 131
sensitivity, overdiagnosis of, 4
sensitized patients, 3
Latex allergy, epidemiology of, 1–13
changing trends of latex sensitivity after latex
exposure alteration, 8–10
epidemiological study determinants, 2–4
allergy prevalence in normal population,
2–3
identification of latex-related symptoms, 3
latex allergy versus hypersensitivity, 2
recruitment of study population, 2

strengths and weaknesses of diagnostic
  tests, 3–4
incidence of latex sensitization or allergy, 8
prevalence in occupational subgroups, 8
risk factors and latex allergy, 4–7
  atopic diathesis, 5
  hand dermatitis, 5–6
  latex and food allergy, 7
  latex glove exposure, 7
  multiple operations and/or indwelling
    latex, 6
Latex-fruit-pollen syndrome, 136
Latex-fruit syndrome, 135–140
  food cross-reacting with latex, 137–138
  latex proteins and, 136–137
  symptoms, 136
LDV, *see* Laser Doppler velocimetry
Leaching, 33
LEAP assay, 73, 74, 78, 79
Leukotriene C4 (LTC4), 250
Leukotrienes, 99
LFD, *see* Low follicular density
Lipids, 168
Liquid latex concentrate, uses of, 219
Local anesthesia, 234
Locobase®, 169
Loratidine, 63
Low follicular density (LFD), 181
Lowry assay, 221
LTC4, *see* Leukotriene C4
Lubricants, 47, 50, 193
Lung function tests, 62
Lycopodium spores, 47

glove hydration and conductivity, 201
glove manufacturers, 201–202
glove regulations, 190–193
  acceptable quality level, 192
  length, 192
  size, 192
  stress at 500% elongation, 193
  tensile strength, 193
  thickness or gauge, 192
  ultimate elongation, 193
protein and allergen levels, 194–195
  allergen-specific assays, 194–195
  assay methods, 194
  labeling, 194
storage stability and expiration dating,
  195–196
synthetic medical gloves, 196–197
  material-specific requirements, 197
  neoprene, 196–197
  nitrile, 196
  polyisoprene, 197
  polymers, 196
  vinyl, 196
Mercaptobenzothiazole (MBT), 29, 121, 129,
  212, 233
Methacrylates, 226
Methylchloroisothiazolinone, 227
Microhelix protein complex, 18
Mimusops balata, 36
MnSOD, *see* Manganese superoxide dismutase
Modified Lowry assay, 73, 93, 221
Moisturizers, 153, 165, 167, *see also* Barrier
  creams/moisturizers
Mold-release agents, 47
MSDS, *see* Material Safety Data Sheets

M

Madison Avenue marketers, term generated by,
  167
Malathion, 181
Malaysian rubber industry, 3
Manganese superoxide dismutase (MnSOD),
  20
Material Safety Data Sheets (MSDS), 198, 218
MBT, *see* Mercaptobenzothiazole
MBTS, *see* 2,2-Dithio-bis-benzothiazole
Medical Devices Directive, 190
MedicAlert bracelet, 63, 254
Medical glove manufacturers, 129
Medical glove regulation, 190–203
  appropriate use of gloves, 199–201
  chemical resistance, 197–199
  donning lubricants, 193–194
    coatings technologies, 193–194
    powdered and powder-free, 193

N

Nail dryness, 142
NAL, *see* Nonammoniated raw latex
National Institute of Occupational Safety and
  Health (NIOSH), 213, 217
Natural moisturizing factors (NMF), 168
Natural rubber latex (NRL), 2
  aerosolized, 225
  anaphylaxis, 58
  commercial harvesting of, 30
  contact urticaria and, 97
  crude, 30, 219
  definition of, 15
  -free environments, 256
  immediate allergic reactions to, 87
  impact on clinical practice, 249
  occupational exposure to, 61

potential sources of, 220
protein(s), 72
  acidic, 18
  allergens, carrier of, 50
  aqueous solubility of surface, 34
  type I hypersensitivity to, 212
Natural rubber latex allergy, 57–66
  case history, 62–63
  everyday exposure to NRL, 62
  fatal anaphylaxis, 61
  occupational exposure to NRL, 61–62
  patients with spina bifida, 60
  surgical and medical procedures, 60–61
  systemic manifestations of allergy, 58–60
    IgE mediated immediate hypersensitivity
      reactions, 59
    sensitization to NRL and development of
      symptoms, 59–60
Natural rubber latex allergy and allergens, *in vitro*
    testing, 67–86
  basis and principles of test development,
    68–69
  evaluating allergenic potential of NRL
    products, 71–80
  methods for measurement of total NRL
    protein, 72–73
  methods for quantification of antigenic
    NRL proteins, 73–74
  quantification of NRL allergens,
    74–80
  future trends, 80
  in vitro diagnosis of NRL allergy, 69–71
    development of *in vitro* tests for NRL
      sensitivity, 69–70
    performance of commercial *in vitro*
      diagnostic tests, 70
    significance of *in vitro* tests in diagnosing
      NRL sensitivity, 71
Neoprene, 37, 196, 223
Nettle rash, 58
Neutrophil chemotactic factor, 99
NHANES III, 7
Nicotinates, permeation of, 183
NICU, *see* Nonimmunologic contact urticaria
NIOSH, *see* National Institute of Occupational
    Safety and Health
Nitrile, 37, 196
NMF, *see* Natural moisturizing factors
Nonammoniated raw latex (NAL), 70, 77
Nonimmunologic contact urticaria (NICU), 98,
    107, 109, 110
Nonlatex alternatives, 209
North American Contact Dermatitis Group, 129,
    216, 217
NRL, *see* Natural rubber latex

O

Occlusion, meaning of, 177
Occlusive effects, man vs. animal, 177–187
  effects of occlusion on barrier function,
    178–179
  evaluating methods, 179–183
    animal models, 179–181
    human models, 181–183
  skin barrier function, 178
Occlusive gloves, irritant dermatitis due to,
    141–145
  occlusion, 142–145
    long-term study, 143
    short-term study, 143–145
  symptoms, 142
Occlusive gloves, predictive testing for irritation
    dermatitis due to, 147–150
  methods, 147–148
  testing paradigm, 149
    exaggerated use studies, 149
    21-day cumulative irritation assay, 149
Occupational exposure, NRL, 61
Occupational health management of latex allergy,
    205–210
  advice to organization, 209
  case management, 207–209
  occupational prevalence of latex allergy,
    205–207
  recognition of cases, 207
Occupational NRL allergy, 113
Occupational Safety and Health Administration
    (OSHA), 190, 198, 209, 227
Occupational subgroups, latex allergy in, 8, 9
Octanol-water partition coefficients, 180
Oil-in-water creams, 154
Oncology Nursing Association, 198
On-line wet-gel leaching, 33
Organic pigments, 130
Organic solvents, 166
OSHA, *see* Occupational Safety and Health
    Administration
OTC products, *see* Over-the-counter products
Over-the-counter (OTC) products, 167
Oxidation-dependent aging, 223
Oxygen-based radicals, 44
Ozone, 46

P

PA, *see* Parathion
PAF, *see* Platelet activating factor
Palaquium gutta, 36
Panallergens, cross-reacting, 214

Paraphenylenediamine (PPD), 129
Parathion (PA), 180
Patatin-like protein, 19, 137
Patch testing, 120, 121, 127, 214
    anaphylaxis due to, 131
    positive, 131
    reactions, 130
Patient management protocols, 228
PBMCs, *see* Peripheral blood mononuclear cells
PCA, *see* Pyrrollidone carboxylic acid
PCP, *see* Pentachlorophenol
PCs, *see* Protective creams
Penetrant lipophilicity, 177
Pentachlorophenol (PCP), 181
Peptides, sensitization processes and, 16
Percorneal permeability, 148
Peripheral blood mononuclear cells (PBMCs), 22,
    23
Permeation, definition of, 198
Personal protective equipment (PPE), 152, 190
Pesticide, 181
Petroleum products, 47
Phenols, 130
Phosphotungstic acid (PTA), 72
Photochemotherapy, 159
Phototherapy, Ultra Violet B, 159
Phthalates, 39
Phthalic anhydride, 109
Pichia pastoris, 19
Pigments, 31, 46
Plant defense system, NRL proteins and, 16
Plasticizers, 31, 37, 226
Plastic occlusion, 158
Platelet activating factor (PAF), 250
Pollens, 135
Polybutadiene, 40
Polyisocyanates, 233
Polyisoprene
    ozone-exposed, 46
    synthetic, 39
Polymer(s)
    coatings, 193
    PVC, 36, 38
    rubber, 34, 35
    strength, 39
Polystyrene block copolymers, 36
Polyurethane, 38, 232, 233, 238
Polyvinyl chloride (PVC), 36, 38, 152, 196
Post cure leaching, 33
PPD, *see* Paraphenylenediamine
PPE, *see* Personal protective equipment
PPPP syndrome, 121
Prevulcanization, 32
Profilin, 19–20, 136
Prohevein, hevein, and prohevein C-domain, 19

Prostaglandins, 99
Protective clothing, 166
Protective creams (PCs), 166
Protective gloves, 152
Protein(s)
    allergy induction, 72
    antimicrobial, 22
    complex, microhelix, 18
    composition, uncertain reproducibility of, 80
    contact dermatitis, 131
    gutta-percha, 235
    -induced ICU, 111
    patatin-like, 19, 137
    recombinant, 80
    reference, 78
    rubber particle, 18
    sensitization processes and, 16
    small rubber particle, 16
    standard, ASTM, 221
    true sensitization to, 24
Pruritis, 98, 212
Psoralen ultraviolet A (PUVA) treatment, 159
Psoriasis, 121
Psychological issues, 236
PTA, *see* Phosphotungstic acid
Pure latex, 131
Purpura, 121
PUVA treatment, *see* Psoralen ultraviolet A
    treatment
PVC, *see* Polyvinyl chloride
Pyrrollidone carboxylic acid (PCA), 168

Q

Questionnaire surveys, 207
Quinolones, 130

R

Rabbit anti-NRL serum, 73
RAST
    assay, 19, 69, 90, 138
    inhibition, 94
Raw latex, 69
Reaction types, 108, 122, 123
Reagent(s)
    IgE-containing, 88, 94
    selection, 68
Recombinant DNA technology, 89, 91, 92
Recombinant proteins, 80
Recurring symptoms, 214
Regulatory agencies, 51
Relaxation programs, 236

Release agents, 47, 50
Rescue medication, 258
Respiratory arrest, 61
Resuscitation Council algorithm, 252
Rhinoconjunctivitis, 3, 102
Root canal surgery, 235
Rubber(s)
    additives, allergenicity of, 47
    allergy, site and cause of, 120
    -based allergies, curative treatment for, 213
    butyl, 40
    crepe, 30
    depigmentation, 121
    deproteinized, 50
    elongation factor, 16
    naturally compounded, 29
    nitrile, 196
    particle protein, 18
    polymers, 34, 35
    silicone, 40
    vulcanized, 223
Rubifacients, 97

S

Sapodilla, 37
SB, *see* Spina bifida
SBS, *see* Styrene-butadiene styrene
SDS-PAGE, *see* Sodium-dodecyl-
        sulphate–polyacrylamide-gel
        electrophoresis
SDT, *see* Sorption-desorption test
SEBS, *see* Styrene-ethylene-butylene styrene
Serological testing, 71
Severe allergic reactions, training patients to deal
    with, 254
Silicone rubber, 40
SIS, *see* Styrene-isoprene styrene
Site-directed mutagenesis, 21
Skin
    abraded, 218
    barrier function, 143, 178
    blood flow volume, 182–183
    capacitance, 171
    cleansers, harsh, 155
    hydration, 101
    hyperhydration, 183
    prick test (SPT), 2, 59, 88, 90, 138, 214
    protective creams (SPCs), 166
    reflectance, 147
    surface roughness, 148
    testing, 77
SLS, *see* Sodium lauryl sulfate
Small rubber particle protein, 16

Soap substitutes, 153
Sodium-dodecyl-sulphate–polyacrylamide-gel
        electrophoresis (SDS-PAGE), 89, 90
Sodium lauryl sulfate (SLS), 142, 148, 155, 170
Solvent exposure, 48
Sorption-desorption test (SDT), 171
SPCs, *see* Skin protective creams
Spina bifida (SB), 16, 59, 76, 92, 116, 256
SPOT analysis, 21
SPT, *see* Skin prick test
Stabilizers, 226
Staphylococcus aureus, 178
Steroid(s)
    absorption, 182
    intralesional, 159
    topical, 158, 217
Stratum corneum barrier integrity, 101
Stress tests, 149
Styrene-based elastomers, 39
Styrene–butadiene ratio, 39
Styrene-butadiene styrene (SBS), 39, 234
Styrene-ethylene-butylene styrene (SEBS), 39
Styrene-isoprene styrene (SIS), 39, 234
Sulfenamides, 29
Sunburn, 217
Surface coatings, 34
Surgery
    anaphylaxis occurring during, 57, 209
    electrocautery, 201
    repeated episodes of, 6
    root canal, 235
Surveillance of work-related and occupational
        respiratory disease (SWORD), 206
Sweat
    -absorbing agents, 229
    glands, 178
SWORD, *see* Surveillance of work-related and
        occupational respiratory disease
Systemic corticosteroids, 159

T

Tachycardia, 59
Talcum powder, 153
TCA, *see* Trichloroacetic acid
T-cell(s), 22
    epitope mapping, 22
    proliferation, 23
TDDS, *see* Transdermal drug delivery systems
Testing
    D5712, 78
    IgE, 122
    in vitro, 68, 75, 77, 237
    lung function, 62

patch, 120, 121, 127, 214
serological, 71
skin prick test, 2, 59, 88, 90, 138, 214
sorption-desorption, 171
strengths and weaknesses of, 3
stress, 149
use, 208, 214
Tewameter™, 147
TEWL, *see* Transepidermal water loss
Thimerosal, 227
Thioureas, allergy to, 130
Thiuram(s), 29, 121, 224
    allergy, 129
    disulfides, 37
TMA, *see* Trimellitic anhydride
Topical corticosteroids, 158
Topical immunosuppressive drugs, 160
Topical steroids, 217
Transdermal drug delivery systems (TDDS), 179
Transepidermal water loss (TEWL), 142–143,
    147–148, 168, 170, 179
Trichloroacetic acid (TCA), 72
Trimellitic anhydride (TMA), 108
T.R.U.E. test panels, 217
Type IV reaction, 49, 102, 119, 151

U

Ultra Violet B (UVB) phototherapy, 159
Unguentum Merck®, 158
Upper airway obstruction, 58
U.S. Consumer Product Safety Commission, 143
Use testing, 208, 214
U.S. Food and Drug Administration (FDA), 2, 48,
    167, 190, 197, 221
    detention, 202

proposal, 231
recommendation, 73
UV absorbers, 234
UVB, *see* Ultra Violet B phototherapy

V

Veterinary medications, 223
Virtual cross-links, 39
Vulcanization, 29, 32, 41, 48, 212

W

Washing machines, industrial-scale, 34
Water-based lotions, 195
Water evaporation rate (WER), 182, 183
Water-in-oil moisturizer, 169
WER, *see* Water evaporation rate
Western blotting, 89
WHO/IUIS Allergen Nomenclature Committee,
    89
Work-related anaphylactic reaction, 208

X

Xanthates, 41
Xerosis, soap-induced, 169

Z

ZDMC, *see* Zinc dimethyldithiocarbamate
Zinc dimethyldithiocarbamate (ZDMC),
    144